Biodynamic

CRANIOSACRAL THERAPY

Biodynamic
CRANIOSACRAL THERAPY

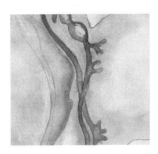

VOLUME TWO

Michael J. Shea, PhD

With contributions from

Carol Agneessens

Sarajo Berman

Raymond Gasser, PhD

Sheila Moon

Alan Schore, PhD

Friedrich Wolf

North Atlantic Books
Berkeley, California

Published by
North Atlantic Books
P.O. Box 12327
Berkeley, California 94712

Cover art by Friedrich Wolf
Cover and book design by Jan Camp

Printed in the United States of America

Copyright acknowledgments begin on page 521

Biodynamic Craniosacral Therapy, Volume Two is sponsored by the Society for the Study of Native Arts and Sciences, a nonprofit educational corporation whose goals are to develop an educational and cross-cultural perspective linking various scientific, social, and artistic fields; to nurture a holistic view of arts, sciences, humanities, and healing; and to publish and distribute literature on the relationship of mind, body, and nature.

North Atlantic Books' publications are available through most bookstores. For further information, visit our website at www.northatlanticbooks.com or call 800-733-3000.

Library of Congress Cataloging-in-Publication Data

Shea, Michael J., M.A.
    Biodynamic craniosacral therapy / by Michael J. Shea ; with contributions from Margaret Scott ... [et al.].
        p. ; cm.
    Includes bibliographical references and index.
    Summary: "A thorough description of the evolution of cranial osteopathic medicine into a new form available to many health care providers, this book presents a technique of touch therapy that is extremely gentle and subtle and gives practical exercises to be proficient in healing physical, spiritual, and emotional conditions"—Provided by publisher.
    ISBN-13: 978-1-55643-591-1
    ISBN-10: 1-55643-591-6
    1. Craniosacral therapy. I. Society for the Study of Native Arts and Sciences. II. Title.
    [DNLM: 1. Complementary Therapies—methods. 2. Musculoskeletal Manipulations. 3. Mind-Body Relations (Metaphysics) 4. Sacrum. 5. Skull. WB 890 S539b 2007]
    RZ399.C73S54 2007
    615.8'2—dc22

                                                                    2006031902

2 3 4 5 6 7 8 9 VERSA 16 15 14 13 12 11

This book is dedicated to His Holiness, the fourteenth Dalai Lama.

If we, ourselves and all the world,
Should wish for unsurpassed enlightenment,
Its basis is a bodhicitta
Stable as the lord of mountains,
Compassion reaching out to all directions,
And a wisdom that transcends duality.

—Nagarjuna

CONTENTS

ILLUSTRATIONS

ACKNOWLEDGMENTS

I must acknowledge the usual cast of characters who have provided the necessary midwifery to bring this second volume to fruition. My wife Cathy has provided impeccable support with her nutritious meals, her tolerance of my absence for long periods of time in the cave of my laptop, and the sacrifice of our play time. In our most challenging moments, she claimed that I had a mistress and her name was Biodynamic Craniosacral Therapy Volume Two. I do have passion for this work that exceeds rationality at times. But, of course, I love my wife more than this book!

Former helpers have fallen ill, unfortunately, and new ones have come forward. The hardest worker has been Sara Dochterman, who, in the midst of getting her Master of Social Work degree, not only formatted the entire book and typed most of the chapters, but also acted as proof editor for the section on trauma resolution. She has been a great gift indeed to sit and work with for many, many hours. Kevin Goulding has lent his usual technical genius and computer prowess to put the entire book together. Jeannie Burns, who helped with the illustrations in the first volume, stepped forward and brought clarity to all the illustrations in this current volume. This includes the drawing of the brain in Chapter 21. Lisa Fay kept my business going while writing this manuscript, and Valerie Gora, my education director, had to nudge me on numerous occasions to return a phone call from a prospective student or do a cranial session with me in order for my brain to decompress.

Carol Agneessens, a highly qualified teacher of biodynamic craniosacral therapy, has contributed greatly to this volume, not only with her poetry, but her skillful editing of some of the chapters regarding how trauma is held in the fluid body. Sarajo Berman, an equally gifted biodynamic practitioner and teacher, has contributed several of her biodynamic poems to this volume, for which I am most grateful. Sheila Moon, a Jungian analyst and poet, through permission via her publisher, brings an awesome interpretation of the Navajo creation myth, which I feel is an accurate phenomenology of the embryonic creation of the human body. I am greatly honored that Dr. Raymond Gasser, professor emeritus at Louisiana State University and co-author with Erich Blechschmidt of *Biokinetics and Biodynamics of Human Differentiation,* has very generously allowed me to reprint three of his early journal articles regarding the biokinetics of the development of the basicranium, the facial muscles, and facial nerve.

I must use the word *honor* again, because Dr. Allan Schore, whom I greatly admire and respect, has contributed a chapter regarding infant brain development that I consider to be a major paradigm shift for working with infants and children; it informs biodynamic practice in terms of the client-therapist relationship. It is a gift to have his mind and spirit in this book. Dr. Schore works at the Department of Psychiatry and Biobehavioral Sciences, University of California at Los Angeles David Geffen School of Medicine.

Barry Williams, a highly skilled Jungian analyst and expert in the field of shamanism, has edited the entire section on mythology and healing. His support for the first volume and this one has been invaluable and heartwarming. He has consistently made himself available throughout the entire process of writing this volume. In addition, his son Rafael has been a great teacher for me ever since his mother Renata Ritzman was pregnant with him. His spirit and love fills this book also.

I am also indebted for the beautiful artwork that Friedrich Wolf has created for the cover of this volume. It shows the early development of the heart in the third and fourth week of embryonic development.

Through this entire adventure, my brothers and sister have supported me with kind and generous words and thoughts. Several weeks before the completion of this volume, all my siblings came to visit me. I was filled with a profound gratitude for each of them by the way they love me. It inspired me to bring this book to completion with joy and happiness. My brother Brian, who is a practicing cranial osteopath, has worked on me frequently to unpack my cranium from the compression of writing, especially at the end when he visited with my other siblings.

I live by the Atlantic Ocean, and she has been the biggest teacher of all. Every day when I could, during the writing of this book, I would approach her and ask for guidance on showing the reader the beauty of her creation and love. She taught me the most about Primary Respiration. During the time I was writing this volume, I also visited the Pacific Ocean, and she taught me about death and dying. I also visited the Adriatic Sea, and she taught me about the mystery of life. Finally, I visited the Mediterranean Sea, and she taught me about joy. I am in awe of the Great Mother.

INTRODUCTION

I can truly say that this Volume Two worked me harder than Volume One. I reached a point in the process where I felt that the book was writing me. The implications of biodynamic craniosacral therapy are so vast and encompass so many disciplines that I found out near the end of the writing that I had enough material for a Volume Three and had to cut the book in half. Volume Two has a bit of samurai warrior in it because of this cleavage so near the end of its making. It was necessary to unfold the information in a correct sequence as I truly feel that the work continues to define a new paradigm of health and healing. It is a paradigm that can offer the deepest healing to our embryo, our infant, our children, and our adults. It is called biodynamic craniosacral therapy.

Volume Two, like Volume One, is divided into five sections. Figure 1 reviews the basic principles of the biodynamic process unfolded in Volume One and that will be elaborated upon in this volume. Each section in this volume goes into greater detail regarding three domains of knowledge informing the biodynamic model covered in the sections of Volume One: Biodynamic Practice, Embryology, and Infants and Children. Two new domains of knowledge that inform biodynamic craniosacral therapy are introduced in this book. The first is covered in the section called Relating with Trauma and the second is the final section, Mythology and Healing. These domains of knowledge give biodynamic practice a more complete picture of the complexity and beauty of the model.

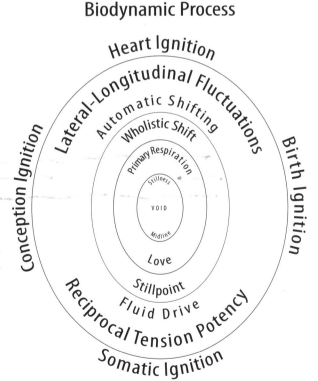

Figure 1. The biodynamic process concept map

xviii ▪ BIODYNAMIC CRANIOSACRAL THERAPY

Several themes are explored throughout the book. The first is introduced as a simple question: What is biodynamics? In each section, the answer to this question deepens until the end, when the discussion turns to the nature of spiritual disease. The second major theme is the relationship of embryology to the healing process and the therapeutic relationship. I am frequently asked by beginning students and other teachers why is embryology so important? One osteopath has said that when a biodynamic practitioner has her hands on a client, she has her hands on more embryology than adult anatomy and physiology. It is this theme of disregarding or bypassing anatomy and physiology and emphasizing contact with the fluids of the embryo that I explore throughout Volume Two. I make the effort to blend the theoretical into a very practical hands-on skill in each section of the book.

A significant aspect of the biodynamic paradigm is an entirely new way of framing the client-therapist relationship. I call biodynamic craniosacral therapy *therapist-centered* therapy. I teach that 80 percent of clinical time with a client is spent by the practitioner in an attunement with her own soma and perceptual process. Thus biodynamic practice is a practice of attunement. How does the practitioner pay attention to the instinctual sentient movement of sense perception going out into the environment, coming back into the body, then back out into the environment in rhythmic cycles? In this way, a major theme of this book is dissociation, distinguishing between its normal and non-normal function and the attempt to depathologize the scourge of our time called post-traumatic stress disorder. As Jerome Bernstein has said in his brilliant book, *Living in the Borderland* (Bernstein, 2006), therapists need to have a greater openness to a transrational reality that does not pathologize states resulting from stress and trauma. As Carl Jung said, disease processes are simply disturbed normal processes rather than an entity unto themselves, although some authors stress the seeming autonomy of the split-off part of the self. Richard Schwartz (Schwartz, 1987), a noted family therapist, has said much the same thing in stressing the need for communication between and among the dissociative affects of our personalities. This is a completely different way of normalizing stress and trauma and in this book is coupled to the consistent theme of the healing power of the slow tempo of Primary Respiration and its rhythmic, balanced interchange with the Dynamic Stillness between the natural world and the soma. Just as the slow-food movement, which started in Italy (Visscher, 2007), has spun off other "slow" movements, the practice of biodynamic craniosacral therapy is the start of a slow-therapy movement.

Another theme explored throughout this volume is the need to get the client involved in his and her own biodynamic process. A wide variety of meditations and visualizations and sensory awareness practices are given here to be taught to both the practitioner and the client, for use before, during, and after a session. How often has a client stood up and asked me what I perceived to be the source of the problem during the session as though I could look in a crystal ball? Out of the sheer need to put the shoe back on the other foot, I developed several processes to help clients get out of the nervous system and into the ocean of fluid experience. Both clinical practice and classroom have shown these practices to be of great benefit.

Section I, called Biodynamic Practice, details the history and evolution of the biodynamic model and then proposes a sequence of principles governing the client-therapist relationship. In this section the basic biodynamic practices are covered to teach to the client as well as the new practitioner. This is a significant departure from Volume One in that I believe the client must participate in the biodynamic process. The practices given in Section I have been worked out in the classroom and treatment room and are yielding excellent results in bringing significant perceptual changes in the client. It will be mentioned over and over throughout the book that the main therapeutic sequence in biodynamic craniosacral therapy is to orient to stillness and synchronize attention to the slow tempo of Primary Respiration. It is the responsibility of both the practitioner and the client to consciously sense Primary Respiration.

Section II, called Relating with Trauma, goes into considerable detail on how to relate appropriately and biodynamically to stress and trauma in the client. A lengthy discussion throughout the section covers how trauma is held in the fluid body. This section is derived from my own personal experience in 1972 when I was a young junior officer in the United States Army and living in Frankfurt, Germany. I parked my car next to what is now called an improvised explosive device (IED). As I went into the building, the terrorist bomb exploded and killed a colleague of mine in back of me. This single experience, being a relative recapitulation of my pre- and perinatal story line, has shaped my entire universe and caused me to spend thirty-five years in a deep study of post-traumatic stress disorder (PTSD).

I learned that the magnitude of PTSD in our culture right now has created a classification of personality that Jerome Bernstein (Bernstein, 2006) calls the "borderland personality." He presents a new perspective that I concur with, in which much fragmentation is no longer a pathology even though it causes an untold amount of suffering. Rather, the borderland personality has embodied the deep split and separation from nature created by the history of our culture's alienation from the natural world. The new character structure is attempting to reconcile the split of body and mind and hold the enormity of the split from nature by resisting a return to outdated Western values, such as the body is a machine. This new client, and many others who have experienced trauma, can be supported by biodynamic craniosacral therapy. Trauma resolution is an advanced training and any of the skills I unfold in this section must be practiced under supervision by a qualified expert.

Section III, called Infants and Children, is about working with infants and children from a biodynamic point of view. My first love is working on young children and infants, and has been for thirty years. I have conducted pediatric trainings internationally and continue to consult at various pediatric clinics and facilities offering therapy to children. The new paradigm detailed in this section is called interpersonal affective neuroscience. It is about the first two years of development with a very basic understanding of how to come into relationship with an infant and the infant's family system using the biodynamic principles of Primary Respiration and stillness. I am very grateful to Dr. Allan Schore, who has contributed the first chapter in this section, which beautifully outlines his entire model in a simple way. At the end of the section I discuss various biodynamic considerations when treating infants and children that can be implemented by practitioners.

Section IV, called Embryology, is about my other mistress—the human embryo. I am greatly honored to have Dr. Raymond Gasser contribute three chapters to this section. The perspective is from a morphological point of view and recent research has begun to verify the scientific validity of morphology (Ingber, 2006; Gasser, 2006). In addition, I help bridge the gap by describing the dynamic movements of the embryo still present in the adult body more into the foreground of the practitioner's hands. This is done through a detailed explanation and exercises regarding the metabolic fields of the embryo.

Section V is called Mythology and Healing. To understand biodynamic craniosacral therapy is to understand the embryo as the symbol not only for origin and transformation, but for the healing connection so necessary to resolve the inherent terror of our contemporary culture and the change process. If the embryo is the symbol for such transformation, then the fluid body is the new metaphor to actualize this symbol in clinical practice. The importance of such understanding of the symbols and metaphors of biodynamic craniosacral therapy is made clear here. This section builds an argument that all disease is spiritual disease and that the biodynamic practitioner is actually doing shamanic work. I do not claim that biodynamic practitioners are shamans, but rather are doing some of the work that a typical shaman does in healing sessions. This requires an understanding of a different sensory language and a different set of rules that at once seem mysterious but are actually completely embodied and present in both the client and the practitioner. Through an understanding of the depth psychology of Carl Jung and mythology, I attempt to give the reader a crucial understanding of the deeper therapeutic dilemma faced by clients in this age we live in. The condensations of chapters by Sheila Moon help reframe the contemporary dilemma using the Navajo creation story. The issue for the Navajo is how the creation of the body comes from below—from the earth rather than heaven. This is the same story as the embryo and must be understood for more effective clinical outcomes. Clients who live in the split and fragmentation of our culture are attempting to make a reconnection to nature, which traditional cultures view as the domain of spirit. Rather than a force to be overcome, nature is viewed in a spiritual context that is resacralized by the biodynamic practitioner as it was by all pre-literate cultures. The practitioner is expected to suspend reason and invoke the inherent power of nature with Primary Respiration and its fulcrum of stillness and bring it to bear in the session of biodynamic craniosacral therapy by rhythmically attending to the natural world inside and outside of the office. Thus the intention of biodynamic craniosacral therapy becomes to reconnect the client with the instinctual intelligence and numinosity of the natural world. Humans share the same tidal body and fluid body with all of nature.

Let me say something about the nature of the language I use in this volume. Figure 2 shows the basic biodynamic language found throughout the book. I made one important change from Volume One: I no longer use the term Mid Tide, but rather the term *fluid body*, as used by James Jealous (Jealous, 2002b). This is prominent in the section on relating to trauma. I also use the term *tidal body* more consistently than before as a synonym for Primary Respiration and the Long Tide (Jealous, 2002a). Consequently, throughout this book I have attempted to use the word *soma* for the actual flesh-and-blood body as distinguished from the fluid body and tidal body. This was not always possible given the context of what I was writing about in any given chapter.

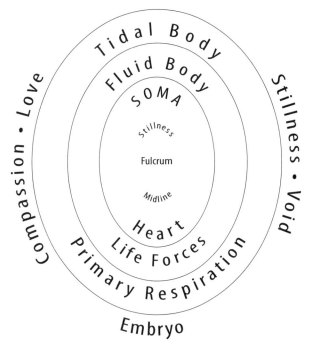

The Biodynamic Model

Figure 2. The biodynamic model of craniosacral therapy

Although osteopathy in the cranial field informs biodynamic craniosacral therapy, its intention is to specialize in working manually with medical pathology as a result of having a medical degree and a medical practice in the United States. There are fundamental differences between these two biodynamic communities. Biodynamic craniosacral therapy does not work directly with a pathological medical model; rather, it is primarily used as a method of mutual exploration of perception, self-development, and integration of developmental experience. That is not to say that clients with medical pathology are turned away because practitioners do not have a medical degree; rather, the pathology is not the focus of a session or in the scope of practice of most biodynamically trained practitioners. Practically everyone who comes into my office these days has a medical diagnosis with some kind of pathology. The contemporary client has already been treated by dozens of other health care providers both in the medical field and in complementary and alternative medicine (CAM). Thus a conscious perception of the whole as the living movement of Primary Respiration and its center of stillness would be crucial to healing. On the other hand, the osteopathic community as a group does not include the trauma resolution paradigm or the affective neuroscience paradigm in biodynamic practice in the way that they are integrated in the biodynamic craniosacral therapy community. Ultimately, both communities share a common bond formed by the perception of Primary Respiration and, I believe, have a lot to learn from each other.

As in Volume One, I "randomize" the use of gender-specific pronouns in different chapters. In one chapter the client will be female and the practitioner male; in the next chapter their genders might reverse. This makes for easier reading. I prefer using the word *practitioner* rather than *therapist* to describe the person in charge of the therapeutic container and attempting to work biodynamically. This is not always possible and in some chapters both words are used for specific purposes, such as the *client-therapist relationship* which is commonly used across professions.

Finally, I urge the reader to learn to sense Primary Respiration. This will aid in reading and understanding this book and the first volume as well. I also believe it will help lead a happier life, as Primary Respiration has taught me to do.

Section I

...

Biodynamic Practice

CHAPTER 1

What Does "Biodynamic" Mean?

I want to reinvent the term *somatic* with this chapter. Somatics comes from a rich experiential therapeutic tradition centered in the lived experience of the body. It is rooted in the philosophy of the phenomenology of the body. It has gradually fallen out of usage in the past decade with the proliferation of many body-centered approaches to health and healing, which actually means it is no longer a marketable term for the masses. I believe however, that the term "biodynamic" is replacing it as a descriptor for lived experience in the body and a therapeutic process that supports awareness of internal aliveness. I would like to define the word *biodynamic* in its various uses for the reader. Then I would like to define the way the concept of biodynamics is used in the context of embryology and how biodynamic is used to describe a discrete therapeutic process in a new manual therapeutic art called biodynamic craniosacral therapy.

To do this I will need to form a bridge to regulation theory in pre- and perinatal psychology. This will include a specific look at how an infant regulates his brain physiologically, how an embryo regulates its growth and development metabolically, and the link between these two developmental periods. I will conclude this chapter with the idea that biodynamic practice is a paradigm shift in the manual therapeutic arts and indeed does have applications for other health care practitioners as well.

To start, it is important to remember that cranial osteopaths and cranial practitioners are not the only ones using the term *biodynamic.* When Franklyn Sills's first book, *Craniosacral Biodynamics,* Volume 1 (Sills, 2001), came out, he got a call from the European biodynamic psychology folks claiming turf. These body-centered therapy pioneers in Europe had developed an approach started by Gerda Boyesen and originally called psychoperistalsis. Biodynamic psychology has a much better ring to it. In my research, I found that the Rudolf Steiner community also uses the term biodynamic to describe an ultra form of organic gardening and soil preparation. Biodynamic farmers reference the myths surrounding Demeter, the female god of all earth and sea, who represents a seminal part of their biodynamic culture. Thus it could be said that biodynamics is a proper course of inquiry because there is also a mythology associated with the biodynamic concept as well as conflict and tension from different communities that use it as a descriptor for their work. Of special note is the fact that the word is used by the founders and developers of osteopathy in the cranial field also in a spiritual context by the use of related metaphors to the Breath of Life, the Master Mechanic, and other such terms found in their literature. Dr. William G. Sutherland himself said that one could consider osteopathy and therefore the Cranial Concept to be religious in nature. Osteopathy in some circles is considered to be a theology of the body in this light. Even the Rolf Institute held a kind of Inquisition around the use and misuse of the word itself and the "right" to use it. Thus the term biodynamic has become loaded with therapeutic, psychological, religious, and mythic overtones. In other words, it is a big story, a very big story.

So what does "biodynamic" mean? The word, as it is specifically used in the cranial community, comes from experimental embryology in the late nineteenth and early twentieth centuries. It simply means wholeness. The question that many biologists experimenting with embryos spent nearly the whole of the last century exploring with their embryonic newts and salamanders was how wholeness is conserved through progressive stages of complexity in the form of an embryo up to an adult human or frog or chicken. It required a whole new paradigm. The conclusion among many biologists was that wholeness was related to biochemistry; nowadays that means molecular genetics. This was a deduction based on an observation. Historically, from a theoretical biology and experimental embryology point of view, biodynamic means wholeness. It is the element of completeness that is seen in each stage of embryonic development.

Biodynamics actually began as a concept and an observation from experimental embryologists at the end of the nineteenth century. It originally lacked a proper description, but that is not the original scientific method. First there is the observation and then a metaphor to describe something, then the experiments, and then the verbal description for a new paradigm. The central theoretical and intellectual inquiry of those early biologists was how the wholeness of the embryo was carried forward in successive stages of development. The embryo became the new metaphor that was concurrently supported by the emerging paradigm of genetics, except for a little detour by a German embryologist.

Along came Dr. Erich Blechschmidt in the 1940s, who in his later writings suggested that the theoretical notion of wholeness was precisely related to the submicroscopic organizing or ordered movements in the fluids of the embryo. He used the term biodynamic to describe the properties of these organizing movements. Dr. Blechschmidt (Blechschmidt, 1977), in the glossary of his first book in English, *The Beginnings of Human Life,* defined the word biodynamics as "a special category of vital phenomena." Then he said, "biodynamics implies biochemistry." In *Biokinetics and Biodynamics of Human Differentiation* (Blechschmidt and Gasser, 1978), he said, "Biodynamics are manifested in submicroscopic developmental movements." In *The Ontogenetic Basis of Human Anatomy* (Blechschmidt, 2004), he described biodynamics as the "dynamic aspects of forces acting in ontogeny, with respect to the fluctuating mechanical equilibrium of metabolic processes in the developing organism." So one has to talk to his colleagues, such as Dr. Raymond Gasser or Dr. I. F. Seidel at the Blechschmidt Museum in Germany and try to tease out a greater meaning. Rather than use the word "wholeness," which experimental embryologists were using at the time, he used the word "entirety." His writings in English imply that he observed submicroscopic movement in the fluids that generate, maintain, and sustain (much like a catalyst) the fields of cellular activity in the embryo that metabolize the raw building materials of the embryo into the structure and function of the body. All of this goes on in the context of the fluid form of an embryo—a water being that over time congeals into the structure and function of the fetus, infant, child, and adult. He went on to say that the genes were not self-activating but needed an impulse coming from the fluids.

To understand and palpate wholeness as a movement is to understand and palpate wholeness as a self-organizing principle in the body. In other words, there is a discrete and palpable movement in the embryo and the adult that generates order as Dr. Blechschmidt said. Both Dr. Blechschmidt and Dr. Sutherland said the ordering movement is located in the fluids. They were saying the same thing except from a different perspective. To make a leap now, I would like to propose that the submicroscopic self-organizing movement in the fluids is the one called Primary Respiration by Dr. Sutherland (because I sense it as a long, slow, subtle breath all around and inside my body). This is no longer a theory but a sensory experience and a clinical observation that I have verified thousands of times. Consequently, the rest of this discussion may seem theoretical unless the reader has sensed Primary Respiration. Furthermore, there is a matrix of form called the human embryo in which the activity of Primary Respiration takes place and is conserved throughout the lifespan. Form is the totality of all structure-function relationships in the embryo at any given time. Wholeness is thus a self-ordering movement and a three-dimensional form in the image of an embryo called Primary Respiration. It is rather hard to wrap your neurons around this until you have a direct palpatory experience of it. It is nonlinear. One has to touch it and feel it in the hands and heart.

Of course, there are many types of movements and vectors in the fluids, but I am specifically referring to a slow one that Dr. Sutherland originally called the Long Tide or Primary Respiration. The discovery that Dr. Sutherland and his students made in the middle of the twentieth century was that something subtle and very powerful was directing the healing process. He originally referred to it as the Breath of Life. It is what I am now calling wholeness, although some would call it love so I will call it love as well. He further observed that it was moving *in* the fluids but it was not *of* the body's fluids. Primary Respiration is a perceptual experience of living, moving wholeness, and perhaps the embryo is the image of love, if I may be so poetic. Some other osteopaths and biodynamic practitioners make distinctions about the perception of the Breath of Life and use other descriptive language, images, and metaphors, all of which is part of the unique perceptual and palpatory experience of the whole. Images and metaphors are extremely useful in describing the preverbal experience of our particular origin in the womb and remember that Primary Respiration reveals itself differently to everyone in the sense of its perceptual sequence.

I personally have had a direct perception of this movement called Primary Respiration and can access it anytime, with or without a client, in my body and around my body. It is a perception of wholeness because of my senses being totally immersed in it and its three-dimensionality out to the horizon and back. It is outside my body and it orients to specific places called fulcrums and axes inside my body. Where does it come from? I do not know. It seems, however, to frequently trade places in my perception with a deep stillness. I am able to sense it in moments of attending to it by evenly suspending my attention throughout my whole body, the total surface of my skin, and then all around me and out to the horizon. But that is not enough because wholeness is a type of breathing, a reciprocal type of breathing. My suspended attention then begins to move back and forth in rhythmic phases of fifty seconds. Out for fifty and in for fifty, or up for fifty and down for fifty, and so forth. I am not attending to tissue but to the image of the contents and surroundings of my body being a fluid medium with multiple currents. This is the new metaphor and the new body-centered practice that seeks contact with the fluids rather than the tissues of the body. What is amazing is how easy it is for students to sense this.

Therefore, I have concluded that wholeness is the movement of Primary Respiration perceived to be occurring in the total fluid medium of the body. It is coming from outside my body when I orient my head and neck to the horizon. It is coming from the earth when I lie supine on the ground, and, most interestingly, I can sense it between my heart and the heart of my spiritual teacher or the heart of my client. I can sense it directing the session of work with clients and its relationship to the deep stillpoint that it dances with and trades places with during the treatment. This is of particular relevance to all health care practitioners and especially manual therapists because of the importance of accessing stillness frequently during any session of therapy for the sake of integration. This makes biodynamic practice a slow therapy.

The way in which the wholeness of the embryo is conserved during a lifetime of shape shifting called development and differentiation is through the 100-second cycle of Primary Respiration, or what is sometimes called the Long Tide, the tide, or the primary respiratory impulse. It is like the catalytic converter of the embryo for the enormous amount of work that the embryo does in its growth. Proportionally, the embryo has a much larger basal metabolism than the adult body. It is working incredibly hard, and it is interesting to note that human embryos spontaneously abort more than the embryos of any other species on the planet. Up to 60–70 percent of all human embryos fail to make it to term. It is hard work being an embryo!

Saying wholeness is a movement is a pretty bold statement and requires perceptual verification by a trained practitioner. As Dr. Sutherland said, "this is not an idle dream" (or, as I would say it, "this is not a new-age fantasy"). To review, the first defining principle of biodynamics is: *Wholeness is the movement of Primary Respiration and its perception as a therapeutic force in the fluids of the body.* I believe that this is what Dr. Blechschmidt meant by "the law of the continuity of individuality." The corollary to this first principle is that the therapeutic force of Primary Respiration originates outside the body and thus exhibits its influence from the outside-in. Several books are necessary to explain these principles properly, which is what I have undertaken with these books I have written. Biodynamics is a whole new paradigm rather than an eclectic therapy.

Let me switch gears now a little bit. You don't have to accept how I am defining biodynamics, but hold it as a possibility because—as Dr. Ida Rolf was fond of saying—"you can't get there from here." But we can at least try to have a basic understanding. The next edge biodynamics explores is to find a contemporary unifying theory to hold all of this information together. It requires a theory that is inclusive of several domains of knowledge and research. Along comes Dr. Allan Schore, who has begun to codify what is called "regulation theory" in infant brain development from numerous streams of literature. He holds the patent on the incredibly complex understanding of the orbitofrontal cortex of the brain. I will talk a little bit about this because it really is groundbreaking work (you can read about it in detail in the section of this book on infants and children). He points out that the fundamental developmental vector in the late fetal brain and the first two years after birth is the self-regulation of the emotions.

Regulation theory derives from an enormous body of research material in the attachment and bonding literature. The new paradigm is now simply called affective neuroscience.

One of Dr. Schore's principles is that the client-therapist relationship is a direct analog of the mother-infant relationship. The client-therapist relationship is the other half of the equation when contacting the fluids of the body. Affective neuroscience describes a process of resonance and attunement that occurs between the right hemispheres of the infant-caregiver dyad. It is the same process when any two people seek proximity to one another or withdraw from one another. It is especially enhanced in any therapeutic relationship involving manual therapy because of the physical contact that a practitioner makes with the client. Recent research has discovered a discrete set of nerve pathways from the skin that go to a center in the right hemisphere that reads the context of the touch rather than the sensory component of it. This context center gets sensitized during infancy as to whether touch is nurturing and loving. This center can be damaged and thus the adult client may misread the contact unconsciously and dysregulate the autonomic nervous system. There is no conscious recall of the touch history because it occurred in the preverbal time of life. The trauma resolution paradigm really speaks to this dilemma.

Recently, the term *neuro-affective touch* was coined by the Schore study group at UCLA. It is a term that recognizes a degree of "palpatory literacy" necessary to hold the pre- and perinatal memories in the client's body. It further implies that the physical contact with a client is gentle, subtle, and synchronized with a slow tempo. I believe biodynamic craniosacral practitioners are using that quality of touch because of the influence on the community of (Somatic Experiencing founder) Peter Levine and other important clinicians like Pat Ogden, Robert Scaer, and Daniel Siegel, who are promoting body-centered trauma resolution work. The reason this is important is because the infant's entire organism, as well as its brain, develops best when it can synchronize with a slow endogenous tempo and be physically held and nurtured by a low-stress caregiver. This describes a biodynamic attachment process as much between a client and therapist as it does between the infant and caregiver because the contact is so slow, still, warm, and tender, mimicking a "secure" attachment.

I have seen this over and over again and write about it in *Biodynamic Craniosacral Therapy,* Volume One. Much of my clinical experience over the past twenty-five years has been with infants and children. I originally had been practicing Rolfing and biomechanical craniosacral therapy with infants who have severe brain damage and evolved into treating infants with feeding problems or complications arising from C-section and vacuum extraction deliveries. Infants are always more responsive when someone in the room is actively engaged in the perception of Primary Respiration or resting in a stillpoint. I have verified this for myself by checking cardiovascular monitoring equipment when I work with medically fragile children. I can see all the parameters—blood pressure, heart rate, and so on—in the infant or child become lower when I am synchronized with Primary Respiration, and the positive affect that this has on the healing process is obvious to me and the pediatric therapists who are present.

Treating someone biodynamically also means that the practitioner needs to spend a majority of the time in a session sensing his own body and accessing a slow tempo. This allows for a biodynamic self-regulation to occur across nervous systems and fluid fields. This creates a resonance that down-regulates autonomic activation or withdrawal states in the client. Biodynamics in this sense is an attunement to these slow tides in the practitioner first, which recognizes the need to remain differentiated in the therapeutic relationship and oriented to a slow tempo in the client. Even psychotherapists are now being coached to sense their own bodies to be more effective biodynamically with their clients. The basic idea here is that the client is trying to learn to self-regulate in two ways. The first is autonomously, or what is called a "top-down" ability of the executive control centers in the frontal cortex of the brain to consciously lower states of activation in the limbic system and body when alone. The second, using the same neural pathways, is through relationship and the way in which I down-regulate states of activation when I am with another person nonviolently or nonaggressively. This corresponds to what Dr. Schore calls "experience-dependent maturation" of the infant's brain, derived from the activity of the caregiver's brain, her gesture and touch, her eye gaze, and sounds being interpreted by the infant's sensory systems and brain. These are the two basic types of self-regulation and are directly related to what Dr. Blechschmidt called an "outside-in influence" in the embryo from fluids to cell membrane to cytoplasm to cell nucleus. But in the case of the infant, the outside influence is the mother's attunement. The underlying metabolic processes in the embryo are directly related to the physiological processes in the infant can therefore be described as biodynamic. Both self-regulatory processes are designed to be slow, purposeful, and well-organized. I believe that the intention of many of the manual therapeutic arts has always been about creating autonomy for the client and thus supporting self-regulation. When this occurs at the same pace and same attunement as the infant-mother relationship, it is biodynamic. This is why I now believe that the term somatic could be renamed as biodynamic.

We have to move infant regulation theory, however, back to the embryo and even the pre-conception time of when the egg originally differentiated in the mother's ovary when she herself was an embryo inside her mother's womb. There are many stages of egg development before fertilization by a sperm, so fertilization is considered to be the next stage of development and not the beginning of life at all. But rather than talk about the genetics of egg development and embryology, as a manual therapist it is more important to understand and then feel the morphology (shape changing) of the embryo. This will circle us back to the discussion of Primary Respiration and fluid movement. The wholeness of the embryo is self-regulated through properties found in its form. Form is defined as the totality of all structures and functions in the embryo. Form involves the following description of fluid behavior: symmetry, polarity, morphology, fields of physical metabolism and tensegrity, character structure (growth as gesture), constitution (heredity), and structure-function relationships. In a biodynamic embryology, the form of the embryo itself is a visible image of wholeness. Fluid behaviors are the behaviors of the whole. In other words, the movement of Primary Respiration takes place in a fluid-form matrix and it generates shapes and structures in the fluid body of the embryo, as one osteopath calls it. The fluid body is the total systemic fluid medium of the developing embryo and Primary Respiration is its brain, so to speak. This is the biodynamic human embryo. This is what I believe Dr. Sutherland referred to as the "blueprint" of form and function carried by Primary Respiration.

A gene responsible for the form and its shaping process that we inhabit has not been discovered yet, and until then this is a plausible explanation because it is a both a perceptual experience and clinical observation rather than a theory. This is a study of the physical laws affecting growth and development coming from "outside-in," whether an embryo, an infant, or an adult. The physics "implies" the biochemistry of the embryo and together they become biology. Biochemistry is about genetics these days, but as Rolf implied with her life's work, I cannot get my hands on the genes. I can, however, sense the shaping processes of the embryo in the fluid body of my adult clients. Hundreds and hundreds of clients report a deeper sensory experience or an image of wholeness from biodynamic craniosacral therapy, as well as from other modalities including Rolfing. The therapeutic experience is reported with different language, images, and metaphors that are uniquely noncognitive because regulation theory is about a time of development that takes place in a preverbal state.

How does one describe the experience of sentient fluids congealing into a specific structure? We need a whole new language and metaphor other than nervous system sensation generated by soft tissue manipulation that travels to the brain and back down to the body. We need something more three-dimensional or perhaps four-dimensional and descriptive of living fluids that were present before a nervous system even differentiated in the embryo. An enormous amount of kinetic metabolism takes place prior to sensory neurons differentiating at twenty-eight days postfertilization, and there is ample literature on the experiences of those first twenty-eight days from regression therapy and analytical therapy from as far back as the 1940s. That preverbal time has what is called a homologous link to adult physiology but needs to be accessed differently by a biodynamic practitioner. Biodynamic also describes the state of mind and body of the practitioner, which is the priority in therapeutic work, rather than the client. What the practitioner is accessing in himself and the client is the behavior of the fluids.

Fluids behave biokinetically, which involves dynamic morphology. Dynamic morphology describes the active shaping processes that occur during each of the first three weeks of embryonic development and weeks four through eight or the end of the embryonic period. During each of these four stages of morphology, the embryo undergoes a different shaping process unique to that week or stage. The purpose of the shaping is to orient the embryonic being to time and space, which are the precursors to a body's orientation to gravity. For instance, this means that in the first week, its morphology has a symmetry that is very inward-directed and thus a significant amount of compression occurs. The first orientation is coming "in" to form. The second week is very outward-directed and thus a lot of decompression and tension. The second orientation is going "out" to make contact with the environment. Such orientation causes symmetry to arise in the structure of the embryo and is necessary for self-regulation at a metabolic level. The orienting embryo must build a system of cavities to create a boundary around its fluids. Think of the early embryo as three concentric spheres of fluid, one within the other and each with its own metabolism and purpose. The boundaries of the cavities generate an inner membrane layer that creates a metabolism of autonomy and an outer membrane layer that is more permeable and open to an exchange with the environment. This permeable layer is the metabolism of relationship. Remember, this is a shaping process and a growth process that is biodynamic as well as biochemical. Dr. Blechschmidt felt there was more physics involved in early growth and development than there was biochemistry. Furthermore, the embryo is free of the influence of gravity and more under the influence of buoyancy or lift in the fluid body for the purpose of symmetrical orientation and metabolic self-regulation. The fluids of the embryo have discrete directions of movement, such as along a longitudinal axis usually associated with a tissue boundary and a movement perpendicular to that axis. Manual therapy that only works with the effects of gravity is perinatal in its application in that the major effects of gravity come on-line after birth. A biodynamic therapy takes into account the biodynamic formative forces in the prenatal time of development as being more important in the clinical process, not in the sense of being better but simply as a correct sequence.

In the beginning of the third week of embryonic development, the symmetry of the embryo becomes oriented to a midline called the primitive streak and then the notochord. With a midline the embryo can orient to the basic directions of right and left, top and bottom, front and back; this is essential as embodiment begins to occur at this time. A middle develops and it becomes the body. The heart and future muscles and bones start to differentiate. I would like to reinforce an important aspect regarding the metabolic function of the midline—that it is a distusion field. This means that the tissue itself is being pulled in opposite directions, and because of its position in the embryo, it is kinetically still. Dr. Blechschmidt felt that this was critically important because all growth and development was oriented to the function of stillness from the beginning and now the stillness became visible in the sense of the stillness shifting from a point in the fluids to an actual cellular structure. Stillness became embodied in the core of the body. This is one reason that biodynamic practice starts by orienting to stillness, which gives the practitioner clear access to observing the activity of these embryonic fields.

Finally, during the fourth week to the end of the embryonic period, an orientation to folding and unfolding becomes possible. Now the human embryo explores freedom, which is a big story covered in Volume One. Of course there are numerous other overlapping metabolic processes happening by then, but orientation to stillness and self-regulation through attunement to a slow tempo are the biodynamic ways that wholeness is conserved through very complex development. I believe that Rolfing is a related field of biodynamics because of its interest in establishing fascial symmetry around a midline. What is fascia? It is thick fluid. It has a different gradient of viscosity in it. Imagine being able to access the less congealed state of the fascia that is not bound by gravity but by the lift of the fluids. This is the embryo, and it is still present in the adult.

Then we have the business of metabolic fields, as I mentioned above—another aspect of biokinetics, also mentioned. A thorough description of all the metabolic fields can be found in Section IV on embryology. Some students think that this business of field activity was Dr. Blechschmidt's idea. But the notion of embryonic fields consisting of differential areas of fluid activity, or "sub-wholes" in the embryo, came into the scientific embryology literature in the 1920s, once again by the experimental embryologists. This is really another aspect of biodynamic practice that is vitally important in the cranial community and manual therapy in general. The eight metabolic fields that Dr. Blechschmidt

described are construction zones in the overall site plan (form)
ing fluid body. They are defined by their different positions, sha
relationships. They are definitely something a practitioner can get
because Dr. Sutherland discovered their homologue in the adult
cally, these movements are described as flexion-extension, compress
sidebending-rotation, torsion-shearing, inferior-superior vertical str
on. When a practitioner orients to stillness and self-regulates biod
these biokinetic fields actually appear as specific shapes and vector
the practitioner's hands as a kind of template subsequent to the four
symmetry and morphology described above; this is done while simul   ...sly
maintaining a wide perceptual attention in the context of the total fluid system
of the body via Primary Respiration, rather than specific end condensations
like the cranial base as is traditionally taught in biomechanical work. These
fields have zones of activity called polarities. One polarity is sensed as different
gradients of density and temperatures in the fluids along or perpendicular to a
membrane axis.

A major polarity begins at the end of the first week, when the first stem
cell lines become apparent. The first two stem cell lines are a division into
two separate bodies. Dr. Jaap van der Wal calls these the "central body" of the
embryo (which ultimately becomes the soma) and the "peripheral body" (which
ultimately becomes the placenta). This type of polarity is more like a bifurcation
of the form of the embryo itself into two wholes that are mirroring one another
but with different bias in their chemical metabolism. There is a certain elegance
here, because the central body projects function to the peripheral body biodynamically (streaming of information in the fluids). In other words, the outer
layer of cells, in contact with the uterine environment, contains liver enzymes
and hormones being produced by the peripheral body and all sorts of interesting movements, areas of stillness, and specialized cells on its inner lining. This
is the metabolism of relationship, because the peripheral body is in contact with
the uterine environment with its outer layer of cells. The central body has no
specific structure called a "liver" or "glandular tissue." It prefers its autonomy
for as long as it can by first establishing two fluid cavities called the yolk sac and
amniotic sac before it connects to the periphery. The communication between
the two bodies is through the fluids biodynamically with the ultimate biological
intention being connected blood to blood. The mother's blood is being invited
to connect to the embryo's blood that is already being produced in the second
week. Blood attracts blood, so to speak. The central body is autonomous and
early on is not even directly connected to the periphery by tissue—only by the
biodynamic movements in the fluids between them.

The process of projecting function by the metabolism of the central or autonomous body to the periphery (until the structure arises internally) becomes a physiological process in the fetus and infant. This means that the infant manages his autonomic nervous system by projecting it to the mother and consequently having it reflected back in a settled state (ideally). Finally, the function of projection becomes psychological in the adult. The strong emotions that I can't handle get projected onto other people around me until I can re-own them with the proper psychospiritual structure. Thus it is natural for the client to project function onto the practitioner, and the practitioner to help build the structure in his body for it to be reclaimed biodynamically by the client with Primary Respiration and stillness. The principle here is that the practitioner simply must stay in contact with his sensory body in a slow tempo. His brain is unconsciously creating the client as a neural network in his brain and body just like a mother does with her baby and just like the baby does with the mother. It is a two-way street, whether in an infant-mother dyad or a client-therapist dyad. Preverbal visitations from the client into the mind and body of the practitioner are constant; likewise, the client is visited by the practitioner's unconscious. It is a two-way street. It is quite real and at times not so unconscious. The client must be able to resonate with a slow tempo in the practitioner to self-regulate the relationship and at the same time generate autonomy.

If a theory is a good one, it will include the spiritual, as the theories of Dr. A. T. Still and Dr. Sutherland did. There are two theologies in the Judeo-Christian world. One is the theology of transcendence, where one projects divinity as something way beyond the horizon of the mind and body to comprehend. The other is the theology of immanence, in which the divine is immediately accessible in and around the body and available in the here and now. I believe this starts with the metabolic function of the embryo having a center and a periphery. The function of projecting to the periphery is maintained spiritually as well, and the connecting link is Primary Respiration—in the sense that the transcendent and the immanent breathe together and are not mutually exclusive. This is the great work of mysticism, Jungian analysis, and countless ecstatic traditions. Please don't think I'm making a case for biodynamic mysticism. I am not. The case here is for understanding the notion of center and periphery and its role in a therapeutic process that does not exclude the spiritual. It is huge. The entire last section of this book is dedicated to exploring the spiritual dimension of biodynamic practice.

Finally, let me say one last thing about the principles of biodynamic practice. Structure-function relationships are quite active at all times in the body, from the first differentiation of an egg cell to the moment of death. I have heard it called "structuring," which describes the structure-function relationship as a unitary metabolic process (build up, break down, and fuel the process of structuring) that is a constant with living bodies. A structure is not a static thing. It is very active. This brings up a particular principle that all adult function is preexercised in the human embryo. For example, Dr. Blechschmidt said that the newly fertilized zygote starts moving with a reciprocal movement in its fluids. He originally called this a "suction field" and said that this was the preexercising of the respiratory function. The respiratory function is the oldest function in the organism and is a high priority to assess therapeutically in biodynamic craniosacral therapy and a first hour of Rolfing. In my Rolf training in 1980 it was stressed that Dr. Rolf believed all change process needed to be supported by an increase in respiratory capacity. The point here is that, embryologically, function precedes structure; but, to avoid this chicken-or-egg argument, a practitioner must be able to palpate, unobtrusively at first, a functioning structure that is constantly shaping and reshaping itself, and to do so requires biodynamic skills derived from the principles stated here and outlined throughout this book. The same preexercising can be said then for endocrine function, autonomic nervous system function, cardiovascular function, and so forth. All of this function is grounded in a slow, developmental tempo with stillpoints all around it. Biodynamic craniosacral therapy is a model of physical metabolism.

In this light, it is possible to understand that the study of a biodynamic embryology is important to manual therapy and especially craniosacral therapy. The embryo is a living whole. It has a form. This living, moving form is the image of wholeness and can be palpated in an adult or a child. Practitioners can synchronize their attention with it and support and augment the healing process of biodynamic self-regulation. All of this is accessible if the practitioner is working at a slow tempo and has a personal relationship with Primary Respiration. This is the meaning of biodynamic. It is much deeper than the embryo itself in my clinical observation. It is first and foremost based on the perceptual and palpatory experience of the practitioner. It describes a unique therapeutic approach to supporting self-regulation of the client from the beginning in the prenatal period of life. It is done through the lens of the practitioner's perception of a variety of events occurring in the fluids of the body rather than the tissues.

The whole process of biodynamic practice becomes deeply instinctual and less mechanical. By less mechanical, I mean less cognitive and more sentient, less intuitive and more instinctual. The mind of the practitioner becomes still, and the slow tempo of aliveness in the fluids becomes the priority, because that is the way it was in the beginning. The biodynamic process then reveals the biokinetic and morphological processes, which then reveal the biomechanical and physiological processes—rather than the other way around. This developmental sequence is honored in biodynamic craniosacral therapy.[1]

Chapter 2

Principles of Practice

Intention of Biodynamic Craniosacral Therapy

Love. The deepest yearnings of the heart with self and other are love and compassion. Biodynamically, love is the felt sense of heat coupled to the perception of openness radiating out from the core of the body to self and others. Compassion is the felt sense and image of someone else's pain and suffering coming into the practitioner's heart.

Differentiation. To differentiate is to become a self-actualized human being, one who is autonomous as a function of wisdom rather than wounding. This is a conception right.

Containment. The practitioner manages the therapeutic relationship through attunement to its midline of stillness. Biodynamic craniosacral therapy is not a release-based cathartic therapy. There is no self-regulation without containment.

Self-regulation. Transformation of emotions both autonomously (withdrawing appropriately to restore equilibrium) and in relationship (contacting another person appropriately to restore equilibrium). This is also a conception right.

Health. The focus of the practice is to orient to and synchronize with the preexisting health in the practitioner's soma, the client's soma, and the natural world that can never become diseased.

Theory—Perceptual Processes

Dynamic Stillness. Awareness of the cessation of movement inside the body and nonlocally (three-dimensionally) outside the body, or both together. All types of stillpoints are related to the Dynamic Stillness. Death (non-existence such as the moment before the egg differentiates) is the deepest state of Dynamic Stillness. Such non-existence is constantly present in a biodynamic process and known by Dynamic Stillness or more deeply as a void state free of any conceptualization.

Breath of Life. A metaphor for love. Biodynamically it is sensed as the "spark" of light or quantum movement in the midline at the beginning of primary inhalation. It is that which causes animation and initiates the life forces of the fluid body. It is known through the presence of love or the felt sense of grace. Love is the deepest imprint in the soma.

Primary Respiration. Together with the Breath of Life, called the tidal body or, in older osteopathic literature, the Long Tide. Primary Respiration is the carrier wave for the spark and the blueprint for the form of wholeness to incarnate in the fluid body and the soma. It moves in 100-second cycles. Together with the Breath of Life, it is an active, numinous intelligence informing, maintaining, and repairing the metabolism of the fluid body and the biology of the soma. The human embryo is the visible form of the invisible but perceivable movement of Primary Respiration. Primary Respiration does not hold stress or trauma. It is known through the presence of compassion or the inherent plan of being. This is the constant heart-to-heart exchange of the practitioner's well-being with the client's pain and suffering at the tempo of Primary Respiration. Compassion is the in-breath and love is the out-breath of the practitioner. See Figure 2.1 for a concept map of the tidal body.

The Tidal Body

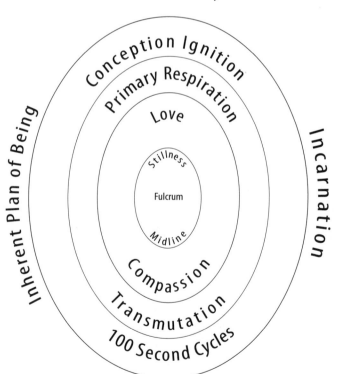

Figure 2.1. The tidal body concept map

Fluid body. Sometimes called the Mid Tide or potency tide. The fluid body represents dynamic whole continuum of living water and protoplasm in and immediately around the form of the body. It has several biodynamic life forces consisting of structured living water and electromagnetism, fluid forces such as longitudinal fluctuation, lateral fluctuations, the reciprocal tension potency (RTP), embodied stillness, and finally Primary Respiration, which is its brain or mind, so to speak. Its activity includes the systemic condensing and breaking down of the protoplasm into the different shapes of the body called embryonic metabolic fields, which ultimately create the structure of the soma. The life forces of the fluid body must animate and maintain every cell in the body. Its movement is a range of possibilities from one to three cycles per minute. The fluid body is also the instinctual intelligence of the natural world that knows how to heal itself. The fluid body holds stress and trauma in a way that is deeper and more fundamental than the way it is held in the tissues of the body, as will be discussed in detail in Section II, Relating with Trauma. See Figure 2.2 for a concept map of the fluid body.

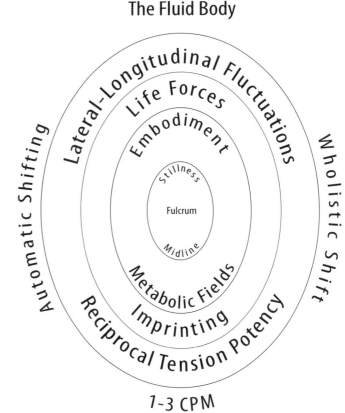

Figure 2.2. The fluid body concept map

Cranial Rhythmic Impulse (CRI). The systemic physiological response of the soma to the activity of the autonomic nervous system, especially its interaction with the respiratory, central nervous, cardiovascular, and musculoskeletal systems. The soma of the client is where the practitioner places her hands and through which a client perceives his basic sensory experience. The soma experiences emotions, conception, and birth trauma, learns to self-regulate, and ultimately dies. See Figure 2.3 for a concept map of the soma.

The Soma

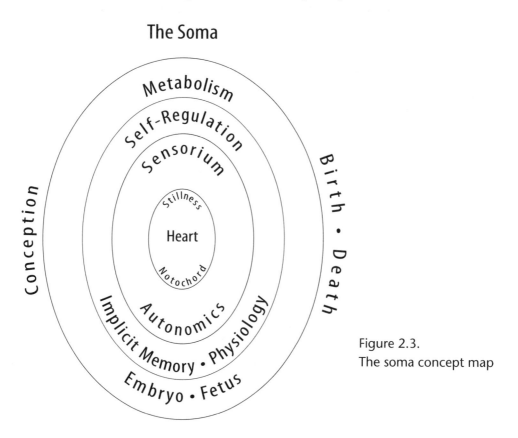

Figure 2.3.
The soma concept map

Midline or fulcrum. Fulcrums are stillpoints of orientation that spontaneously arise in the embryo, especially during the first two weeks of development. Midlines are still axes of orientation that arise spontaneously in the third week and beyond of embryonic development. All growth and development in the soma, as well as all perceptual states of the PRS, are oriented to a midline or a fulcrum. The terms midline and fulcrum are used interchangeably. Clinically, the practitioner works with the simultaneous perception of movement and nonmovement (stillness-midline) through divided attention until the movement peripheral of the midline and the midline become well related or unified as a single continuum or whole. The first function of the midline is to maintain one's connection to sacred space, which is a foundation principle of healing in biodynamic craniosacral therapy. See Figures 2.4 and 2.5 for a description of the fulcrum and the midline referenced throughout this book.

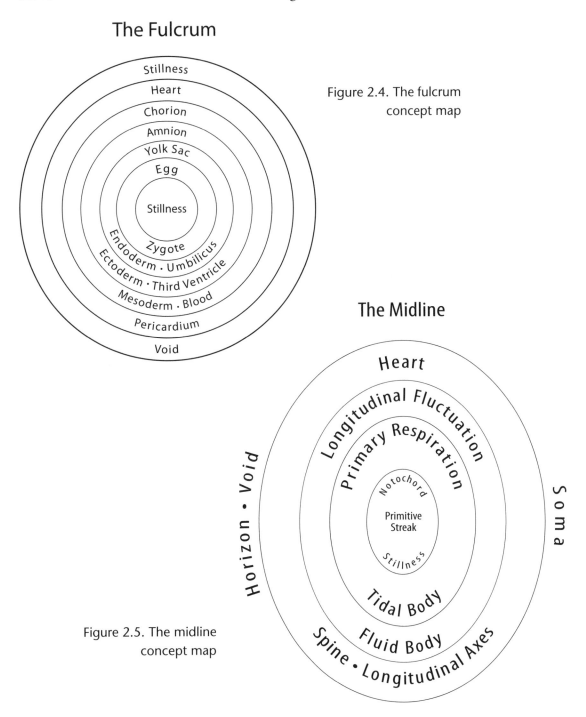

The Fulcrum

Figure 2.4. The fulcrum concept map

The Midline

Figure 2.5. The midline concept map

Sentience. All processes in the PRS represent sentient activity outside the control of the brain. Thus, they are considered to be an instinctual intelligence found throughout nature and intrinsic to the fluid and tidal bodies of the PRS. It must be remembered at all times that our biology and perception is the subject of this fluid intelligence rather than this intelligence being subservient to the practitioner's will.

Basic Clinical Relationship Skills —Establishing Safety and Trust

Communication. Verbal skills with the client for the acknowledgment of pain and suffering include resourcing, acknowledging, and mirroring. All other bio-dynamic skills are nonverbal and perceptual (sensing and fluid shaping), ima-ginal (images and mythic stories), or instinctual (in common with the natural world).

Orienting. Sensing stillness in the fulcrums and midlines of the body of the practitioner and three-dimensionally in the environment without overtly focus-ing on the client is the starting point in the therapeutic process. This establishes the practitioner as a therapeutic fulcrum in the relationship rather than the cli-ent being an "identified patient." This requires the practitioner to consciously disassociate from the contemporary world outside the office.

Synchronizing. Sensing the slow tempo of Primary Respiration inside and outside the practitioner's body, two-dimensionally and then three-dimensionally. It moves away from or toward the fulcrum and the midline.

Buoyancy. Allowing the hands to float and be transparent when in physi-cal contact with the client. They seem to be submerged in liquid up to the elbow. Gradually the hands disappear, or, alternatively, a second pair of hands or benevolent presence is perceived to be leading or assisting the session.

Receptivity exchange. The pain and suffering of the client is acknowledged nonverbally at the beginning of a session, as follows: Initially, the practitioner dwells on an image or memory that produces tenderness, sadness, and warmth around the area of the heart, lungs, and rib cage. This produces a felt sense of heat in the core of the body and possibly the face and eyes. Upon initial physi-cal contact with the client, the practitioner receives the flow of the client's PRS with a heart-to-heart connection of compassion moving at the tempo of Primary Respiration. The practitioner imagines that her whole body is one large heart that can take in the totality of the client's dilemma. When this tide changes direction, the practitioner gives the client unconditional love at the same tempo. It helps for the practitioner to also imagine that this movement not only has a felt sense of warmth but is the color red—the color of blood. The infant seeks to have the caregiver receive its love and for the caregiver to acknowledge that love and return it in kind. This is the same in the client-therapist relationship. Through compassion, pain and suffering are transformed into the original condition of love. This entire process of receptivity exchange is inherent to the heart and brain of every human being. It is well documented, especially in babies. All other palpation skills mentioned below are secondary.

Disengagement. Hands are instinctually removed at the conclusion of a segment of work or the end of the session. Knowing how to end is as important as knowing how to begin.

Pacing. A biodynamic session of work is divided into three parts. There is a beginning, in order to establish the container. There is a middle, where therapeutic forces tend to manifest in the session if they choose to. Finally, there is an ending period of time, when the practitioner and client gradually and mutually withdraw attention from each other. There is no set timing for these phases. Each session is unique and reveals its own timing based on the principles stated below.

First Principle of Perception—How Systemic Organization Is Witnessed in the Practitioner

Autonomy. The practitioner establishes the ground of autonomy by sensing the interplay between stillness and Primary Respiration in her own self first. Dr. Rollin Becker called this rhythmic balanced interchange—the practitioner's perception of Dynamic Stillness changing places with Primary Respiration. This takes an unspecified amount of time to establish at the beginning of a session and forms a clinical baseline of perception for the whole session. This is how the midline is established in each session. By doing so, the practitioner self-ignites her instinct for empathy and compassion. The conventional world fades and dies for a brief period of time. This builds a container for a natural therapeutic engagement between practitioner and client. The practitioner remains as the therapeutic fulcrum for the session.

Attunement. The practitioner gradually and consciously attends to the cycles of stillness exchanging places with Primary Respiration, both outside and inside her body. The cycle of attunement includes discerning pauses, breaks in continuity of perception, activity of discursive thinking (mental chit-chat), and the precision and timing of the rhythmic balanced interchange of stillness and Primary Respiration in one's self and then in the client. Attunement requires equanimity of heart, mind, and body for self-observation of subtle fluid phenomena.

Symmetry. Capacity to witness unobtrusively the activity of the midline and the fulcrum in relationship to the whole. This includes the symmetry of growth exhibited in the four stages of embryonic morphology detailed in Volume One and includes the movement of the whole in the tidal body of Primary Respiration and the systemic activity of the fluid body.

Resonance. This is both the initiation and fruition of one of the deepest therapeutic processes. The practitioner automatically and unconsciously metabolizes stress states in the client through the biodynamic processes. The client automatically and unconsciously seeks coherence with the practitioner's slow tempo and ability to be still. Coherence requires a relatively noiseless mind (non-neurotic), which is a function of autonomy. At this level of understanding, the practitioner becomes a valuable therapeutic fulcrum for resolving stress in the client, as a function of the practitioner's perception rather than using a manual skill (which comes later, if necessary).

Nonlinear. Biodynamic perception is not a linear process. Rather, it is dynamic and mutable. The practitioner consciously disassociates her attention from the contemporary world into the sacred world of stillness, love, and compassion. Session work with biodynamic craniosacral therapy rarely has logical sequential processes. There is a starting point and an ending point because of the clock. Everything in between is nonlinear; consequently, the biggest job of the practitioner is to become comfortable with not knowing what the next step will be. It is revealed as a function of the practitioner's perception of the rhythmic balanced interchange of Dynamic Stillness and Primary Respiration.

Horizon. The movement of the practitioner's perception is oriented to the Dynamic Stillness at the horizon or the far edge of the natural world. The perception of the outside presence of Primary Respiration must be established between this location of the Dynamic Stillness at the horizon (biodynamic) and the practitioner's midline of metabolic stillness (biokinetic) in order to establish sacred space.

Second Principle of Perception—How Order and Organization Are Witnessed in the Client

Pendulation. As a foundation principle, the practitioner spends the majority of time in a session sensing her own PRS rather than that of the client, until both become one unified field. Pendulation describes how the practitioner gradually and periodically attunes to the interplay of stillness and Primary Respiration in and around the client while in physical contact with the client after establishing this quality of perception in herself. Secondarily, when the fluid body manifests its therapeutic activity in the client, the practitioner must be oriented to Primary Respiration in herself in order to resynchronize the fluid body of the client to its temporary therapeutic fulcrum in the practitioner. Through pendulation the practitioner gradually returns the normal fulcrum of the fluid body which is Primary Respiration back to the client.

Center-periphery. The next foundation principle regarding the client-therapist dyad is based on the dual bodies of the embryo as being one unit of function described in the dynamic morphology of the human embryo. Please refer to Chapter 24 describing embryonic visualizations. The client begins as a peripheral body and practitioner as central body. The hands and arms of the practitioner are the connecting stalk and then the umbilical veins and arteries. The principle of center-periphery includes frequent role reversals in the client-therapist relationship, just as the embryo turns itself upside down and inside out as a frequent gesture of growth and development. The practitioner constantly exchanges her body-mind with that of the client's body-mind as a single metabolic field of mutually related activity. The base tempo is always within stillness and Primary Respiration.

Stillpoint. A broad category of self-correcting phenomena in the PRS. The biodynamic function of a stillpoint is to kindle the ignition processes of the PRS and allow heat to permeate the soma of the client. The stillpoint may be the only healing dynamic available in or around the client or the practitioner for the entire session. At this second level of healing principles, the stillpoint is related to the Dynamic Stillness as an embodied awareness of its presence inside or around the practitioner or client and close to the therapeutic container, such as trees or clouds rather than at the horizon. It is an indication that something is dying and coming to an end perceptually. This is called transmutation.

Movement of the whole. This is an important principle after the autonomy of the practitioner has been established. The practitioner disregards localized movement in the client and initially attends only to movement in the whole in or around the client's body. This is a perception that will be greatly augmented by asking the client to use his imagination of his internal fluid sense, fluid image, and fluid shape.

Communion. Progressive stages of perceiving Primary Respiration and its fulcrum of stillness are described in Volume One and in this volume. Gradually the practitioner comes into a unified sense of the client (whole)-therapist (whole) relationship breathing as one entity. This is a deep therapeutic process and is still dependent on the practitioner maintaining autonomy. Communion ignites the therapeutic potential within the relationship.

Client participation. The client must be taught to participate in accessing his fluid body and tidal body. Guided meditations are taught both during a biodynamic session and afterwards, to enhance the healing process. They allow the client to step out of his nervous system and uncouple from trauma with the aid of Primary Respiration. Results are much quicker and more recognizable by the client. Chapters in this section of the book go into detail on client participation.

Third Principle of Palpation Skills—Hand Placement and Focus of Attention

No structure. All adult anatomical structure must be considered (visualized) to be non-existent and in its original state of protoplasm in the first two weeks postfertilization, both in the practitioner and the client, to be therapeutically effective with one's hands biodynamically. At the same time, the knowledge of anatomy is temporarily used for locating specific hand placements and then quickly forgotten. The practitioner imagines that the client's body is a transparent, dynamic water being in the form of a human during its first two weeks of development postfertilization.

Precision. This skill specifically refers to the exact location of the hand contact on the client that initially requires knowledge of surface and internal adult anatomy. In addition, the quality of touch is so neutral and unobtrusive that its intention is to circumvent the corticolimbic system as much as is possible in a contemporary client. The specific intention of the physical contact is first to be the connecting stalk. The second intention is to connect with the skin as a metabolic field that developed under water for nine months. Third, the intention is to orient to the stillness in the capillary beds of the vascular system subdermally. The fourth intention is for the hands and arms to become the umbilical veins and arteries between the placenta and the embryo and subsequent fetus.

Alignment. The practitioner aligns her soma and her physical contact with the client's soma at the beginning, middle, and end of a session to touch both sides of the client's soma and the top (head-shoulder) and bottom (feet) if possible. Starting at the side allows the practitioner to sense the movement of the whole in the client's tidal body with ease and the least amount of reactivity. Starting at the feet or head allows the practitioner to sense the midline of the client and is not as subtle as working from the side. Caution is necessary when at the top or bottom of the client's midline. The movement of the whole from the side is the priority before sensing the movement on the midline.

Windows. Contacting specific areas of the client's body from foot to head at the beginning of a session in order to determine which hand placement (window) allows the perception of the most movement. That location(s) becomes the starting place for deeper observation. The practitioner's decides how many hand placements are made; there is no set protocol for where the hands are placed.

Respiratory entrainment. The practitioner senses the first function of respiration in the client while the hands are under the thorax of the client. This is sensed as prehistoric movement. Students are asked to identify a reptile, fish, sea sponge, or bird associated with the movement of the thorax rather than specific structure and function.

Vascular entrainment. The practitioner may visualize the developing cardiovascular system of both the practitioner and client as a shared system while in physical contact with the basic embryonic positions of the connecting stalk (dorsal, caudal, and ventral). The hands and arms of the practitioner are the connecting stalk that allows the client to be able to "root" in the periphery of the practitioner. This is described in detail in the embryology section of the book.

Neuro-affective touch. The practitioner must be aware that visually looking at the client's face and body mutually engages the right hemisphere of each and especially when making eye contact. Neuro-affective touch includes awareness that light physical touch also activates the right hemisphere of the client, which unconsciously interprets the context of the touch as nurturing (or not) based on preverbal experience before and after birth. Because many contemporary clients, both adult and children, have an uncoupled, nonreciprocating autonomic nervous system, the possibility of non-normal dissociation and its effects must be contained by the practitioner. The focus needs to be on the relationship of Primary Respiration to stillness as a way to heal the autonomic nervous system and create a flexible and normal dissociation for the client. All biodynamic palpation skills support neuro-affective touch.

Embryo. Numerous other embryological perceptual explorations are taught in class to image while in physical contact with the client. These enhance the notion that Primary Respiration has a visible form in the image and morphology of the human embryo. Some of these explorations are given in Chapter 24 on client-therapist visualizations. Any contemplation taught in class is to be used in the clinical situation when appropriate.

Seams. Contacting specific morphological derivatives of the embryo, such as the pharyngeal arches and floating ribs. The embryological seams are important windows to view the activity of the metabolic fields and the structuring process that are being catalyzed by Primary Respiration.

Germ layer derivatives. Typically used in pediatric practice where the practitioner focuses on the endoderm derivatives first, mesoderm second, and ectoderm third. This term specifically refers to assessing the suck-swallow-breathe reflex and heart-liver-lung relationships first rather than the infant's cranium. These instructions are detailed in Section III on infants and children.

Wait, watch, and wonder. Attunement and resonance in a session always start with the autonomy of the practitioner, as described in the section above on perception by the practitioner, and returns there whenever doubt arises in the therapeutic process. This is frequent in biodynamic practice.

Fourth Principle of Process— Witnessing the Forces of Origin

Foundation. Relating to the following forces is dependent upon maintaining a majority of one's attention on, first, the practitioner's own systemic organization, and, second, the order and organization of sensed phenomena in the client. Biodynamic and biokinetic therapeutic processes cannot manifest without the practitioner maintaining autonomy, pendulation, and palpatory precision.

Ignition. Five types are perceived: heart, conception, birth, soma, and death. These are associated with the creating, maintaining, and repairing of structure and function with Primary Respiration and stillness as the source. All rates and rhythms in and around the client are ignition related. All levels of ignition except death are concerned with the generation and permeation of heat in the body. This includes its actual perception and all of its different implications metabolically, physiologically, and psychospiritually. Consequently, heat is the most important effect of a biodynamic treatment, beginning with the autonomy of the practitioner.

Regarding death ignition, it must be stated that in biodynamic practice visualizations are taught to see the client as nonexisting in the sense of the time just before his egg differentiated. In addition, to be conceived is to encounter time and space, which means the soma enters a terminal condition biologically and will ultimately die. At all times in growth and development the soma has an inner corpse that is constantly dying as millions of cells die every second. The states of dying and nonexistence must be acknowledged and ignite the deepest level of compassion in the practitioner.

Void. This is the fulcrum of Dynamic Stillness, a deep stillpoint in which the practitioner rests her attention without cognition or thought. The desire to perceive the movement of Primary Respiration is eliminated. This is the realm of greatest potential for creation and the domain of shamanic healing because it is outside the domain of rational thought and normal sensation. The distinctions between practitioner and client dissolve. This mimics death and for a short time the soma of the practitioner and the client is forgotten and may disappear altogether, which is valuable. This is discussed in detail in Section V, Mythology and Healing.

Dream body. This is the normal dissociation from the rational mind. Frequently, practitioners see images in and around the client, and vice-versa. This is the nontemporal dimension of Primary Respiration displaying a therapeutic process. It may or may not be related to non-normal dissociation. It is important, however, that students be taught embryology from a visual image point of view to augment this aspect of the therapeutic process and normalize the effects of a non-normal dissociation. The embryo is the visible and tangible manifestation of Primary Respiration.

Healing. An infinite variety of biodynamic healing processes are in the PRS. This whole volume of work is therefore inherently limiting. One must allow the client's uniqueness to reveal itself biodynamically or biokinetically in each session, for in every session something new is to be learned. Recall that the first and second principles described in this chapter are more fundamental to the healing process. Since the healing process is nonlinear, one can always join unexpected circumstances in a session to Primary Respiration and the stillpoint. Subsequent directions will then be revealed to the practitioner on the spot directly from the circumstances at hand, and these may or may not relate to what is described here.

Fifth Principle of Observation— The Structuring Forces in the Fluid Body

Heat. The fluid body lacks an ignition of heat (see sphenobasilar synchondrosis, below). When a practitioner narrows her attention on the fluid body, it is for three purposes: first, to sense the movement of its whole; second, to witness the coherency of its midline; and third, to observe the permeation of the life force associated with heat in the fluid body to and from its midline in the fluid body itself. All three purposes relate to the thermodynamic activity of the PRS. Heat is the most vital of all biodynamic phenomena. Various skills are taught to explore these three priorities in the context and importance of heat in types of ignition. Recalling the principles of autonomy and pendulation, the practitioner maintains her personal perception on Primary Respiration and stillness in order to observe the emergence of the therapeutic and biodynamic function of heat in the soma.

Active resistance. From a biokinetic point of view, the client-therapist relationship also represents two metabolic fields of activity. Initially, these two fields actively resist each other normally through the autonomy of the practitioner.

Resistance and its honoring is essential. Resistance takes on many forms in the adult; in the embryo it is essential for differentiation to occur. It represents real work as it builds potency and resources the fluid body. It is also the driving force of freedom and the unfolding of the human spirit as seen in a late-stage embryo. Primary Respiration allows pathological resistance to uncouple and normalize. In no way does biodynamic craniosacral therapy attempt to break down resistances in clients.

Metabolic fields (eight in number). These are spatially ordered growth and metabolic movements in the fluid body of the embryo. They cause the originally indefinite course of the individual parts of the embryo to become definite and specific and, furthermore, cause this to occur in compliance with an organized pattern. Thus the structure of the soma is formed. These metabolic fields in embryology require an understanding of the organization and ordering forces of form and the increasing complexity in the timing of growth and differentiation because of the spontaneity of their arising. Their relationship to specific positions in the embryo (space), hierarchy of structuring the tissues and organs of the body, and transformations over time must all be imaged as a moving whole and understood in its morphology. Metabolic fields have gradients of density and direction and differentiation centers in which the specific properties of movement and density drop off in intensity as the distance from the center of the metabolic field increases, but in which any part, within limits, may represent any other because the fields are related to each other by contact and proximity. This is covered in detail in Chapter 28 on metabolic fields.

Metabolic fields arise from fluid body condensations or prestructuring of the future structures of the soma. They are governed by the principle of *active resistance* between each other, which changes their shape and thus their fate structurally. Such relationship resistance causes growth and development because of a state of stillness that automatically arises where the resistance is equal in all directions. Biology seeks stillness for growth. Stillness is an intrinsic part of all metabolic fields because of the principles of symmetry and orientation. The client and therapist are two unique, self-regulating metabolic fields, just as a mother and her newborn baby are, which requires access to a stillpoint for self-regulation to occur. Both self-regulatory processes of the autonomy of the practitioner and client and the relationship between the practitioner and client must be balanced through the embryonic process of attunement to active resistance and its opposite, which is a sense of opening, relaxation, and spaciousness.

Metabolic field palpation. In general, the metabolic fields exhibit a reciprocal breathing type of motion within different densities on a continuum from living water to living bone, as described in detail in Chapter 28. The rate is in the range of the fluid body and fields are always in relationship to adjacent field(s). Here is a brief description of the levels of perception for metabolic fields:

- Fluid breathing oriented to a fulcrum of stillness

- Sponge breathing. On the exhale fluid is squeezed out of the sponge and on the inhale the sponge rehydrates.

- Tissue boundaries dissolving and subsequent disengagement

- Stillness through tension resistance

- Fulcrum compression-decompression and midline compression-decompression

- Systemic shearing, torsioning, and sidebending of membranes. All motion at this level of perception is generally three-dimensional with multiple motions overlapping.

Primary Respiration is the catalyst for maintaining order and organization in the metabolic fields.

Stillpoint. At a more dense level, the palpatory sense of the metabolic fields in the adult may typically manifest unusual and localized shape changes in different regions of the body and within the density of the physiological fluids (blood, lymph, and so on) of the soma. This includes the shape of tissues and bones in relation to their organizing fulcrum of stillness. In other words, the subcompartments of the fluid body, including tissues, breathe eccentrically in response to held imprinting in the fluid body. Consequently, it must be remembered that all metabolic fields are oriented to stillness located in the fluid body, the soma, or around the outside of the soma (including inside someone else's soma), and must be re-related to the outside presence of Primary Respiration breathing out to the horizon and back in order to restore normal motion and uncouple from held stress in the fluid body.

Sphenobasilar synchondrosis (SBS). These fields are occasionally reciprocal in their motion as they literally breathe each other into existence. Consequently, some of them came to be called the classical patterns of the sphenobasilar synchondrosis (SBS) before literal knowledge of metabolic fields was known to early biodynamic practitioners. Consequently, the SBS patterns became linked to the technology of stillpoint, which was correct to a degree mechanically but too narrow in focus. It is now known, for example, that the SBS originates from at least three metabolic fields. The eight classic biomechanical patterns of the SBS are to be sensed in the fluid body rather than the CRI as systemic and whole rather than localized to the SBS. Transmutation of shape and density in the fluid body depends on the mutual arising of both biokinetic stillness and growth resistance under the catalytic guidance of Primary Respiration.

Stillpoints at this level of understanding build heat systemically in the fluid body. Heat is the main effect of the reassociation process of the fluid body to Primary Respiration from the ignition process.

Midline. The practitioner senses the movement in the whole fluid body as a priority in this principle. The fluid moves as a whole; this reciprocal tension potency is detailed in Section II, Relating with Trauma. Then the practitioner senses the therapeutic activity of the midline of the fluid body called the longitudinal fluctuation. What follows from here are secondary considerations in the fluid body.

Wholistic shift. Also called the Neutral, this is a pause in the non-normal dissociation of the soma and its CRI (the autonomic nervous system) just long enough to allow the soma and fluid body to ignite a reassociation with Primary Respiration. This may also ignite a reassociation of the fluid body to its orienting midline of the longitudinal fluctuation and other discrete therapeutic processes unique to the relationship of the soma to the fluid body.

Automatic shifting. This form of therapeutic activity following the wholistic shift in the soma and fluid body is described in the early cranial osteopathic literature. It is the fluid body reassociating with the soma as the autonomic nervous system begins to thaw from held stress and trauma. It is frequently visible as shaking and trembling in the client's extremities or core or both, which the client is usually unaware of since he is either unconscious and sleeping or deeply relaxed. A balanced equilibrium between the soma and the fluid body is being achieved under the direction of Primary Respiration as trauma is uncoupled.

Inherent treatment plan. Dr. Becker described a three-step healing process in the fluid body during the early 1960s (Becker, 1997). It is synonymous with automatic shifting.

Tensegrity. Shape changing of the whole fluid body happens in response to the activity of the metabolic fields within it. Tensegrity describes the systemic network of dynamic living compression and tension-decompression in the fluid body of the embryo and adult. Dr. Jealous (Jealous, 1993) calls this "reciprocal tension fluids." Tensegrity involves areas where the tension and compression zero out each other's influence. Thus the "zero sum" areas are dynamically still and cause for normal growth and development.

Polarities. These are densities and gradients of structured water activity on or around the midline and the fulcrum in the whole fluid body in relationship to the differential activity and location of the metabolic fields.

Imprints. Systemically held stress and trauma in the fluid body cause non-normal dissociation from Primary Respiration. Imprints are generally prenatal and, more important, embryonic in origin. The ground of Primary Respiration and stillness must be available to the practitioner for imprints to uncouple and normalize.

Expansion tide. This very long inhalation of the fluid body is usually related to the fluid body reassociating to its wholeness and breathing midline of longitudinal fluctuation via Primary Respiration. The term may also refer to an aspect of Primary Respiration moving only in one direction for prolonged periods of time.

Trauma. The fluid body is rarely the starting point in a session. It is the greatly wounded instinctual intelligence of the body in the contemporary client. It holds trauma systemically and is dissociated from Primary Respiration. The practitioner must wait for the fluid body to reveal its instinctual healing activity and help reassociate it to its mind and brain—Primary Respiration. And then to orient both to their fulcrum of stillness.

Adjunct Clinical Skills

Containment of shock-trauma requires extensive specialized training and is usually not within the domain of biodynamic craniosacral foundation trainings. Synchronizing with the movement of the whole rather than fragmentation is the key.

Containment and processing of prenatal and perinatal imprinting requires specialized training.

Relating with syndromes such as TMJ requires specialized training.

Relating with disease process such as cancer and death and dying requires informed consent and specialized training.

Using functional and biomechanical skills on tissues is appropriate only in the middle of a session, and then only briefly. These skills are not usually within the domain of a foundation training.

The CRI is rarely worked with in biodynamic practice as it is nonexistent in the context of ignition, Primary Respiration, and stillness.

Code of Ethics—Boundary Management

See Appendix A for a complete code of ethics that I have written, based on my experience of more than thirty years of clinical practice.

Community Service

Donation of time and talent is crucial. Give sessions without financial remuneration to those in need in your community, especially children, their mothers, and their fathers.

CHAPTER 3

Midline Review

The midline implies service to my body and the body of the world by learning to self-regulate. To mature and self-regulate requires that I listen to my body and respect it. In this way the body itself is the midline.

The core of the midline is Dynamic Stillness. It translocates from the core of my body out to the horizon and back.

The midline builds tolerance by developing the ability to hold diverse and complex sensations, images, and shapes with peace of mind.

The midline occurs when I witness my sensations with nonattachment and learn to rest my mind in the stillness out to the horizon and back.

The midline emerges when I move with my instinctual fluid body by allowing Primary Respiration to be the guide.

The midline evolves in my spiritual longing for a connection with spirit.

The midline manifests out of my body and mind in symbolic form through dreams, emotions, fantasies, sensations, behaviors, images, and so forth.

The midline arises after the fallacies that imprinted me, such as what my mother and father died of, my childhood wounding, my felt experience of stress, democracy, the media, and so forth are seen through and reframed as initiations.

The midline reveals psychological integrity. Integrity is the capacity to affirm the value of life in the face of death, to be reconciled with the finite limits of one's own life and the tragic limitations of the human condition, and to accept these realities without despair. Integrity is the foundation upon which trust in relationships is originally formed, and upon which shattered trust may be restored. The interlocking of integrity and trust in caretaking relationships completes the cycle of generations and regenerates the sense of human community that trauma destroys (Herman, 1992, p. 154). Integrity implies self-regulation, autonomy, and a sacred view of life.

The midline incarnates when stillness and silence are brought to the foreground of perception as simple awareness without a reference point. Thus the midline is both two things (me and my awareness of it) and no thing (no me, no it) at once.

The midline is the center of sacred space. Healing is not possible without it.

The midline and the fulcrum are interchangeable concepts. Can you see the midline in the rest of this page below?

CHAPTER 4

Guiding the Client on the Table

This is the process that I use at the beginning of each biodynamic session. I verbally guide the client for five or ten minutes into a gradual awareness of the inner ocean of her body. This is exceedingly important so that the client has a reference point for the work and a way of discussing any sensations and feelings she has from the session. I tell the client that I want to guide her into the memory of the first two weeks after she was conceived. This was a time when her embryonic body was totally fluid and clear like glass.

To help the reader, I have written this narrative as though I am speaking it. When the word "pause" appears in the text, the practitioner is reminded to literally stop speaking for several moments.

1. Breathing and sinking. As you lay there on your back, I'd like you to get in touch with your respiratory diaphragm. Bring your attention to your inhalation and exhalation. Now, as you exhale, I'd like you to allow your feet and legs to sink into the table. Pause. Now, as you exhale, I'd like you to allow your pelvis to get heavy and sink into the table. Pause. Now, as you exhale, I'd like you to allow your spine and rib cage to sink and get heavy into the table. Pause. Now, as you exhale, I'd like you to allow your head, neck, arms, and shoulders to get heavy and sink into the table. Pause.

2. Sensing the skin. Now I would like you to bring your attention to the surface of your skin. We are going to try and get a sense of the total surface of your skin as though it were one continuum. Begin to notice all the skin that is in contact with the table, from head to foot. Pause. Now begin to sense all the skin that has clothing on it, from head to foot. Pause. Now begin to sense all the skin that is exposed to the air, like your face and your hands. Pause. Is it possible to sense more and more of the surface of your skin from the top of your head to the bottom of your feet and all the way out your hands? Pause. Can you sense, as you inhale and exhale, the total surface of your skin expanding and contracting like a living balloon? Pause. Your diaphragm is like a great wave-making machine in your body. Pause.

37

3. Disappearing the body structure. Now bring your attention to the inside of your body. We will gradually disappear all the structure of the body until all that remains is the living water that's clear and transparent and moving with tides and currents. Pause. Bring your attention to your face and head. Imagine that there are no bones in your face and head. Pause. Bring your attention to your spine, from your neck down to your pelvis, and imagine it is no longer there. In its place is just clear, living water. Pause. Bring your attention to your ribs, shoulders, and arms, and imagine there are no bones there, just transparent, clear, living fluid. Pause. Bring your attention to your pelvic bones and sacrum. Imagine they are no longer there. All that remains is clear, living water. Pause. Now imagine the bones of your legs and feet are completely gone. Just clear, living, transparent water. Pause.

4. Disappearing the muscles. Now bring your attention to the muscles of your face and neck and imagine they are no longer there. Pause. Bring your attention to the muscles of your back and trunk. They are no longer there. And all that remains is a very clear liquid. It is living and streaming. Pause. Now bring your attention to your shoulders, arms, and hands. Disappear all the muscles. Pause. Let your body become buoyant. Let your body float inside the ocean that it is. Pause. Bring your attention to the muscles of your pelvis and legs. They are no longer there, just living water. Pause.

5. Disappearing the inner organs. Now we will bring attention to your innermost organs, starting at the top. Beginning with the brain, imagine that it is no longer there and the entire cranial cavity is filled with a relatively viscous fluid similar to the texture of liquid soap in your hand. It is very alive and moving slowly. Pause. Now bring your attention to your lungs and your heart. Imagine they are not there. All that remains is clear, living water, just as it was in the first two weeks of embryonic existence. Now bring your attention to your abdomen, the liver, the stomach, the intestines, and let them go. Completely disappear the organs of your abdomen. Pause. Now get in touch with the organs of your pelvic floor, the kidneys and bladder, the uterus or prostate, the rectum and sigmoid colon. Completely and thoroughly disappear all those organs, even the ovaries. All that remains is clear, living fluid. Pause.

6. The sea sponge in the ocean's tides. Imagine now that the inside of your body was like a tubular sea sponge and the ocean is moving through you from the top of your head down through the pelvic floor and out your arms and legs. Pause for fifty seconds. Then, just like the tide in the ocean, this inner ocean changes direction and comes in through the pelvic floor and up the core of the body, just like a mountain stream or the heat of the Gulf Stream in the Atlantic Ocean. As I place my hands on you now, see how this big ocean responds to my hands as though they were a rudder or the oars of a boat coming into the ocean that you are. Allow yourself to notice how the currents and tides change inside your ocean as I rest silently in my own inner ocean, meeting your inner ocean. As I place my hands now under your shoulder and leg, see if you can sense how your inner ocean shapes itself around my hands and all through the session as well. Then we will compare notes at the end of the session.

It is very important for the practitioner to move through this sequence very slowly with each client. The entire sequence is rarely done at one time with the client. Practitioners may find the need to change the language, especially with a word like *disappearing*. Some clients will respond better if the practitioner suggests that the client "allow the inside of the body to become fluid." Another reason for going slowly through this process is to determine whether a client lives more closely in and around the body or around and further out of the body. There is a natural habit of proximity closer to or further away from the body that everyone develops over the lifespan. Since this sequence is specifically oriented to locating the client's attention in and around the body, it may prove to be challenging or even reactive to those clients whose habit is to be attending to the space that is further away from their body. By going slowly and taking time, the practitioner can discover with the help of Primary Respiration where the client lives in the soma and whether the client has a friendly relationship with inner sensation.

A further note of caution must be added in that some clients may have had a near-drowning experience and such imagery as suggested in this chapter could possibly retraumatize the client. Therefore, it is crucial on your intake with a new client to discover if she has ever had a near-drowning or other negative experience with water.

This is the typical sequence that I go through with each client at the beginning of a session. Of course, it can be modified as need be. Rather than having the client ask you at the end of the session, "What did you do?" or "What did you feel?" the dialogue can shift into a biodynamic discussion that empowers the client to uncouple from her nervous system and reassociate to the fluids of her embryo. This particular practice is also done in conjunction with teaching the client Primary Respiration, as detailed in the next chapter.

CHAPTER 5

Teaching Primary Respiration

As biodynamic practitioners, it is necessary to find a way to get clients involved in the perception of the contents of their body being one fluid continuum. This client contemplation is a guided meditation done verbally by the practitioner when his hands are in contact with the client. I recommend trying it at the beginning, first in order to settle the client and then later I can ask the client to reference that fluid perception if appropriate.

I like to start by taking a few minutes to ask the client to take a few deep breaths and settle into the table very slowly with each exhalation. Then I ask the client to get a sense of the total surface of her skin that is in contact with the sheet and the table. Then I ask her to sense the entire front surface of her body and even how the air feels against her face and arms, and how her clothes feel on her body. Then I remind the client that the entire inside surface of her body is one fluid continuum and, even though the books say that there is anatomy present, the living anatomy is actually all living liquid like the embryo.

Then I negotiate contact with the client. Yesterday, when I did this with my last client, I started by putting my hands under her feet. Then I asked the client to think of a fluid image such as a body of water that she may have been swimming in or next to in her life that left a very satisfying and nurturing impression on her. I ask her what that image might be. Then I slowly ask her to get in touch with that inner ocean (if the ocean was her image). I start at her head and have her imagine the contents inside her head and neck are very liquid and without very firm structure. Then I ask her to go down into her trunk and arms and maybe sense the movement of the heart as a fluid pulsation and the movement of the diaphragm as a wave-making machine. Then I ask her to go down into the abdomen and pelvis as though it was just thick fluid. Finally, I guide the client down into her legs and feet as completely fluid filled.

Next, I ask the client to connect the two surfaces of her skin, the back and the front, with the total fluid volume inside of them from the top of her head down to her feet as one single liquid-filled container. Then I take several minutes to settle myself back into Primary Respiration or a stillpoint. This may be all that is necessary to initiate a transition from the autonomic nervous system in the client to the fluid gel and protoplasm that preceded the development of the brain.

At this point, I ask the client if she has a sense of a fluid shape or movement in her body, even if it's just her heart beating. This only takes a couple of minutes at the beginning of a session and greatly facilitates the possibility of the wholistic shift and automatic shifting in the fluid body. The other biodynamic game I like to play with my clients, once they've had several sessions and we've done this brief guided meditation early in the session, is to ask them, as they get settled on the table and before I put my hands on them, to imagine that my hands are like the oars of a rowboat and when I put my hands on the client, that the body of water inside of them is a moving stream, and when the oar of my boat comes down into their stream to describe the sense of how the stream accommodates or changes to the oars submerged in their stream. Many clients are able to respond with different sense images and metaphors. It is important to encourage the use of images and metaphors, which are the sensory language of the fluids.

Frequently, I will ask the client at the beginning of a session, after doing the meditation above, to take a sensory snapshot of the entire shape of her body from the inside. I might ask the client to describe the shape that she senses her body inhabits. Then at the end of a session, as the client is slowly coming back to be able to sit up, I remind her of the snapshot she took of her original shape and ask her if there is any change in her fluid shape. Remember, whenever making contact, to keep attention on your hands, arms, trunk, and heart as being very receptive to the stream of protoplasm in the client moving into your hands.

The first contact with the client biodynamically is the actual quantum shift that is necessary to synchronize your Primary Respiration with that of the client. Initially, they are not in register with one another, even though they are the same. The quantum shift occurs when the practitioner is able to stabilize his perception on Primary Respiration or a heart stillpoint before the first contact. Then, when contact is made, the practitioner automatically changes his perception of Primary Respiration to starting anew at the moment of contact rather than a continuation of the pre-contact perception of Primary Respiration. This means that it is not enough that the practitioner knows personally where his cycle of Primary Respiration is located and to begin making contact either at the initiation of inhalation or exhalation. It is only necessary to know that you are in Primary Respiration and not which phase. Knowing phase changes in Primary Respiration is important later on in the session. Thus when you make your first contact with the client, let a new phase of Primary Respiration begin at that point, because it is necessary to be synchronized with the receptivity of the practitioner's heart. Open to a flow coming from the client. This is what Paul Pearsall (Pearsall, 2007, p. 18) calls "interpersonal cardiovascular systems." Synchronization at this point means a quantum leap facilitated by the practitioner in receiving the protoplasmic streaming of Primary Respiration coming from the client. A bridge is made by the practitioner's hands and the flood gates must be allowed to open instantly, in the direction of the practitioner rather than the client. This avoids the chance of provoking a reaction and a false fulcrum.

This means that fifty seconds later the practitioner's sense of Primary Respiration will start streaming from his heart and arms back to the client and I recommend that initially the streaming of Primary Respiration going back to the client not be done with the intention of it going into the client, but rather *around* the client as though supporting the sphere or egg shape of the client in the great ocean around us. Gradually, there will be a sense of an inner fulcrum or midline in the client, toward which Primary Respiration is oriented. But this takes time and should not be done at the beginning of the session, but rather allowed to reveal its own timing in order to get to a unified sense of Primary Respiration being one field of living, moving wholeness in which practitioner and client are a part.

Now let me walk you through one version that you can adapt as you see fit with any of your clients.

1. Sitting and grounding through pelvis with a sense of weight. The practitioner uses his hands to gently cue the client. At this point, gently sliding the hands under both ischial tuberosities and verbally asking the client to relax through the floor of her pelvis is most helpful. I generally like to ask the client to inhale and imagine that she can breathe into the floor of her pelvis.

Alternatively, I may ask the client to find the diamond of her pelvis. I have her put one of her hands on her pubic symphasis and reach behind with the other hand and touch the tuberosity on the right. I ask the client to sense the transverse lengthening occurring between the two hands. Then, while maintaining one hand on the right tuberosity, the other hand reaches behind and makes contact with the coccyx. Now the client is asked to sense lengthening between the right tuberosity and the coccyx. The next step is to change hands so that the hand that was on the tuberosity on the right now goes to the coccyx. The hand that was formerly on the coccyx now goes to the left tuberosity. Again, the client is asked to sense space between the two hands. Finally, the client makes contact with the left tuberosity and the pubic symphasis again. This is the last part of the diamond in which the client can sense lengthening and overall spaciousness in the floor of her pelvis. With each hand position, I ask the client to breathe gently into her hands and allow more space in the floor of the pelvis.

2. **Sensing surface of skin, under the surface or outer surface.** This instruction takes several minutes. I usually touch the top of the client's head very lightly and with my other hand down around the knee for a few seconds. This is another cue for sensing three-dimensionality in the client's body. I ask the client to sense the total surface volume of her skin. Sometimes I ask her to imagine that as she breathes in, the whole surface of her skin, from head to foot, is expanding, and then contracting as she exhales. I might gently touch the surface of the client's skin in two or three places with as broad a span that I can reach on her body. This means one hand touching the toes and the other hand as far up on the back as possible, and so on. I might only use three or four gentle hand placements in order to help the client sense her skin three-dimensionally. I then dialogue with the client about what she might be sensing, either on the surface or under the surface of her skin. One intention here is to activate the right hemisphere of the client in terms of its spatial awareness of wholeness and three-dimensionality. It is important in the perception of Primary Respiration that the capacity for three-dimensional perception is awakened early in the practice. Sensing the skin facilitates this process.

3. **Cueing to midline and fulcrums, especially the heart—moving up the body.** This step involves gently placing my hand around the umbilicus and the opposite hand around the middle of the lumbar spine. I like to ask the client to tell me how many inches she thinks are in the space between my two hands. I then ask the client to gently allow her breathing to expand and contract between my two hands. Next, I move upward to a hand placement on the top of the sternum and the middle of the thoracic spine. I ask the client if she can sense the movement of her heart and, if so, what the felt sense of that movement is around the entire trunk, neck, and abdomen. Finally, I delicately place the pads of my fingertips on the client's forehead and the opposite fingers on the external occipital protuberance. I ask the client to close her eyes and gently roll her eyes up for a few seconds and just sense the space in the middle of where her brain is located.

4. **Locating the VOR (Vestibular Ocular Reflex) for a sense of space in middle of head.** This is a continuation of step 3. I like to very gently make sure that the client's head is actually sitting on top of the cervical spine in a way that makes it possible for the eyes to be on a horizontal plane. I am also careful not to make too many adjustments around the position of her head, as this may cause discomfort, even though the client may look straighter with her posture. The inner sense may be quite awkward and feel unbalanced. It is important to make simple micro-corrections and solicit the inner comfort and ease of the client. Ultimately, as the client begins to practice this meditation on her own,

the entire atlanto-occipital joint space will self-correct. So there is no need to make big corrections, since Primary Respiration will do the work once the client catches on to it and begins to practice. It also helps to have the client roll her eyes up slightly again to the middle of her forehead. This places a slight tug on the third ventricle via the optic chiasm. It's important to tell the client to only hold her eyes up for several seconds and then to relax them.

   5. Opening or closing the eyes. This whole practice can be done with eyes open or eyes closed. I frequently tell my clients to try it both ways, depending on where she is located, either inside or outside her house, out in nature or at her office.

   These first five steps are the foundation and generally do not need to be repeated in the later stages of the perception of Primary Respiration. The following steps are the core of the practice and are repeated once the client is able to synchronize her attention more regularly with Primary Respiration.

   6. Directing attention to the horizon. The VOR orients the entire nervous system and body, especially the head, to the literal horizon of the planet. It is very helpful if the client can be looking out the window while you are teaching this practice in your office. The VOR is also called the head-righting reflex and is related to the orienting reflex spoken about in the trauma resolution community. Thus, this practice is potentially curative for some types of shock and trauma that involve a disruption of the orienting reflex. While the VOR orients the nervous system to the horizon, the same neurology facilitates the orienting reflex, which is the capacity to turn the head and eyes to greet stimuli perceived auditorially or sensorially.

   An aside: As I was flying in Europe this past summer, one of the in-flight magazines had an article entitled "Horizon Therapy." It described a stress reduction technique at some European spas that involved sitting outside and simply gazing at the horizon. It was found to be very restorative for many clients at these spas.

   What I am adding here is a sense of embodiment and synchronization with a specific slow tide that moves between the body and the horizon in regular intervals of fifty seconds in one direction and fifty seconds in the other direction. At this point, it is important that you, as the practitioner, sit down and begin doing the practice with your client as you talk her through it.

   7. Buoyancy—letting go of attention, senses, brain, and eyes, and imagining them floating out and back. This is the fun part: You instruct the client to let go of her eyes and her brain and her senses and imagine that these structures are floating out to the horizon for fifty seconds and then flowing back in to the head for another fifty seconds. This may take some time to get accustomed to it. Sometimes, I use imagery like visualizing that you are unzipping the front of your face in a way that even the bones and the muscles float out to the horizon or that these structures are breaking down into floating molecules. There are no precise verbal instructions to give the client at this point. You need to be creative and adapt your language to the sensibility of the client.

8.   Sense of turning—a tidal movement coming from the horizon and moving eyes and brain back into the body. All the body parts are put back together inside the body cavities, especially the brain. Perhaps one of the biggest challenges with this whole procedure is to be able to sense how Primary Respiration changes directions and begins moving from the horizon back into the body and, in this particular practice, into the orbits of the eye and the cranial cavity itself. It's important to use images of the molecules of the parts of the body floating in this Long Tide so that there is an image and a metaphor that can be linked to a sensation. Oftentimes, both the practitioner and the client space out and start having a lot of mental chatter. I like to tell the client that she might notice when the chatter stops; at the same point Primary Respiration is changing direction. Somehow, the client needs to find her way with this and give feedback with her own language, image, and metaphor.

9.   Finding tempo—the sensation of moving in and down or up and out. It is important to point out to the client that in this practice, if one does not perceive this slow tide, then one is actually sitting in its source, which is the Dynamic Stillness. In other words, I tell the client that she is either in a stillpoint or the Long Tide, and that they exchange places with one another. Thus it is not unusual to actually sense Primary Respiration and then feel like it has been lost. In reality, the stillness has come forward into one's perception and simply changed places with Primary Respiration. The instructions at this point are to wait and listen for the sounds of stillness and allow the slow movement of Primary Respiration to spontaneously reveal itself. Gradually, as the client is able to sustain attention on Primary Respiration, its perception grows and expands deeper into the body, beyond just the head, face, and eyes. The whole front of the body begins to open, and even the organs and spine go out to the horizon and come back. The client needs to be reminded that this is a possibility and to watch for any signs or signals that Primary Respiration is moving elsewhere in her body. The perception of Primary Respiration is unique for everyone, or reveals itself to everyone in a slightly different sequence. The practitioner needs to have a listening for that uniqueness in himself and as it is reported by the client.

10. Discovering the quality of being breathed by the intelligence of nature. This is a little bit tricky in the sense that it could be perceived to be a little too New Age or pseudospiritual for some folks. The basic idea is that the forces of nature are bigger than us singular human beings and that Primary Respiration is one of these larger-than-life, yet subtle, forces. It has been said that Primary Respiration knows more about us than we know about it. This simply means that one could have an attitude of humility and patience because Primary Respiration is not given; it is revealed by the quality of our respect and reverence, not for it as some kind of deity but rather as a larger part of the natural world, which in traditional cultures represented the divine.

This practice needs to be done ten times a day for at least several minutes at a time. It can also be done standing or lying down in bed. It works well for insomnia.

Chapter 6

Meditation on the Great Mother

Once the client has begun to sense the slow tempo of Primary Respiration moving between her body and the horizon and back, the following contemplations are possible. These contemplations involve more active engagement and perception of the three embryonic fulcrums. The three meditations are: first, on the umbilicus and umbilical cord connection; second, on the heart-to-heart connection between two people or between someone and a spiritual teacher or friend; and third, the perception of movement from the third ventricle to the horizon and back (which I detailed in the last chapter). Now we will begin to work more closely with the umbilicus and heart. These contemplations can be done seated or in a side-lying position. They can also be practiced in bed.

Umbilical meditation. I have discovered that this umbilical meditation is particularly valuable if a client has lost her mother. This meditation can formally dissolve the umbilical cord between the mother and child and reconnect the umbilical cord to the Great Mother of the Earth or Ocean. I usually have the client either lying on the side on the table or seated, depending on the comfort level of the client. I ask the client to visualize her mother sitting close by, and proceed as follows (in narrative form, again, with "pause" inserted to show where the practitioner gives the client a few moments of time).

Now I would like you to bring your attention to your umbilicus. Pause. I'd like you to sense the whole space and shape of your abdomen as though it has only a very warm, living fluid in it. In the middle of this fluid is a slow movement going toward your umbilicus. Pause. Imagine there is an umbilical cord connected between your umbilicus and your mother's umbilicus. Pause. Perhaps your umbilical cord actually goes from your umbilicus into your mother's womb. Either way is fine. Pause. Which image works for you in terms of sensing the connection to your mother? Pause.

Begin to sense the stream that moves for about a minute out through your umbilical cord into your mother. Pause. Let's wait until it turns direction and now the movement of this slow, nurturing tide comes from your mother deep in her core through the umbilical cord and into your belly and body. Pause. Originally all sorts of nourishment came through to you from your mother. Her own cells and molecules and even her genes floated into you through this cord. Likewise your cells and genes floated into your mother in this unspoken communication.

Now let's repeat this cycle at least three times, sensing this slow tide of sharing food and parts of each other through the cord. Pause. Now I'd like you to imagine that this umbilical cord is starting to dissolve at a point that is halfway to your mother. In this way, your umbilical cord is now suspended in space and your mother slowly disappears. Piece by piece and part by part she fades away. Let her go because her cells and genes are still inside of you and you no longer need her to feed you. Pause.

Where does this umbilical cord attach itself now? Does it go down into the earth? Pause. Does it go down into the ocean? Pause. Let it go into the Great Mother, either the earth or the ocean. Allow the earth or the ocean to send its flow of love and generosity through the umbilical cord very slowly into the depths of your belly and body. Pause. Now sense your whole being as a fluid entity streaming out the umbilical cord, perhaps with bright colors going right down into the earth or ocean. Pause. Repeat this cycle three times. Pause. Now wait for the stillness and let yourself rest in the greater womb of Mother Earth or Mother Ocean.

Meditating on the heart-to-heart connection. The next meditation is a heart-to-heart connection, again using Primary Respiration. I like to sit with a picture of my spiritual teacher, His Holiness the Dalai Lama, on a table directly in front of me. I then settle myself into a stillpoint. I find this stillpoint surrounding my heart in the pericardium or deep inside the heart between the atrium and the ventricles. It is the deepest stillness in the body, centered in and around the heart. This is the starting point. Next, I allow myself to feel a genuine sense of warmth as generated by the heart and circulated by the blood. Here is the narrative.

Imagine love and affection as though your own spiritual teacher is actually present. Now imagine that your chest cavity is slowly opening, exposing your entire heart, and imagine the color red moving like a slow ocean current in a canal or channel directly to the heart of your spiritual teacher. Pause. Wait for this spiritual blood transfusion to switch directions and allow the blood of your spiritual teacher as the color red to move slowly into your heart and surround and support your body. Imagine the deepest love possible, even more profound than that of a mother for her child, a love that seeks only your total spiritual fulfillment. Pause. Let more and more of your chest cavity open, all the way down through the abdomen to the pubic bone.

Surrender all of the contents of your body, starting with the heart, as the color red moving toward the heart of your spiritual teacher. Pause. At the tempo of Primary Respiration, this tide of blood changes directions and begins to move into your body. Allow the entire inside of your body to be completely rebuilt and renovated with the highest known spiritual principle of loving kindness and compassion. Pause.

Repeat this cycle three times. Pause. Wait for a deep stillpoint to emerge and fill your body and space all the way out to the horizon. Imagine the very edges of the universe as clear light.

This completes the sequence of chapters on teaching the client Primary Respiration.

CHAPTER 7

Ignition

By Sarajo Berman

I have known Sarajo Berman as a student, colleague, and friend for almost a decade now. What she brings to biodynamic practice and education is the essential embodiment of the work. During a foundation training we were teaching in Vancouver, British Columbia, Sarajo was inspired to write the poem that appears here and the one at the end of the book. Sometimes the only way that a practitioner can express her perception of Primary Respiration in the therapeutic relationship is through poetry. I introduce you to the beauty and eloquence of Sarajo's embodied experience.

IGNITION

Again.....
For the very first time ever
A warm vibration ripples out

I am sinking.......
Sinking below the earth into an unknown dance
A dance of unknowing
Deeper and deeper
Weightless and yet so heavy
I am unable to move any portion of my body.
My lungs....taking...feeling.....emptying air
My eyelids opening and closing
Settling over floating irises

I feel rather like the flow of a body of water
My belly rides a wave
An arching wave so large my head seems to rear back
    in slow motion

my lips are being pulled apart
I can almost taste the thick sweetness of the air
One quick involuntary jerk
The entire center of my body…..trillions of molecules pull
            Apart…..together

I am dropping fast
Seconds, minutes …a lifetime passes

I can see myself
Liquefying, disintegrating into formlessness
I am entering another world
A world where the rules are different
A world of no rules
Calmingly familiar, mysteriously comforting
moving….stillness

Ghost sensations of the past brought to the present
Leaving the outside world in a fog just out of reach
Yet, its' sounds and energy remain clear and pronounced
Fear…..curioity…..anticipation

A warm vibration ripples in

Something telling me….
I am still alive
And in this world I know and love
I dance a dance of unknowing.
A dance of ever flowing Love.

SECTION II

. . .

Relating with Trauma

CHAPTER 8

In Search of a Quiet Place

I commend you for your actions on the evening of 11 May 1972 when a terrorist bomb exploded at the Officers' and Civilians' Open Mess in Frankfurt, West Germany. Your presence of mind and self-assured manner contributed to the orderly evacuation of the mess and were instrumental in preventing panic among the employees and patrons.

—Lt. General Willard Pearson

Once or twice a year a bomb goes off in my head. I am dreaming, of course. It is the middle of the night. The startle is deafening and shocking. My heart is pounding and racing and, without a voice, I cannot scream. I lie in bed sweating with my eyes fixated on the ceiling fan, chest heaving, gasping for oxygen. I am moving, therefore I am alive. I find my breath consciously. My lungs are screaming like a pump on too high an idle. I begin to slow down my respiratory diaphragm as I keep talking myself down from the roller coaster— "hold on, hold on, ride it through." I look for awareness to return to different parts of my body as I breathe slowly into them. One by one I go through my legs, then my pelvis, my abdomen, my rib cage, and finally my head, neck, and arms. It takes me an hour of this focus to return my body to neutral. Then all that remains is the fear. It is bone-chilling, numbing terror. I almost died again. I was on the edge. I now breathe into my fear. I breathe into my bones and organs. At last I breathe into my inner terrorist mind. Slowly it melts away with each exhale. I yawn. It has been over an hour now since the bomb went off in my head, and I can return to sleep now. I roll over and get closer to my wife until I fall asleep. She never heard the bomb go off, she never saw it, because it is all inside of me.

Now it takes an hour to decompress from the improvised explosive device (IED) in my nervous system and body. However, for the first ten years after the original blast my breath, body, and psyche were alien to me. The compulsive need to avoid government buildings, sweating profusely while waiting in line at the post office and getting anxious next to any public garbage can were constant companions. So were the bad marriages, the inability to hold down a job, and the drinking and drugging, all new friends in this inner world of terror. In my heart I felt I was a coward, even though I was given a citation. In my mind I could have done more to help the man in back of me who was killed, just three days before he was to retire from the army, with his wife and children who were waiting inside the officers' club for him.

I parked my car next to the bomb. I got out of my car and went into the front entrance of the officers' club. I walked right by a suitcase full of plastic explosives. Two other bombs went off first across the street in front of the building I worked in. Then the big one went off as I turned the corner and walked into the dining room. The ceiling collapsed down on me, every window was blown in, and glass flew everywhere. Major structural damage occurred to the façade of the building. Lieutenant Colonel Smith, however, was walking between my car and the bomb when it went off. He was decapitated. We tried to lift him into a car to get him to a hospital, but his head just wouldn't stay on. Parts of him ended up in the back seat of my car. As things settled several hours after the blast, I simply walked home and went to bed exhausted. Then I lived with armed combat infantry soldiers surrounding my ground-floor living quarters for two months as a grim reminder of the fickle nature of being in any Army anywhere during "peace time."

No one in the military checked on my well-being then or subsequently. I simply went back to work the next morning inwardly freaked out. My boss laughed and asked me immediately how I liked my first "taste of action." I do not remember my answer because I do not remember much for the next couple of years. I had a good case of post-traumatic stress disorder (PTSD). Since I was not treated early for it, I became numb, eccentric, and obsessive. It was never part of the conversation with anyone, not even my parents, when I was released from the Army. I loved being numb and I did behaviors that supported being numb. I was always searching for a quiet place inside of me. I was always searching for a quiet place in the space around me. My PTSD became chronic. Then I finally got psychotherapy for ten years and lots of bodywork to reawaken my senses. And one day I woke up. It happened in 2001, the week after 9-11 in New York. I was not a coward. I was not fat, dumb, and ugly. I could trust life. As a therapist of mine said, "Your illness is wasted unless you are transformed by it." I had already created a new life, a new career—one that is much different than I could have ever imagined. I come from a family of lawyers and I was supposed to go to law school. That was not meant to be.

PTSD is like a long dream you never wake up from, and every time you think you have awakened, you are in yet another dream. It is real, but unreal, confusing and self-absorbing. I had a very deep secret and a very rich inner life that I never talked about. I was convinced that people didn't know nothing about life but I knew some stuff. I would try to control the uncontrollable and rage inside at my failure. Then I would feel guilty and get depressed. I would repent and bargain with an invisible demon in my head, over and over and over. Rage, depression, and repentance—that was the cycle I felt locked into, but the boundaries were hard to see and still are.

PTSD is right in the middle of a spectrum of what are called dissociative disorders. At one end of the spectrum is simple dissociation. I space out, day-dream, have vague feelings of unrealness. The constant images of violence and horror on TV and in the media create dissociation and post-traumatic shock called virtual violence. Let's watch the twin towers go down, let's watch Iraq being invaded. The way the nervous system deals with shock and trauma is to numb the senses and fragment the experience, shunt it into different parts of the brain and body. These are the quiet parts of the body and the nonthinking parts of the brain.

I could not watch TV or read the newspapers for two weeks after 9-11. Then one night I did and I cried and I shook and I had to breathe again and again. My bomb was in a suitcase and their bomb was in a plane. The bombs have gotten bigger and more powerful over the years. The Pentagon calls them "asymmetrical weapons." And the university scientists, sociologists, and psychologists all line up to do their research, as if it would change the military establishment. The story will read, in years to come, that those close to Ground Zero in New York were seen to have a rise in suicide, broken marriages, drug addiction, alcohol-ism, and joblessness. There will be transformation too, as the victims search for the quiet place inside them and find an adventure beyond belief. It is a lifelong adventure. I believe in a miracle of spirit for the victims of 9-11 and Katrina and now Iraq and Afghanistan. I read the death notices in our local paper of all the soldiers killed in Iraq for the first three years of the war. I wrote poetry about IEDs and the dust of Baghdad below. Then I stopped, because the bombs stopped going off in my own head and body. I became a student of the Dalai Lama and both my parents died. It was the end of a long family conversation and the beginning of another one deeper than can be imagined. I can feel the dilemma of every returning soldier from Iraq in my heart rather than my mind. I have an explosion of heart that does not disintegrate. This is my new jihad, to hold the returning soldiers and their families with heart in their missing faces and lost limbs. I found mine.

Iraq

by Michael J. Shea

I smell your blood
I taste your bullets
I hear your smoke
I see your screams
I touch your mind
All of it
Every moment
Every cell
The hatred of intolerance,
Jihad, fatwa
The folly of ignorance and
Precision bombing
Car bombing
Suicide bombing
Civilian shields and
Mosques for munitions
The greed of politicians
Media fear and Middle American
Values
Ooze through an open wound
As shrapnel in my psyche
A soldier's stigmata

February 2004

CHAPTER 9

Release-Based Cathartic Therapy: Cautions and Considerations

With regard to individuals who have been the victims of trauma, the classical analytical model of working through the defensive structure of the patient "on the way to" addressing the core trauma itself usually is counterproductive and is contraindicated. Too often this approach will reactivate the trauma, derailing the therapy and in extreme cases, seriously damaging the therapeutic relationship, as well as retraumatizing the patient. When the therapist is perceived as trying to access the core trauma wound, patients sometimes tend to naively drop their defenses—as they did as a child—thus opening themselves to retraumatization. (Bernstein, 2006, p. 143)

This chapter takes a close look at the theory of emotional release and proposes a shift in focus away from emotional release therapies. I would like to begin by discussing the definition of emotion. Emotions have many meanings. They represent a visceral change in terms of the physiology of the gastrointestinal system (Donaldson, 1971). Emotions are neurological events (Ekman, Levenson, and Friesen, 1983; Heller, 1990). Emotion is an observable behavior. It is a feeling realization from a desacralized culture (Bernstein, 2006). It is a need. It is an instinct and many people are instinct impaired. It is an intelligence (Goleman, 1995). It is a significant experience. It is an energy. It is meaning (Hillman, 1997). It is a developmental process. Emotions are both organizing and disorganizing forces. Emotion is a hypothetical construct (Lewis and Haviland, 1993). Emotions are held in one's posture and structure (Keen, 1970; Rolf, 1978; Feldenkrais, 1949). Emotions are social interactions (Schachter and Singer, 1962). Thus, there are many meanings to emotions, how they are perceived, and even their purpose.

Fundamentally, emotions are vital sources of information about self-identity and individual needs as well as behaviors necessary to get those needs. Emotions can motivate one to act in self-correcting ways. Whatever emotions might be, they are certainly a source of connection between the mind, the soma, and the stimulus to act (Dafter, 1996). Theorists have suggested that the number of primary emotions vary from six to nine, from which there is a wide range of more subtle affective experience (Plutchik, 1980). Furthermore, infants are now considered to have a full complement of emotions at birth and able to express them. Infants are now being taught sign language to express their emotional needs.

It is important to make a distinction between an *emotional release* and an *affect.* An affect may be an emotion, a behavior, a feeling, a mood linked to an image, usually from a traumatic experience. Further distinctions must be made between those terms and *abreaction,* which is the shorthand of its equivalent *emotional release.* A stronger form of emotional release is *catharsis,* which includes experiencing specific memories and reliving an event in present time. Emotional release is usually accompanied by crying and/or body movement. It also has an equally important cognitive component (Safran and Greenberg, 1991). I am neurologically wired to perceive feelings and sensations. Perception is the link between sensation and emotions. I perceive the feelings generated by sensation underlying my emotions. Emotion is rather the tip of the iceberg. Feelings and sensations are usually unconscious and, with help, can be made conscious before emotions emerge.

Next, it may be necessary to *communicate* what I perceive. This is one key to self-regulation of emotions, which is the choice to contain and transform the emotion or transform it through expression in relationship to another person. Processing feeling states with others may be crucial to healing. The research is not really clear about this. It gets down to personal preference and learning the value of appropriate suppression from time to time.

Finally, I may need to *understand the meaning* of my feelings and emotions as a way to change the memory of a stressful situation for future self-regulation and reframing the past. Consider that there are no negative emotions. There are only blocked emotions, which are considered by some to be an impediment to health and healing (Spiegel, Bloom, and Kraemer, 1989).

Any single act of emotional release or catharsis only provides a temporary release or brief pleasure. It is important to understand how physical energy stagnates in the soma and how there are sophisticated processes for redistributing and organizing it. Later in this section of the book I will go into detail on the physiology of the autonomic nervous system, where stagnation is rooted. This physiological process then corresponds to the complex of motivations, values, and beliefs that clients have and the increasingly complex situations in which they are involved (Schafer, 1970). Please bear in mind during this chapter that the point of view being presented is that a majority of health professionals question the validity of catharsis (Biaggio, 1986). Sigmund Freud and Carl Jung came to the conclusion in the later stages of their careers that catharsis and emotional release were not primary factors in the therapeutic treatment, but rather a secondary component (Jackson, 1994).

Craniosacral therapists often witness their client's emotional experience. This often leads to the desire to encourage more emotional release due to a lack of understanding emotional process and the underlying psychophysiology. This is difficult territory to traverse without some depth of training and knowledge in at least the psychology of client-therapist relationships and the neuroscience of emotion. Readers should refer to my first volume and, in this volume, Section III on infants and children for an in-depth discussion of affective neuroscience. There are many sources for cathartic discharge of emotions—listening to opera, going to an inspirational church service—and techniques, including special types of breathing exercises such as used in holotrophic breath work, Reichian therapy, and bioenergetics or rebirthing therapies. While catharsis therapies were an important part of therapy during the era of rigid bodies after World War II, these therapies often lose their relevance on the contemporary client without more understanding and training. The soma of the contemporary client is much more complex than the clients I was seeing ten years ago and radically different than the clients I was seeing thirty years ago. Training in the self-regulation and containment of emotions rather than release, discharge, and catharsis of emotions is greatly needed.

Concept Over Simplicity

Some body-centered therapists have adopted an old belief called the *hydraulic theory of mind* (Nichols and Zax, 1977). This theory postulates that there is an excessive amount of fluid behind a client's eyes that needs to come out and it's up to the therapist to facilitate that release. A view of clients as having pathologically dammed up, unexpressed emotions only impedes the therapeutic process (Warme, 1980).

Emotional catharsis was historically associated with purging the soma of emotions for spiritual purification. Aristotle was the founder of the cathartic method. He wrote about the catharsis of one's passions, especially pity and fear, through listening to music and viewing tragedy in the theater. There is a rich history in religion, theater, psychopharmacology, and music for the release of emotions as a communal event (Scheff, 1979). It was not until the nineteenth century that psychologists began to reinterpret what Aristotle meant by catharsis.

In the nineteenth century the roots of the current practice of provoking emotional release can be found. Then people like Pierre Janet created a treatment for the *mental disinfection* of traumatic memories by *mental liquidation* (Jackson, 1994). These treatments were specifically designed for discharging emotions and were called a *moral fumigation.*

There are four categories of catharsis: abreaction, integration, inclusion, and significance or spiritual catharsis (Blatner, 1985).

The catharsis of **abreaction** is the experience of reliving a traumatic event along with its associated memories. It is an essential principle in facilitating catharsis that a client not be simply reexperiencing the original trauma by abreaction. Rather, the practitioner must anchor the emotional awareness in the context of *right here and right now.* Hyperarousal from past trauma is experienced in the nervous system as a current event in present time, not as a memory. If a client has a catharsis with me, I look to see if she can witness her experience dispassionately rather than being totally overwhelmed by the emotions. "Can the adult in you see the experiences you are having right now?" This is a question I often ask my clients. "Where are you within all of that?" is another question I ask.

Integration is an expansion of the sense of self-regulation to include new experiences that have previously been overactivating. I cannot reject my past or purge myself of it by surgery or therapy. I can only transmute it to a higher level of functioning through containment and self-regulation. To thoroughly understand integration requires knowledge of the coping mechanisms and the variety of defense strategies that a client uses to shield from inner lived experience.

The catharsis of **inclusion** includes the need to feel love and friendship. It is a deep and powerfully significant part of psychosocial functioning. Any therapist, whether psychologically or body-centered, must never underestimate the need for inclusion as a source of motivation for the healthy and unhealthy self-regulation of emotions. My sense of self naturally expands beyond my skin to include whatever groups or individuals I identify with in my life. For whatever reason, people often feel alienated from others and this brings them to therapy. The therapeutic exchange of "helping and being helped, self-disclosure and empathy and forgiving and being forgiven are some of the components of the greater process of inclusion" (Slavson, 1951).

My experience has taught me that many of the currently popular approaches to healing trauma provide only temporary relief at best. Some cathartic methods that encourage intense emotional reliving of trauma may be harmful. I believe that in the long run, cathartic approaches create a dependency on continuing catharsis and encourage the emergence of so-called *false memories.* Because of the nature of trauma, there is a good chance that the cathartic reliving of an experience can be traumatizing rather than healing. (Levine, 1997, p. 10)

Spiritual catharsis is the fourth type of catharsis and occurs when a client perceives a greater degree of wholeness, unitive consciousness, God, a higher power, a deeper power, the numinous, and so forth. These states have historically been referred to as religious conversion, ecstasy, receiving the Holy Spirit, being saved, mysticism, an epiphany, and so on. However, it must be emphasized that these states be integrated into daily life and the ordinariness of everyday existence. A client may have an extraordinary realization and still abuse her kids when she gets home. It is important to help clients work through or discover the meaning of such events and how to maintain the numinous experience on their own (Scheff, 1979). The last section of this book goes into this in detail.

Emotional release work has two aspects: first, the somatic element, and second, the cognitive element (LeDoux, 1989). When a practitioner focuses only on somatic sensate level, the work is only half done. The same can be true in psychotherapy, which tends to focus on the cognitive (abstract) aspect of the emotions and leaves out the felt sense of the soma. Ideally, then, a therapy that offers deep insight into change processes would make available somatic self-regulation and cognitive integration. However, emotional release work is sometimes viewed as a quick fix and as a substitute for ongoing psychotherapy or more appropriate body-centered approaches. Thus it becomes a very mechanical process, like getting your oil changed in your car regularly.

The expression of affect in therapy becomes an end in itself, rather than a welcome by-product of the process of resolution of intrapsychic and interpersonal conflicts and their self-regulation. Patients are encouraged and even exhorted to vent their feelings and express their impulses. At worst, unconscious conflicts and urges unacceptable to the patient are exposed triumphantly as soon as they are recognized by the practitioner, partly in an attempt to elicit as much affect as possible and thereby *drain the psychic abscess.* The highly questionable implicit assumption is that catharsis contributes to internalized, lasting change. There is a danger that the coping mechanisms the client has built over a lifetime will be overwhelmed and not simply breached. This has very adverse therapeutic results. The side effects may last a long time, such as a prolonged regression or even more intense psychological symptoms, or worse yet, a dependency on the practitioner. Frequently this can translate into various forms of acting out (such as sexually), which consequently have adverse effects for not only the client, but others related to the client (Lowy, 1970).

Increased Consideration for Individual Differences

> In the case of individuals who encounter … trauma, the clinical picture is more complicated. They too have come into the world with their "origins story" in place at birth. However, the impact of their traumatic experience(s) overlays a new and powerfully charged story—a trauma story—which, because of its impact on the self, takes on numinosity *as if* it were their "origins story." [It] tends to leave the individual cut off from his pre-trauma "origins story" with which he came into the world *as if it never had existed.* (Bernstein, 2006, pp. 146–147)

As Jerome Bernstein has pointed out, the trauma story becomes the most prominent story line that the twenty-first-century client presents in clinical practice. As numerous researchers have pointed out, the trauma story needs to be told, held, and contained by a witnessing therapist. Such is the case with a client of mine. Recently I was called in to consult with a twenty-eight-year-old woman, a school teacher who had to quit working. She suffered from chronic pain, trigeminal neuralgia, and migraines. Before I could begin talking with her, she handed me a document that contained information on more than forty health care practitioners she had seen, what each had diagnosed, and what each had prescribed. This amazing document was a completely new experience for me—now it is common with every client. There was no technique or method I could use with her that had not been tried already. I had to absolutely be with her on her own terms. I had to listen to her very deeply, which apparently no one had ever done. When people know they are being heard, they can begin to relax. Because I listened, we mutually discovered that she had lost her ability to pray, to connect with something or someone larger than herself. She needed a gentle reminder of the spiritual dimension of healing. She was reminded that she had a heart and could look to her heart for healing and guidance.

While each client is completely unique, with her own autobiographical narrative and metaphor, as the reader will see in the last section, Mythology and Healing, it is the origin myth and embryonic narrative that needs to be listened to by a perceptive practitioner. Thus the practitioner holds the trauma story and the origin story in a container of love and compassion. It is crucial to suspend the use of protocols, formats, and techniques as often as possible because they usually alienate the client even further. One of the results of not considering the individual differences in clients is a lack of understanding of just how deep the difficulties are that many clients have and the incredible frustration for the practitioner of not being able to fix someone on the spot. John McPartland (McPartland, 1996) described in an article entitled "Craniosacral Iatrogenesis" the ill effects of craniosacral therapy that does not honor boundaries or individual differences. This is iatrogenic disease. Iatrogenesis is defined as *physician-induced disease or disorder* (Illich, 1976).

> To the degree that such therapies attempt to undo the effects of trauma and developmental neuroses originating in childhood, notwithstanding language that directly addresses and proclaims such matters, they often fail at any more than superficial amelioration or fictive redirection *unless* they energize a whole complex which then unconsciously sinks to the source and transmutes it—and in that case the activating mechanism is the power of therapeutic touch, not concomitant psychological language. As long as that language is literal, linear, and posed in the terms of sociocultural metaphors of abuse, traumatization, low self-esteem, and past-life history, it is unlikely to enhance the treatment, and it may well serve to clutter or confuse it. (Grossinger, 1998, p. 93)

There is an important distinction between retraumatizing the client and driving the trauma deeper. Any body-centered practitioner may inadvertently retraumatize a client by an act of omission—going too fast, going too deep thoughtlessly, inexperienced communication skills, and so on. Even experienced body-centered therapists can retraumatize clients quite by accident. The skill is how to recognize this breech and repair it. However, driving the trauma deeper is not only a retraumatization, but a deepening of the insult—the client is more easily dissociated, more symptomatic, or more easily moved into hyperarousal. The practitioner, in effect, becomes a perpetrator, an abuser, according to Judith Herman (Herman, 1992). Whether conscious or not, and many practitioners would disavow even a remote possibility that they could or would drive the trauma deeper, the abuse of power is inherent in the client-therapist relationship. When a practitioner retraumatizes a client, he is part of the problem rather than part of the solution. When a practitioner drives the trauma deeper, he is a false god, a charlatan (Guggenguhl-Craig, 1971). Trauma does not really end when its source from the outside is finished. The trauma that resides in the right hemisphere of the brain and soma perpetuates itself and continues unabated in the mind and dreams of the trauma patient, according to Donald Kalsched (Kalsched, 1996).

What is truly bizarre about trauma is that the victim of trauma regularly and repeatedly finds herself in life situations where every attempt to improve a relationship is undermined and frequently destroyed by something more powerful in her mind and soma. This frequently shows up in dream material as a devil or a demon or intense and paralyzing states of fear from unseen figures and deep anxiety in waking life.

Emotional release work often violates a client's boundaries, which is unethical at best. The practitioner needs to have a clear contract prior to the session with the client. This contract must specifically spell out that emotional release work is involved and that the client identifies the issues that he or she wishes to process. The practitioner then receives permission from the client to proceed with the work. The practitioner must also be clear that if, in the middle of a session, the issues change, the client is informed and additional permission received before proceeding. These are essential, ethical guidelines for emotional release work (see Appendix A). Without negotiated boundaries, there is no safety or trust. Safety and trust do the healing, not the technique.

How do we really know if catharsis is of any value? It may just be that the client has a good cry to indulge the practitioner or that crying is learned behavior. How do we even know whether a client integrates this type of emotional experience? In body-centered psychotherapy training, such as somatic experiencing, sensory-motor psychotherapy, and body-centered psychology, much time is spent on the theoretical and experiential components of ego defense mechanisms, transference and countertransference issues, and theories of personality. This is a minimum standard: equal time for theory and the development of correct understanding of the emotional dilemma.

The same technique cannot be applied to every client. It depersonalizes the relationship (Meares, 1986). It only serves the needs of the practitioner, robs the client of intrinsic meaning, and dooms the healing relationship to failure. The practitioner takes power from the client. Not only does this disempower the client, but it is unethical (see Appendix A). The very reason my clients come to me is to get their power back, the power to heal themselves, and for me to listen to their disturbance without interference. I focus on finding the health of the system and listening for that. This is a deep listening and acknowledgment of pain and suffering. Repetitive technique (doing the same thing to the client every session) may retraumatize the client. It reinforces fragmentation and emotional wounding. Even though a client may report feeling great, this can be what is called *euphoric dissociation*. Inevitably such clients relapse into old symptoms within several weeks and are back to square one.

When touch therapists deliberately enter into the psychological world of their clients, they are creating what is called a *dual relationship*. This is performing the role of both a manual therapist and a psychotherapist. Dual relationships of this kind are considered unethical (see Appendix A). Massage therapists must consider obtaining more background in psychology if they intend to work psychologically with their clients and perhaps be licensed as such. According to Judith Herman (Herman, 1992), the therapist can frequently participate in a reenactment of the original traumatic event and actually fulfill the role of the perpetrator, as I mentioned earlier. Specialized knowledge and experience must be obtained because the client frequently desires a rapid cure, and this all too often is not possible. This is one of the many reasons why I like biodynamic craniosacral therapy because of its *modus operandi* being slow and still.

Differentiating Vitality Affects, Sensation, and Feeling from Emotion

> Feeling realizations bring with them a somatic embodiment of emotion. We have not learned—yet—to shut down our body sensations the way we have learned to shut down our thinking and rational process. And for increasing numbers of us, when we do try to shut down our body processes to avoid frightening truths, we become ill—literally—with everything from depression to psychosomatic disorders to environmental illness. So, from whence does this notion of self-extinction derive? (Bernstein, 2006, pp. 43–44)

Affect is defined as a feeling, emotion, and desire linked to sensations and images. Important in determining thought and behavior, affect relates to one's disposition or moodiness, character or personality, and personal appearance. As such, affect may also mean to have an emotion or to display likes and dislikes, or adopting or following other people such as movie stars, athletes, or cultural or political notables. Affects produce an effect. Effects manifest as mental states and thinking processes, as well as feelings of affiliation and approach, or withdrawal and rejection. Affects are one of the ways someone communicates to someone else. The effect on the people around a person with a happy affect is a joy to behold. The reverse is also true. An affect of anger and irritation is difficult to be around. Affects are mannerisms that may imply an excess or uniqueness but do not suggest insincerity. My wife is a good example. She is the happiest person I know. It took me years to settle into her affect of happiness because I somehow felt uneasy, as though it would end and not be real. Now I am able to adjust my behavior to support her happiness because it and she are just great to be around even when I am grouchy and grumpy. The essential basis of one's personality is affect, such as my wife's happiness.

Affect is a central organizing principle of the inner psychic life because it links together the various elements of the body-mind complex (sensations, ideas, memories, judgments) by lending feeling tones to them. Strong affects such as love, joy, depression, and irritability are natural and transform themselves into the world of emotion in the image and story of character and personality. In other words, affect becomes autobiographical.

According to Carl Jung, the essential basis for our personality is affectivity. As the central organizing principle of psychic life, affect links sensations to ideas to memories to judgments, as I mentioned above. What's important here is the sensation underneath the feeling and the feeling under the emotion and the process of linking or coupling the different components of body and mind. When we have a strong experience, such as shock-trauma from 9-11, it is usually accompanied by a strong affect such as fear, and attention will accumulate around this affect. Typically what happens is that then the fear organizes around an archetypal core, which is some universal characteristic seen in a myth such as war stories in the Middle East or even a strong emotion such as anger and rage. The strength of the affect creates images and meaning that are clearly discernible throughout history in mythology and religion, which I will discuss at length in Section V, Mythology and Healing. Very strong affects can become transpersonal or spiritualized or otherwise amplified in the mythic dimension. The world of affect, as it grows in strength, leads to religious experience, clearly one of the defining aspects of being human. It is the power inherent in the strong affect that touches the numinous and is necessary for healing.

Vitality affects are illusive qualities and are concerned with how a behavior is performed, not what the specific behavior is (Heider, 1974). Each person has a style of expressing vitality affects. This is called *gesture* in embryology. There are people with explosive feelings, people with long and drawn-out feelings, people who are very reclusive with their feelings, people who have fleeting emotions, people who take a long time to reach a crescendo with their feelings. These qualities are both separate from and connected to one's emotions at the same time. This is why emotions seem so paradoxical at times—everyone has had the experience of laughing while crying (I hope). They involve a person's basic constitution and personal preference. They are what make us unique and vital. Perhaps anxiety and depression are essential affects and maybe they are an expression of something that is healthy rather than pathological. Jerome Bernstein (Bernstein, 2006) calls this the "borderland personality"—one who holds and carries the tension of the cultural split from body and nature and at the same time is attempting to reconcile the split in a new way. Donald Kalsched (Kalsched, 1996) warns against manual therapy in that it may release too much oversomatized energy without the ability of the strong emotions being contained and transformed and ultimately understood for healing. Strong emotion that resides in the soma must reach the level of meaning. In the world of biodynamic craniosacral therapy, this means accessing the stillness of the midline. The work of manual therapy must necessarily include the reestablishment of a functioning midline in the client. The possibility of transmutation may be lost without the midline.

Meaning and Problem Solving

The normally integrated components of experience include both *somatic* and *mental* elements—affects and sensations from the body, thoughts, images and cognitive mechanisms in the mind, as well as a mysterious "meaning" dimension which has to do with whether something can be integrated as a part of one's personal identity and narrative history. Related to this dimension of meaning, and rarely discussed by clinicians, is that animating *spirit* at the center of all healthy living. This spirit, which we have described as the transcendent essence of the self, seems to be compromised in severe trauma. (Kalsched, 1996, p. 37)

There is a continuum of fluid communication that emotions can provide:

- This continuum starts with my ability to sense what I am sensing as a fluid being

- Second, it involves my ability to trust the feeling shapes that arise from fluid sensations

- Third, it involves giving voice or expression to feelings inwardly or outwardly with fluidity in the tempo of Primary Respiration

- Then it involves problem solving and finding the biodynamic midline of stillness

This biodynamic continuum of emotional responsiveness is undermined when one element or aspect of it is focused upon or left out altogether. Health care practitioners must understand that it is unethical to not offer self-regulation skills with the performance of emotional release work. Self-regulation derives from an inner witness who has the ability to watch bodily experience nonjudg-mentally and nonpreferentially. It is the ability to stay in present time and rest in a slow tempo or stillness. When emotional release work is used by a practitioner, it often will dissipate the charge that a client is processing before she is able to learn from it or make meaning of it. It is clear that blocked or repressed emotions are there for a very intelligent reason. They should be left in their state until the client learns how she got there, becomes aware of the attitudes that surround the contraction, and whether there is any value in removing the contraction.

Self-regulation of one's emotions is an essential part of stress reduction. A client needs to learn when certain thought patterns lead to specific behaviors that are stress and anxiety producing. Clients must begin to recognize the problems that racing thoughts produce and begin to learn the power of spiritual con-templation and stillness. Cognitive restructuring is a self-regulating discipline employed when I sense negative thoughts that will ultimately lead to arousal or a strong emotional state. I consciously rebuke those thoughts and disown them. I head off the emotional storm at the pass by not entertaining them. There is an old Tibetan expression about negative thoughts: "Do not let the pig into the house." Cognitive restructuring is equivalent to building a containment barrier. A variety of self-management strategies—meditation, prayer, progressive muscle relaxation, time management, mental focus, and so on—are essential adjuncts to cognitive restructuring. Formal relaxation training, regular sleep, and the development of an attitude of compassionate nonattachment are building blocks to a more stress-free life. Happiness is a birth right according to His Holiness the Dalai Lama. Finally, self-regulation may involve these four elements (Safran and Greenberg, 1991):

- Experiencing compassion for one's self
- The completion of an interrupted emotion or motor sequence in the muscles
- The generalized attention to muscular tension and heartbeat
- Cognitive restructuring, as detailed above

Learned Behavior

Donald Kalsched cautions that trauma victims "will [often] present themselves as innocent victims seeking support, but they are really unconsciously engineering self-damaging situations that they inwardly enjoy. Until they realize this and break the self-destructive pattern, supportive psychotherapy will not help them." It is precisely at this point—when … the therapist has the relief of knowing that now *the patient himself* knows that the trauma story is inauthentic as his "origins story"—that both therapist and patient are at risk. … A kind of trickster energy waits until defenses are down and then pounces to reinvigorate the trauma story. (Bernstein, 2006, p. 148)

How many of us used tears to get what we wanted from our mom or dad, husband or wife? Very often clients will perform a similar emotional release for the practitioner. This is implicit memory and subsequent learned behavior from infancy in order to get what one needs from one's parents. Once again the practitioner is put in the unconscious role of the powerful parent and the client acts out the emotion for the practitioner. Emotions set up a chemical dependency in the brain and soma from prolonged overuse of dopamine (Lemonick and Park, 2007). In essence, we become addicted to feelings and emotions and it becomes one of the primary ways to get our needs met unconsciously. This addiction keeps the underlying imprinting in the right hemisphere of the brain locked in place and well-hidden.

Emotions are used to manipulate the environment and others. Emotions become a performance. That is another reason why emotional release work is most often a short-term solution, offering little long-term value in a person's life. Emotional release work is but one option among other complementary and alternative medicine (CAM) practices as well as mainstream therapies that may be more valuable. Arousing emotions during a treatment has no advantage over many other possible methods, which casts doubt on abreaction as essential to therapy (Horowitz, 1970).

Crying is never a cure. It is an archetypal necessity of the child. What does the cry suggest from the deep inner experience? What is it saying? "I want to be alone"? "I need help"? Is it a primary or secondary process? Is it a learned behavior or a nervous system discharge? What is the history and the story line? What is the affective process that is running the emotion? Is it something I cannot learn, someone I cannot love, a situation that is hopeless? Is it an expression of helplessness? This is where the child is hidden in the adult. Very often strong messages from the unconscious are misunderstood as sentimental feelings about childhood and in this way a much romanticized image of childhood is developed.

It was Sigmund Freud's point of view that the conscious mind was superior to the unconscious and therefore one cannot let go into the archetypal imaginary realm because it is associated with childhood and therefore inferior. This inferiority is equated with insanity, vulnerability, and weakness by the culture.

My emotions and my crying are threatening to me because they break into the primitive realm of childhood and I do not know how to separate the real child from the archetypal child. The tendency is to dump one's feelings and emotions on the literal child that once existed. This makes personal emotions impossible and intolerable. Since that child is no longer real, it consequently puts pressure on the archetypal child. This archetypal child of creativity, freedom, and artistic expression was never meant to be abused with so much embodied emotion and feeling (Hillman, 1975).

There is way too much focus in our culture on emotional release, according to Rachel Remen (Remen, 1995). The culture continually defines a person by how much he or she feels and, consequently, this creates a gap or a gulf between a midline connection with spirit requiring a middle man to sort it out. Western man lives in his head and is having a feeling realization from the imbalance and cut off from body sensations and nature. Body sensations are nature. With a functioning biodynamic midline however, a client's emotions do not have to fully process the pain and suffering of being alone and feeling disconnected from life. This is the traditional job of nature herself, and by this I mean the natural world. With the help of nature, emotional turmoil can be considered impermanent and transitory, rather than a deep, long-lasting wounding, such as a mother complex. The mother complex is the belief that something is deeply flawed on the inside of one's mind and soma. The midline allows certainty and connectedness to nature and the numinous in which self-regulation is spontaneous and instinctual and not dependent on a middle man to process it.

Clinical Supervision

Most psychotherapists receive supervision once a week, from another psychotherapist. The supervisory relationship involves discussing difficult or challenging clients and getting unbiased feedback. It helps determine where the stuck areas or blind spots are in a client-therapist relationship. Any body-centered practitioner who finds himself immersed in a client's emotions would be wise to receive supervision regularly from a qualified psychotherapist. This is an essential, ethical consideration (see Appendix A).

Therapeutic cleverness can rob the client of self-discovery and, worse yet, the client may feel that her thoughts and feelings have been stolen. The client may have within her a system of ideas or memories that are highly valued and very emotionally toned. Although it might be a secret, the client has a large preoccupation with these internal body-mind mechanisms. The practitioner should in no way impose his own sense and sensibility upon the client's experience. This is a futile attempt to manipulate a client's experience, which can only be done by helping the client to learn to self-regulate.

Emotional release work often depersonalizes the client-therapist relationship. This means that the client's inner state does not really match the practitioner's interpretation. Interpretation becomes a curse put on the client. This mismatching diminishes the boundary experience. A heavy emphasis on overcoming the client's defenses to secure an emotional release and believing that this release is of primary importance in the life of the client is the principle deficiency of many body-centered therapies. This overemphasis has become obsessional with many body-centered therapists who continue to insist that clients cry in order to experience healing or telling clients that they have deep-seated emotional problems if they won't cry for them.

Clients need to be guided toward an ownership and self-regulation of their inner experience as it is rooted in the fluid body biodynamically rather than their emotional body, as it has been called. The emotional body is the continuum of the soma, autonomic nervous system, cardiovascular system, and corticolimbic system. It is essential to form a relationship between the preexisting health in the fluid body via Primary Respiration and uncouple from one's imprinting in the emotional body. I must give freedom and space to that process. I must be able to distinguish between genuine and habitual affect and between the fresh and the stale part of my personality. This is the essence of self-regulation.

Emotional Intelligence

Daniel Goleman's (Goleman, 1995) book *Emotional Intelligence* is a great read. He summarizes a significant amount of research on emotions. The following are some of the major qualities that make up healthy emotional intelligence biodynamically and also support self-regulation from research literature cited in his book.

- **Self-awareness.** I need to be able to recognize a feeling as it is happening. I need to be able to tune into somatic markers. These are gut feelings, sensations, and a felt sense of my soma and fluid body. To do so, I orient to stillness in the biodynamic midline and synchronize my attention with the slow tempo of Primary Respiration all day long and when I can't sleep at night.

- **Mood management.** I have to get a handle on my negative thought patterns. I need to be able to recognize the types of thoughts that, when left unattended, lead to a negative shift in my mood. This is the *cognitive restructuring* described above. Once I see negative thoughts begin, I make a conscious effort to shift to another train of thought or pleasant activity.

- **Self-motivation.** Whatever I can do to gather feelings of happiness and confidence is crucial for my life. I may be predisposed to a positive or negative outlook by my genetics or early attachment experience, but it takes a hostile negative environment to trigger my own hostility and negativity.

- **Impulse control.** The essence of emotional self-regulation is the ability to delay an impulse in the service of a goal such as peace of mind, a sleeping baby, or happiness. This is not to be mistaken for the neurotic qualities of denial and repression.

- **Empathy.** To get along in life, it is crucial to know how other people feel. I transmit and catch moods from others on a subtle, almost imperceptible level, from heart to heart and right hemisphere to right hemisphere. I live in a day and age where I am networking and communicating with more and more people. This calls for greater interpersonal skills, tolerance, empathy, and sociability.

The following questions are important to ask as a body-centered therapist and biodynamic practitioner in regard to working with emotions.

- How comfortable am I with witnessing another person's feelings, both within and outside of my professional role? Have I witnessed fear, sadness, and anger being expressed by a client?

- How comfortable am I with my own emotions? Have I experienced fear, sadness, and anger in myself lately?

- What, if any, are the noise limitations of my office setting if a client should begin to cry loudly?

- How well do I know this client? What do I know about his or her history that may be an indicator that I need to refer the person on to a psychotherapist or other skilled health care provider?

- Am I aware of what triggers me (or upsets me) when I am with somone who starts to experience emotions? Do I know how to contain my own feelings while dealing with a client experiencing his or her feelings? (Traer, 1992)

It is simply not possible to know what clients are experiencing. This is because it is frequently hidden to clients, which is why they are in therapy to begin with. The only way practitioners of any type of therapy can know the experience, and I mean the deep inner experience of a client, is by placing a considerable amount of attention on their own sensory experience in their own soma. This is the meaning of therapist-centered therapy. The practitioner of biodynamic craniosacral therapy spends the vast majority of any given session in direct observation and perception of his own feelings and sensations. Only then can there be a more direct experience of the relationship of two people whose bodies and minds are in resonance with each other. This is not an intuitive process. It is a deeply experiential and instinctual, gut-level process.

Emotional Release, Breath Work, and Spiritual Process

Breath work is not only the gateway into the spiritual realm, according to various religious traditions, but also the psychological realm. All shock and trauma that the soma experiences are in some way connected to the respiratory mechanism (Levine, 1976, 1990, 1997). The most common response to shock and trauma is to hold the breath or to breathe shallowly until the danger passes. Unfortunately, some clients forget to let go of the held pattern or the danger is sustained for a long time and inappropriate respiratory patterns are adapted. As a skilled biodynamic craniosacral practitioner begins to relate to these restrictions, some of which have been there since the embryonic time, changes may begin to occur in the nervous, endocrine, and soft tissue systems (Selye, 1976). All shock and trauma has an element of fear imprinted with it and that can begin to trigger strong emotions such as rage, grief, despair, bliss, or joy.

I remember my surprise in my early experiences of practicing massage and Rolfing. I had no conscious intention to invoke such reactions; I just wanted my clients to breathe better! As my clients began to breathe more freely, I noticed how the breath was used to facilitate opening in the soma. Old tight, restricted areas could be breathed into and restriction would just melt. I also noticed how this psychological, physical opening often gave birth to a deeper spiritual meaning in one's life. Just to make a connection within one's self about the power of physically holding onto an old, useless pattern produced a richness and peacefulness in my clients that at times appeared to be profound, mysterious, and transcendent. One of my teachers once said that the goal of health and healing ought to be peace of mind. This is the stillness of biodynamic practice. When I see clients achieve this through biodynamic craniosacral therapy and then see the impact that this experience has in other dimensions of my clients' lives and mine, it is nothing less than spiritual, which I speak to in depth in the last section of this book.

Clients have a wide variety of responses to any body-centered practice. A normal response to safety and trust being available in the therapeutic relationship invokes relaxation. It has been my experience that no client will open up to her deeper, inner experience and self-regulate emotionally until the practitioner and the client are properly relaxed around well-negotiated boundaries. Students often express hesitation when I mention the possibility of spiritual crises or emotional catharses. It just does not happen without a context of readiness on the part of the practitioner or client when the intention is noncathartic. The practitioner might not know that he is ready, and that is okay. It is not a cognitive process but rather a very nonlinear one. The rule of thumb is always "seek not, forbid not" when it comes to a client's emotions. It is not so much that the practitioner needs to do anything once one of these processes have been initiated; it is that the practitioner needs to be present to witness and, yes, at times, guide the process for the client in order for the client to learn to self-regulate. Above all, keep breathing and maintain contact either verbally or with Primary Respiration. I think that what is truly important to understand about this discussion is the logic that if someone develops a spiritual crisis from body-centered work, as mentioned in Volume One, then it follows that the client has a spiritual illness and is in need of reestablishing a biodynamic midline of stillness.

In conclusion, I have presented some of the relevant literature and some cautions when body-centered practice evokes clients' emotions. We live in a psychologically based culture that puts a prize on feeling emotions, mentalizing spirituality, recapturing the past, and romanticizing it. Emotional release therapy is a temporary cure. When emotional release work enters the therapeutic environment and a body-centered practitioner feels equipped to handle it with minimal or no training, there is a great potential for quality control problems and retraumatization. This has been aptly pointed out by John McPartland (McPartland, 1996) in an excellent essay on craniosacral iatrogenesis. The practitioner becomes part of the problem. A culture of emotion-centered therapy has created an atmosphere of psychological consumerism that lacks boundaries and ethics. It seems that we have moved away from the Stone Age regarding longevity, witch hunts, crusades, and public executions (Stone and Church, 1968). But on the other hand, the newspaper headlines tell us that the health care system is failing and we indeed remain in the Stone Age in the Middle East. The loss of contact with the symbolic nature of life, with nature and the environment, and especially the midline, is damaging beyond belief and even suicidal, according to Jerome Bernstein (Bernstein, 2006). Emotions are not the issue and perhaps never were.

> Ultimately, the abhorrence of nature as *the* enemy became a characteristic of the western ego and of western culture itself, resulting in what I have come to call a "fragmentation complex." Characteristically, a fragmentation complex leaves one with a feeling of disintegration or ego fragmentation in the face of powerful irrational forces that cannot be explained, psychologically split off, or rationalized away. ... It is a feeling that can leave one in abject terror, a feeling that can be experienced as even more frightening than a perceived physical threat to one's life. (Bernstein, 2006, p. 36)

CHAPTER 10

Shock, Trauma, and the
Primary Respiratory System

These discoveries made by exploring the inner world help us to explain two of the most disturbing findings in the literature about trauma. The first of these findings is that *the traumatized psyche is self-traumatizing.* Trauma doesn't end with the cessation of outer violation, but continues unabated in the inner world of the trauma victim, whose dreams are often haunted by persecutory inner figures. The second finding is the seemingly perverse fact that *the victim of psychological trauma continually finds himself or herself in life situations where he or she is retraumatized.* (Kalsched, 1996, p. 5)

We live in the age of post-traumatic stress. In the United States, September 11, 2001 was a vivid confirmation of this fact. We see it written on the bodies and imprinted in the fluids and brains of our clients. It is epidemic and invites biodynamic craniosacral therapy to become one antidote to the overwhelming experiences that are held in the mind and the soma. This is the new dilemma found almost universally in all clients. In this and the next few chapters I will define terms from the field of trauma resolution and then look at how to integrate this new information into biodynamic practice.

- *Trauma* is a challenge to the coping mechanisms of the mind and body. It triggers a variety of responses in the autonomic nervous system of the brain and body.

- *Shock* occurs when body-mind resources are overwhelmed.

- *Traumatization* is repeated shock that is driven deeper and compressed into one's body and brain. This creates an implicit memory of distress in the right hemisphere of the brain, which is accessed unconsciously in the future.

- *Shock affects* are the cyclic expressions of embodied shock and trauma. They occur over a lifespan, as a disruption of the cohesion among parts of the self, especially sensation, imagination, behavior, emotion, and memory (Levine, 1997). The cumulative pattern of shock affect in a person is called a *trauma schema.*

- *Resources* are anything brought to a situation involving traumatic stress that help alleviate it, especially a slow tempo and stillness. Biodynamic craniosacral therapy is a crucial resource in the treatment of shock and trauma.

- *Ignition* is the body's constant attempt to reorient to stillness and Primary Respiration. Please refer to Volume One for a complete discussion of ignition.

Traumatization held in the fluid body and soma of the client is the result of shock and trauma being recapitulated over the lifespan. Over and over, again and again from conception onward, the fluid body and then the soma are subjected to repeated stress and trauma. Research suggests that the original trauma is from the prenatal and perinatal time of life. For some clients conception is the first shock. Then there is a traumatic birth or, worse, the surgical shock of a Caesarian section. Then perhaps there is a misattuned attachment. Later there is a broken arm in childhood, car accidents in adolescence, and so on, all of which may represent an ignition of the fluid body and soma to heal the core shock. These repeated traumas are layered throughout the soma and nervous system and keep the autonomic nervous system in an activated state. Life force in the fluid body is allocated to containing the effects of trauma in the fluids. The natural ability to cope, or to be resourced, and to orient to nature and the environment is greatly diminished. One's freedom to respond appropriately and self-regulate under stress is significantly restricted.

Resources

Certain affects simply cannot be processed with the normal resources available to the ego, and "deeper" resources need to be marshaled. These deeper resources are the life-saving defenses of the Self and they block the ego's path at those traumatic times when, as these defenses can apparently "see" in their wisdom, the psychic circuit-breaker needs to be thrown, so to speak, so that lightning does not burn up all the circuits in the house. (Kalsched, 1996, pp. 41–42)

All work with trauma is resourcing work. Trauma cannot uncouple from its speedy physiology without the proper resources. A resource can be anything that helps the uncoupling process. The foundation resources in biodynamic craniosacral therapy are Primary Respiration, stillness, and life forces in the fluid body, especially the longitudinal fluctuation and the stillpoint in the reciprocal tension potency (RTP). Some natural resources are: safe places in nature, church for some, safe friends, the practitioner, reading books, meditation, and comfort food.

Biodynamic resources, as suggested in the first section of this book, become invaluable in uncoupling from trauma gracefully. The discovery of available client resources must be assessed before treatment begins when the client presents a history of shock and trauma. Then the client must be taught biodynamic resources such as Primary Respiration. In this way, if the inertial forces of the trauma schema are encountered in a session, the client has a reference point or enough buoyancy in the fluid body to uncouple or automatically shift away from the trauma.

The practitioner's voice is also a resource, as well as the practitioner's ability to maintain orientation to Primary Respiration, to slow pacing and remain in present time. The pendulum of attunement and attention swings back and forth between the biodynamic resource and the shock affect, with the help of the practitioner's containment. Slowly, this integrates the hemispheres of the brain and sends a *top-down* signal from the cortex to the deep limbic system to self-regulate. Remember that any professional touch therapy can create a *bottom-up* signal from the body to the limbic system that may trigger the trauma schema, which is well below conscious awareness in the client. This is one of the essential points about resources. The practitioner's verbal skills of facilitating access to the fluid body rather than the autonomic nervous system, as well as his attunement skills act as a set of external resources for the client to resonate with.

Here are some questions to evaluate a client's resources. They are important considerations as the practitioner talks to the client and reviews the intake form.

• What is your general sense of the client's distress level at home?

• What is your sense of your client's tendency toward depression or anxiety? Remember, this is just a feeling tone you might have about the client or it could be an actual disclosure on the intake form.

• What is the overall sense you have of the client's physical health?

- What is your sense of issues that the client may have around safety and trust with you?

- How successful is your client in her chosen career and relationships?

- Is there an overall sense of success in life?

- What are your feelings about the client's ego strength? This relates to her courage and religious faith. It includes a sense of some potency underneath the symptoms and, especially, a sense of humor, which is an indication of self-reflection and perspective on the irony of life.

- Does the client's personal life feel stable to you?

- Is the client receiving support from family and friends, and can the client identify a particular resourced friend or family member?

Resources are frequently lost in cases of sexual abuse, rape, surgery, car accidents, and orthopedic injuries. Even witnessing violence on TV, such as millions of people did on September 11, 2001, is shocking to the nervous system; this is called virtual trauma. Primary Respiration and stillness are the most important resources in biodynamic craniosacral therapy. Biodynamic resources are preexisting within the tidal body and fluid body of the PRS, as well as within one's social and cultural milieu. Another key resource therapeutically is safety. *Safety,* as a perception of flow and connectedness and sensation as a comfort in the body, is lost in trauma. Therefore, the most important resource is safety and anything that can restore safety, especially a therapeutic container with healthy boundaries, is critical to the healing process.

Another type of resource is called a *survival resource.* It is much deeper and more primitive than the soma's usual resources. A survival resource is a primitive defensive strategy originating deep in the brain and far below conscious awareness, such as normal dissociation and hyperarousal. These survival mechanisms are found deep in the limbic system of the brain or in the tissues and fluids of the embryo before there was a nervous system. The survival resource is normal and a preexisting gesture of sentient fluid activity in the body. It must be respected by the practitioner.

As a principle, biodynamic craniosacral therapy looks for the survival resource of stillness and Primary Respiration without challenging the traumatic effects of hyperarousal and non-normal dissociation that can lead to retraumatization of the client. Practitioners must have a deep understanding of the preexisting resources, no matter what they look like in their clients, especially the value of stillness and Primary Respiration. Biodynamic craniosacral therapy is a valuable adjunctive therapy for helping to resolve some cases of traumatic shock. It is not a panacea, however—some clients must be working with other experts in the field of trauma resolution such as somatic experiencing, while others must really be under the care of a psychiatrist and medicated or be in psychotherapy.

Finally, resources arise in the context of past experiences, present experiencing, and future expectations. Often, if a client had an experience of overwhelm in the past, she may be able to visualize someone or some place at the time of the trauma that could have been resourcing for her. This is also true in dealing with present time or recent trauma. Ultimately, the client will need to build biodynamic resources to navigate through any future experience that could be traumatic or reactivating for her. This is why I believe it is critical to teach the client to perceive Primary Respiration before she leaves the practitioner's office.

Autonomic Nervous System Activation

When the soma's protective mechanisms are overwhelmed, at least three physiological events occur. We'll inevitably see hyperarousal, dissociation, and withdrawal of one's physical energy.

Hyperarousal

The first physiological affect is *hyperarousal.* The sympathetic nervous system speeds up the right hemisphere of the brain, activates body memories, and triggers strong physiological reactions, such as the fight-or-flight response in the body. Emotional flooding, claustrophobic thinking, and confusion characterize the internal experience of hyperarousal, since the right hemisphere is nonverbal and information to the rational left brain is greatly diminished. The right hemisphere is where memories of shock and trauma are stored and consistently get activated when someone reexperiences traumatic stress. Past traumas and shocks are stacked like poker chips in the right hemisphere of the brain as compressed experience. It is hard to find a client with only one trauma in her life, given its pervasiveness in the culture. When the emotional intensity of a shock or trauma memory begins to flood the body, it may have the effect of retraumatizing the client by placing her once again in a situation where she feels helpless and overwhelmed. Therefore, it is vital to come into appropriate relationship with shock and trauma without intensifying it. The client already lives in trauma and does not need to be taken there for resolution. States of activation and associated processes are all viewed as biodynamic ignition processes. They need to be held with loving kindness and compassion via stillness and Primary Respiration, which allow the client to uncouple gracefully from the affect.

I often let myself visualize the client's trauma and breathe it into my heart at the rate of Primary Respiration, as described in Volume One. I exhale perfect health back to the client as a light color. I sit in stillness and wait for Primary Respiration to manifest its "unerring potency" for healing that which I cannot know anything about in the client. When a practitioner is able to hold the client's totality in his heart, the client can spontaneously create a container for different healing possibilities that are known only by Primary Respiration and the Dynamic Stillness.

Dissociation

The second affect involves *dissociation.* Dissociation is typically defined as being stuck inside a body that doesn't work so well and is full of painful sensations, or outside the body unable to contact the lived experience of the body through sensation. I will cover this topic in detail in the next chapter. Dissociation involves a profound activation of the parasympathetic nervous system in the soma—this is usually a learned response to prenatal and perinatal traumatic stress. The common definition of non-normal dissociation described in psychological literature is a partial or complete loss of the normal integration between memories of the past, lack of awareness of self-identity in relationship to others, intrusion of intense body sensations and a misinterpretation of them, and loss of control of bodily movements, thoughts, and emotions. Biodynamically, however, I define non-normal dissociation as a loss of flexibility in one's ability to shift conscious attention between the midline of the body and the horizon at the tempo of Primary Respiration, as the reader will see in later chapters.

Dissociative disorders and the study of its neurobiology are important for at least two reasons. The first is because of the overwhelming speed and volume of information that confronts the body and nervous system in the modern world keep non-normal dissociation constantly kindled. The pilot light is always on for fear and terror. The second reason is the sheer magnitude of prenatal and perinatal neglect and abuse that contribute to varying degrees of insecure attachments between infants and their primary caregivers.

The first dissociation is an effect of modern culture, with multitasking and unlimited access to the world of high-speed Internet, instant messaging, and fast food. The second dissociation is developmental—set in place before, during, and after birth. This means that the body and behavior have maladapted because of shock and trauma, from a time when brain development was primarily focused on the dyadic regulation of emotions with a primary caregiver. This was the time when the right hemisphere of the brain was developing. As we will see in the next chapter on the value of dissociation, this damages a person's ability to self-regulate the autonomic nervous system, not only with other people but also when alone, throughout life. Furthermore, there is a much greater susceptibility to post-traumatic stress disorder and psychopathology in adulthood. When hyperarousal and dissociation are prevalent aspects of a client's experience, the touch of any cranial practitioner, biodynamic or otherwise, requires more skill and supervision than many practitioners have. Trauma resolution work requires advanced training and necessitates that the practitioner is active in his own self-development.

Withdrawal of Physical Energy

The affect related to the contemporary definition of dissociation is the parasympathetic nervous system response of a strong withdrawal of one's physical energy. Such a withdrawal causes either a freezing response in the soma systemically or a collapse and lack of tone in the tissues of the body.

Whether one gets stiff or goes slack is genetically programmed in the individual as a preference to stress. It is a survival response generated by an overactive limbic system, especially the amygdala, which I wrote about in Volume One. This is an overactive parasympathetic nervous system. In addition, both the sympathetic and parasympathetic nervous systems may be uncoupled from their reciprocal function and can be simultaneously overactive. These conditions in the brain cause the soma and mind to fragment and lose cohesiveness. Mental and physical experience becomes disorganized. Furthermore, this causes a loss of contact with the world and cognition because of diminished left hemisphere activity. Life feels unreal and hopeless and causes significant changes in behavior. Basically, the parts of the soma and the world don't feel like they fit together. Typically such withdrawal causes immobilization to occur in the extremities of the body, the arms and legs. It is here where the fight-or-flight mechanism is thwarted. Clients may report parts of their body being numb or having no sensation at all. Other clients may report brief episodes of intrusive pain and sensation.

Permission to Touch the Client

Understanding the psyche as half-bodily—half spiritual (or mental) entity has some important implications. … A danger of pure body-work is that it may release much somatized energy without this raw affect becoming available to the mind in the form of images or words that would enable it to be understood. If affect from the body cannot be expressed in verbal or symbolic language between people, it cannot reach the level of "meaning" which is where the psyche is. So bodyworkers can also lose the psyche and if this happens, the possibility of truly transformative work is also lost. (Kalsched, 1996, pp. 65–66)

How does a biodynamic craniosacral therapy practitioner work with trauma appropriately? It is important to establish a verbal contract regarding the use of touch with a client. The pressure of the touch, its duration, and locations of the hand positions on the client's soma must be described to the client and it must be said especially that the client does not need to remove any clothes. Biodynamic practice is done with the client's clothes on. This provides a healthy boundary for the relationship.

The next ethical principle in trauma work is informing the client of the practitioner's exact training and experience and how it will be brought to the therapeutic relationship and under what circumstances (see Appendix A).

Further, it is essential to enter into a dialogue about the quality of the touch and what feels comfortable. I regularly ask clients, "Are you comfortable?" Could my hands be in a different place that would be more comfortable?" In this way, the practitioner is able to assist the client in reassociating to resourced sensations that underlie emotional states. This integrates the right hemisphere with the left hemisphere, which is responsible for maintaining an accurate connection to outside reality.

Sensation

The most interesting current theory about trauma's effects on the psyche takes into account how difficult it is for us humans to *process* certain aspects of our experience. Work by clinicians have combined to help us understand that "whole" experience is a unity of many factors and that *integrated* experience is not always easy. One researcher (Braun, 1988), for example, describes four aspects of experience along which dissociation can occur, namely *behavior, affect, sensation* and *knowledge*—otherwise known as BASK model of dissociation. In dissociative disorder, any of these aspects can be split within itself or the usual links among them or between them can be severed. (Kalsched, 1996, pp. 36–37)

The uncoupling of shock and trauma from debilitating affects comes about through reassociation to fluid sensation and fluid image in the biodynamic relationship. Therefore, exquisite attunement to both the practitioner's and the client's state of sympathetic and parasympathetic activation is required in the first three sessions of biodynamic practice. This also includes the ability of the practitioner to attend his own felt sense of stillness and Primary Respiration that were present before the autonomic nervous system came to be in the embryo. This is one principle of biodynamic practice that must be emphasized and that is the focus on the fluid body of the client's embryo prior to the development of a nervous system. The practitioner automatically resonates with the client's nervous system and soma as well as his own because it is the first line of defense from the outside world in the adult soma and practitioners are simultaneously touching it and the pre-nervous system state in the fluid body. The practitioner needs to be attuned to both his own autonomic soma and fluid body continuum while with a client who has a trauma history. One osteopath calls this divided attention. The client's trauma is like a virus and can infect the practitioner during the treatment. This is just normal brain and autonomic soma resonance between two people, which is greatly augmented during a session. I wrote extensively about this in Volume One.

Biodynamic craniosacral therapy helps the client reassociate to the sense, image, and shape of the fluid body around and underneath the survival resources in the soma. This has the ability to normalize the survival resource and have it be more fluid. It means that, rather than obsessing about emotions or impulsively acting them out, a client identifies with the sense, image, and shaping experience of her fluid body at the tempo of Primary Respiration and is able to talk about it from a witness perspective or stillpoint. This uncouples the sensation from the intensity of the emotional state and realigns it with Primary Respiration and the fluid body of the embryo. There is a big difference between saying "I'm angry" and "I'm noticing the sensation of anger coming up right now." I ask the client to focus on the edge of her skin and disappear the structure of her body so that all that remains is a living ocean inside the soma, just as it was during the first two weeks after conception. The client can then witness her experience and be supported by the ocean as the mother of all creation.

Pacing

Pacing and slowing in biodynamic craniosacral therapy require the ability to attune to the mutually unfolding perceptual experience of both the practitioner and the client during the session. This *attunement* skill becomes an artistic ability to wait, watch, and wonder with the presence of stillness and Primary Respiration. This is the compassion to bear witness to the client's pain and suffering. A deep attunement to one's own body and the client's also involves sensing the stillness and ocean of Primary Respiration in the office space, which means the practitioner moves his sense attention all the way out to the horizon and back. This quality of attunement is called establishing *right distance* and creates a matrix for stillness to interchange with Primary Respiration in the therapeutic relationship. Attunement in this way decompresses the client's nervous system and is a critical antidote when encountering shock and trauma. The practitioner moves his attention up to the third ventricle of the brain and shifts his attention out to the horizon and back until a stillpoint manifests. The horizon is the deep stillpoint that is invited to move into the foreground of the therapeutic milieu by approaching it in the tempo of Primary Respiration.

Healing is a slow process, whatever the diagnosis, prognosis, and cause might be. Only the soma gets diagnosed in contemporary medicine. The fluid body and tidal body are virgin territory for biodynamic practice. Healing involves working with the client slowly and at the pace of Primary Respiration. I am frequently asked if one is ever able to successfully resolve trauma. The answer is: resolve no, transmute and reframe yes. It requires love to rewrite the story of life and understand its perfection from the time the egg differentiated. In this way trauma does not disappear forever from the soma and the brain, but rather that the memories and physiological states lose their debilitating power to subvert behavior. I still avoid proximity to public garbage cans because of my own terrorist bombing experience, but I do not go into fight-or-flight. Rather, I see it as an honoring of my past and a small reminder of my interconnectedness to everyone with PTSD symptoms. I no longer feel like a prisoner in my own soma. To get to that place has involved growing and developing resources over time.

Gradually the antidotes for traumatic stress become more manifest and the client is empowered to lead life to a fuller potential, with happiness and freedom of mind. This empowerment not only is reflected in her own life and dreams, but also radiates out to those around her and ultimately to the society as a whole. Life in any dimension takes courage to navigate. It is about awakening a loving and compassionate heart. Healing trauma further involves arresting it at its source with better prenatal care, saner birth practices, and teaching parents to be better at what they do, by being better resourced. Together, these measures will improve our capacity to love because, after all, love heals all things, especially shock and trauma. Love *is* the greatest resource. Ultimately, shock and trauma are not laminated in the body nor is the nervous system the main layer of traumatic imprinting. Shock and trauma are disturbances in the whole person and the whole environment. Biodynamic craniosacral therapy treats the whole through the portal of love.

Chapter 11

On the Value of Dissociation

> The psyche's normal reaction to a traumatic experience is to withdraw from the scene of the injury. If withdrawal is not possible, then a part of the self must be withdrawn, and for this to happen the otherwise integrated ego must split into fragments or *dissociate.* Dissociation is a normal part of the psyche's defenses against trauma's potentially damaging. ... Dissociation is a trick the psyche plays on itself. It allows life to go on by dividing up the unbearable experience and distributing it to different compartments of the mind and body, especially the "unconscious" aspects of the mind and body. (Kalsched 1997, pp. 12–13)

Everyone has dissociation. It is normal. I define dissociation as a diminishment of reciprocal contact with nature and normal sensory processing of the body. There is an element of withdrawal from the ordinary way of experiencing the outside world and the inside world with the body's perceptual systems. My contention is that everyone has a natural form of dissociation with normal phases of social and self detachment that are valuable and not pathological. These phases are actually extra-sensory and quite valuable in a therapeutic relationship.

Dissociation exists on a spectrum of disorders from mild to severe. I was trained in graduate school to work with multiple personality disorder, which is now called dissociative identity disorder. This is a severe form of dissociation as defined by the psychological community—something that most craniosacral therapists are unlikely to see in their office, and if they do, need to do so under supervision and with special training. I recognize the severity of the problem as defined by the medical community in some people; these people are usually "in the system," being medicated and not available to the alternative community of biodynamic practitioners. Throughout this book, I am suggesting a total reframing of the dissociation "problem."

I have this point of view because I was in a terrorist bombing attack while in the military and have been in therapy for PTSD (post-traumatic stress disorder) for many years. I knew about improvised explosive devices (IEDs) thirty-five years before they became a household term from the current Iraq war. In addition, many of my clients and students have experienced sexual or physical abuse, and I have learned from each of them for the past thirty years. The field of pre- and perinatal psychology suggests that the roots of PTSD are in the preverbal time of life. I have thrown myself at that literature and therapy as well for the last decade. Given what I know to be true of this preverbal time in my own life, coupled with a terrorist bombing and the standard American diet of virtual violence through television, media, and movies, I consider myself an expert in dissociation. One of my ex-wives, among others, claims I had multiple personalities, so I also have witnesses to my claim. The most difficult part of my rehabilitation and wounding is choosing carefully who I can work with professionally. It is even more difficult to observe a student coming into relationship with her own traumatic issues and at the same time learning a system of therapy that is not specifically oriented to resolving traumatic stress. All the while she is putting her hands on practice clients and managing her own process. Bearing this in mind, I would like to continue now with a historical perspective on the subject of dissociation. I would then like to build a bridge into biodynamic craniosacral therapy and its ability to uncouple from the non-normal effects of dissociation.

Dissociation is a buzz word for many therapeutic communities, from the mainstream field of psychology to complementary and alternative medicine (CAM) practices such as craniosacral biodynamics (Sills, 2001), somatic experiencing (Levine, 1997), sensory-motor psychotherapy (Ogden, Minton, and Pain, 2006), Hakomi therapy (Kurtz, 1990), interpersonal nervous systems approach (Siegel, 2007), and others. These are just a few of the approaches that work with traumatic stress in adults. Likewise, there are many differing ideas about dissociation, spanning the Diagnostic and Statistical Manual (DSM-IV) from neuroscience to the biodynamic craniosacral therapy group of schools and practitioners. I will continue to refer to the definition that I gave above. Any discussion on this topic, however, should include a history of dissociation or, as the philosopher George Santayana said, "Those who cannot remember the past are condemned to repeat it."[2] Dissociation first came on the therapeutic radar screen, so to speak, during the Industrial Revolution in Europe, and especially France. It was originally called hysteria (Scaer, 2005; Herman, 1992; Spiegel, 1994) and considered to be the scourge of the latter part of the 1800s. Its characteristics were similar to the etiology of the Black Plague in the Middle Ages in that it was felt that hysteria came from "an unsanitary mind and body." Gradually it was discovered that the roots of hysteria were in the rampant physical and sexual child abuse of the time. The enormity of that discovery and its consequences were not readily understood by a male-dominated therapeutic and medical community. According to Judith Herman (Herman, 1992), Freud had little choice but to conceptualize it as a repressed sexual neurosis in the patient herself.

Following World War I, dissociation took on a new identification, as "shell shock." Soldiers who were directly exposed to being shot at and next to bombs going off, plus having the constant sight of bloodied and dead comrades, sometimes were unable to return to action the next day. The ones unable to return were called "shell shocked." But dissociation is always two things; it is experienced at both personal and societal levels. There was actually a point during that same war, when 55,000 British soldiers lost their lives in one day due to mustard gas. The casualties so traumatized England and the European culture that research into dissociation was effectively thwarted until the late 1930s. It disappeared from the literature. Of course, the great loss of lives at the battle of Gettysburg in this nation's Civil War nearly half a century earlier traumatized Americans. Remember, as I go along in this discussion, that of the two ways in which dissociation is experienced, there are methods to treat the personal trauma but not the societal type. This in itself is a tragedy that I will address in the section on mythology and healing.

Shell shock, however, at a personal level is something encountered every day during a war, whether it be World War I, the Iraq War, or the "global war on terrorism." It was a stigma on the soldier to not be able to return to battle immediately after being shell-shocked. He was branded a coward. A good example of this is in the movie *Patton,* which depicts General Patton entering a military hospital ward and severely berating a shell-shocked soldier. This attitude permeates the military-industrial complex in such a way that the devastating effects of dissociation and its current metaphor, PTSD, must be denied—and still are as of July 2007. No political system can acknowledge the severity and damage of traumatic shock in a theatre of war because it would necessarily change the nature of war itself; political and military leaders would be less likely to put troops in harm's way, or would be mandated not to do so, if they acknowledged the long-term effects psychologically, physically, and socially of being shell-shocked.

What about those of us who have a steady diet of watching news of the war, or the effects of hurricanes, or sadistic violence depicted nightly on television. This is virtual violence and results in the same affect of dissociation as if being there. Dissociation anesthetizes the outrage at the carnage and wasted lives constantly being viewed today. It allows a population to be manipulated for political purposes by its government. Wilhelm Reich was the first to say this in the 1930s; Al Gore and others are saying it in 2007.

Historically, this is both a cultural problem and an individual problem. Together, the two ends of the spectrum of dissociation create a tension or a polarity through the entire fabric of society and the planet. The therapeutic community, at its own level of understanding, recognizes the damage of traumatic stress and the non-normal affects of dissociation. The military-political complex has to deny it in order to make effective warriors who can win battles. They break, we fix. I watched the hearings on television in June 2007 regarding the poor medical care that American veterans are receiving as they come home from Iraq. This includes denying claims for PTSD and an enormous backlog of up to 55,000 soldiers who need immediate care for PTSD, but are not receiving it. The politics of dissociation permeate the therapeutic community is not only by denying adequate care, but by offering only a modicum of care when absolutely necessary. Lloyd DeMause (DeMause, 2002) further suggests that if our culture could recognize the enormity and prevalence of traumatic shock, we would then see its roots in the aggression of the way babies are birthed in the medical system. His research points toward the need of aggressive societies to have aggressive birth practices to build strong armies and police forces.

> I will be using the word "trauma" to mean any experience that causes the child unbearable psychic pain or anxiety. For an experience to be "unbearable" means that it overwhelms the usual defensive measures. … Trauma of this magnitude varies from the acute, shattering experiences of child abuse so prominent in the literature today to the more "cumulative traumas" of unmet dependency-needs that mount up to devastating effect in some children's development. … The distinguishing feature of such trauma is what Heinz Kohut (Kohut, 1977, p. 104) called "disintegration anxiety," an unnameable dread associated with the threatened dissolution of a coherent self. (Kalsched 1996, p. 1)

The default position, without adequate personal care, is medication, which may be necessary to stabilize a patient who is in a hyperactive state. But medication is frequently overprescribed and keeps emotions from erupting, which makes the staff's work easier. Consequently, patients are unable to break the cycle of dissociation—they are like a billboard I saw in an airport recently that said "Hamsters spend their whole life running in circles." Dissociation is already addictive at a physiological level because of the constant activation of the body's opiate-producing system. Drug addiction truly robs people of seeing their political choices clearly and consequently exercising their free will, as opposed to the free, unresolved anger that permeates trauma patients and frustrates their therapists. "Going postal" is the term given to employees who finally snap and go berserk at the workplace; it is derived from the post office killings in America in the last several decades. Consequently, the care that now arises out of such an unconscious attitude in the mainstream is barely palliative, in the sense that it is designed only to stabilize patients so they can maintain an effective work ethic from 9 to 5 on their jobs and when they get home and are on their own. Inner happiness, lasting change, and self-discovery are for pansies and flower children (get back to the battle!). As long as the bottom line keeps improving, employees with PTSD just have to pass a random drug test and not scare the other employees.

Dissociation is not culturally sanctioned in a cosmopolitan society that demands clarity and effectiveness in the workplace, at school, or on the ball field. Many traditional cultures use dissociation for healing purposes and in healing rituals. This outcome and efficacy flaw within the therapeutic community is unconscious. It is built into the history of the military-industrial complex. It also permeates complementary and alternative medicine practices, including the trauma resolution community. CAM practices are unconsciously allopathic. Attempts are made to stabilize clients in the short term, which is good, but without a long-term plan for change process, self-discovery, and transformation over time. These long-term objectives are part of the design of life: to integrate previous life experience over the lifespan by changing the memories, reframing the past, and entering the mystery of life and death without fear. The spiritual component is relegated to the Moral Majority. People are now "coached" to be effective at work, in relationship, while driving, or in raising children. Forget the fear, forget preparing to die—be effective! Effectiveness, as I use the term here, is defined as any behavior that will improve the bottom line—usually someone else's rather than mine, as Mark Twain remarked. To stabilize someone physiologically is incredibly important in the beginning phases of treating dissociation and PTSD. Eventually, the client has to make meaning out of his life and reestablish a midline to this meaning-making capacity. I believe this is where biodynamic craniosacral therapy is quite valuable in assisting the client in reassociating with the midline and its metabolism of stillness as a dynamic and spiritual potential, rather than a pathological dissociative effect of traumatic stress.

Along with the history of dissociation comes the advent of psychosomatic medicine in World War II, as well as Reichian therapy and its spin-off called bioenergetics after the Korean War. Any discussion of dissociation necessarily includes the body and the sensory awareness of one's body. Almost every alternative practitioner and trauma resolution expert would now agree on this principle. This is the hallmark of trauma resolution therapies in general—to facilitate embodiment in clients. The healing is in the feeling, or in this case, the sensation. Wilhelm Reich and some medical authorities during the late 1930s and '40s began examining the psychosomatic body more closely. Thus, the history of embodiment practices with a psychological edge to them began during the 1930s. At the same time a completely different community of academicians and mainstream psychologists rediscovered dissociation and its devastating impact. Consequently, different researchers were exploring aspects of traumatic stress and were not talking to one another even if they were in the same university until the past decade. This I would call academic dissociation.

Now there is a collusion or cross-fertilization of sorts among all of these fields as they together and try to make sense of dissociation (no pun intended). Their methods and focus are consistently placed on the recovery of the sensory body and maintaining embodiment in general. This is commendable, given the history of the body-mind split as it has been called, which offers a rich philosophical history and discussion of dissociation as a splitting of the masculine and the feminine. I believe this focus, however, has become almost compulsive regarding the internal experience and perception of the body. It needs to be reexamined, especially in light of advances in affective neuroscience and an embryology that is morphologically based rather than genetic. Reassociation to sensation perpetuates the crisis of fragmentation. Sensation becomes friendlier but the whole sensory body as a single continuum in relationship and shaped by other sensory bodies is left out of the therapeutic equation.

Biodynamic practice focuses on contact with the movement of the whole in the practitioner first and then the client. It is a reciprocal relationship of moving attention in and out and between bodies. This is the top priority of biodynamic practice. I would like to state for the sake of the reader that for as long as I've studied embodiment practices, and my doctoral work was in somatic psychology, I've never been able to maintain embodiment. I've tried, I really have. I have more embodiment workshops under my belt than anyone else. Honest. It has always felt to me like I was working on the parts and not the whole. Some days I cannot even pull a shirt over my head. I was able to discharge some strong affects over the years with the help of some great teachers, but in reality was frequently left euphorically dissociated, but by God, I could feel something in my body! I even became quite good at euphorically dissociating my Rolfing clients. This was the learning process as it was in the experimental years as I cut my New-Age teeth in a new calling. There is no blame—becoming whole is a developmental process, after all. It took years to discover wholeness piece by piece. It was not until I studied biodynamic craniosacral therapy that I came to the realization and perception that the design of our organism, starting with the embryo and going through the entire lifespan, is to maintain a flexible attention and attunement at a tempo that moves from the outside of the body. It moves through it, changes directions, and goes out from the midline of the body to the horizon of the planet. This is called Primary Respiration. This is wholeness first in biodynamic craniosacral therapy.

Classical dissociation is a state of either being oversomatized or undersomatized. This is someone who has lost sensory awareness and spends a lot of time spaced out of his body unconsciously. Dissociation in mainstream practice is called a spectrum disorder, in the sense that there are many degrees of intensity with over- or under- somatization effects. In the past couple of decades, however, the definition of dissociation has begun to include the possibility of having too much sensation in the body and thus being oversomatized with "intrusive sensation." Thus the flexible movement of conscious attention and attunement is lost and such people remain fixated or stuck in their body or outside of their body. The job of Primary Respiration is to help clients uncouple from this fixation and consciously begin to breathe their attention more flexibly in and out of the body. Dissociation does not go away, but its normal function is restored with Primary Respiration.

I would like, however, to offer one possible insight into the etiology of dissociation that is coming from the field of pre- and perinatal psychology. It is called affective neuroscience. Birth processes, attachment distress, and neglect in infancy are strong indicators for future dissociative problems. Likewise, prenatal distress, either nutritionally or with traumatic stress coming through the mother, can also result in dissociation later in life. Fundamentally, at this pre- and perinatal level, the organism's primary response to stress is going to be to withdraw. That is normal sentient behavior. At the same time, the neurological system is building an autonomic nervous system that is attempting to learn how to approach and reach out as well as to withdraw from contact—again, normal growth functions of the developing brain and body systems. This is now called attunement and is the subtext of this entire volume.

Attunement is the ability to be conscious of the cycling of contact and withdrawal. Attunement to approach and withdrawal behaviors is the hallmark of a healthy attachment between a caregiver and an infant. Lack of attunement causes what Alan Schore calls an *autonomic set point* to be determined. The set point is that level of stimulus in the autonomic nervous system that, when reached, would cause an episode of sympathetic excitation and approach behavior and then the reciprocal activity of parasympathetic withdrawal behavior. Again, the set point will cause normal behavior in a low-stress attunement but aberrant behavior in a misattuned parenting process. Either way, this needs to happen thousands of times for it to be wired into the infant's neurological circuits and have potential long-term damage for hyperarousal and dissociation.

Biodynamic craniosacral therapy attempts to circumvent the non-normal affects of dissociation by a focused attunement on the movement of the whole in the fluid body and tidal body—Primary Respiration in the practitioner and the client. This focused attunement is called neuro-affective touch, because it is not the intention of a cranial practitioner from the neurological point of view to stimulate the client, but it happens by a function of subtle physical touch. The moment the practitioner makes physical contact with a client, with even with the greatest amount of compassion, the touch itself can trigger implicit memory in the right frontal cortex, which reads the context of the touch, rather than the sensation. If the context center for love and nurturing in the prefrontal cortex of the right hemisphere has been compromised during the third trimester, birth, and the first two years after birth, then the touch itself may trigger a well-compensated reaction, which will usually be dissociation. This reaction is normal and rooted in the preverbal time of life. Consequently, the client will likely have no conscious recall of that time of life. The practitioner must be attuned to this possibility and stay focused on the movement of Primary Respiration. Even stillness is suspect if it loses its dynamism and the practitioner succumbs to the numbing intensity of the affects of dissociation. Primary Respiration must be clear and able to exchange places with stillness for normalizing dissociative affect. It is not the therapeutic intention to get rid of dissociation. The intention is to normalize it and use it constructively to reconnect with the midline.

The natural state of perception is to have phases of withdrawing attention from either the inside of the body and going out, or withdrawing attention from the outside world and going in to the mind and body. It is a cycle and biphasic. It is about seeking contact and then withdrawing slowly from that contact. This is the essence of embryonic metabolic behavior. It is called sentience and even single-celled organisms display attunement. The hardest work in the world, because of early imprinting, is to see outer reality and inner bodily reality with any kind of precision. The capacity to withdraw from the outside world is a normal and natural response. It is the foundation for autonomy, wisdom, and a direct personal experience of a personal connection to spirit. This is half of the self-regulation matrix that an infant's brain and body is focused upon during gestation and in the first two years of life. The other half is the relationship itself with its own embryonic bodies, as I explained in Volume One, and then the caregiver as a fetus and infant.

Cultures and affinity groups have difficulty supporting autonomy, as Wilhelm Reich said. It is easier for authorities to control behavior through the pathologizing of withdrawal and calling it dissociation and giving it metaphors such as numbing, fragmentation, splitting, projection, freeze, collapse, bipolar disorder, somatoform disorder, ADD, depression, autism, and PTSD. These are all evolutions of hysteria, shell shock, and, worse yet, cowardice in the face of the enemy! These are all labels for a cultural inability to contain and transform such affect. The process becomes rigidified, oversomatized or undersomatized, and driven by speed and a fear-based media.

This results in a loss of sentient behavior and basic attunement to the need for both contact and autonomy. Misattunement suppresses the natural instinct to heal oneself and creates a speedy mind and an equally speedy body that is alienated from nature and spirit. Projection, on the one hand, is normal and natural, but becomes a solidified transference because of a relentless demand for relational and rational effectiveness. This completely misses normal relationship approach and withdrawal behaviors. It is this part of self-regulation that a practitioner builds in any client-therapist relationship, because the first foundation for healing dissociation is safety and trust. This is built upon normal attunement.

Reassociation to sensation is not enough. People with traumatic stress issues—the majority of the population—need a different strategy, and that is to contact the metabolic dynamic that preceded the development of the brain and the central nervous system during the embryonic time. This requires a different metaphor that embraces the ocean, the blood, the rivers and streams of the vascular system, and the living waters of the human body. It requires participation on the part of both the practitioner and the client to contact this fluid reality and sense the resonance and exchange of two oceans uniting in the tempo of Primary Respiration. This is normal dissociation.

> We must remember that for the person carrying around a dissociated trauma experience, integration or "wholeness" is initially experienced as the worst thing imaginable. … Work with them, therefore, must involve "softer" techniques. … Great attention must be given to the creation of a safe physical space and a safe interpersonal environment within which dreams and fantasies can emerge and be worked with in a more playful, open-ended fashion. … All forms of the so-called "creative-arts" psychotherapies are extremely helpful toward this end and often these will open up traumatic affect much faster than purely verbal exploration. (Kalsched, 1996, pp. 26–27)

CHAPTER 12

Relating with Trauma Biodynamically

Many of us have lost access to a ritualized "world center" where deep healing and rejuvenation can occur. … Our prophets speak from television sets. We require our children to stay in school from age five [or before] to twenty-five or thirty if they get professional degrees, but rarely in this education do we make room for the integration of psyche in ritual. … The end product can be a dissociated adult who has been taught more about correct behavior, competition, and conformity than about inner wholeness. (Schulman, 1997, p. 173)

Biodynamic craniosacral therapy works with the forces outside the nervous system, specifically Primary Respiration and the fluid body. It also influences the nervous system and, consequently, stress and trauma held in the implicit memory brain and soma.

This chapter elaborates on additional practitioner skills for relating with trauma imprinted in the fluid body of the Primary Respiratory System (PRS). I have attempted to condense what I feel are the necessary advanced skills a practitioner must have, when encountering the interface between physiological states in the soma and their fluid body imprints. The biodynamic practitioner uses her hands to listen to the story in the fluids as the first priority. Trauma is very magnetizing and seductive, especially in the aberrant behavior of fluid body. Trauma is said to be contagious in this way, as a practitioner can get lost in the dissonance that a client's trauma creates in the practitioner's brain and soma. What is missing is the link to the creation story of wholeness in the embryo called Primary Respiration. Primary Respiration is the mind of the fluid body, and the fluid body forgets that relationship in shock and trauma. Consequently, the biodynamic practitioner reacquaints the fluid body with its brain.

Witnessing

Witnessing includes the ability to be reflectively and alertly attuned to the practitioner's own or another's experience, without judgment or expectation. This is done first with the heart, which is the most fundamental attention center for empathy and compassion. Then attention rests in the third ventricle of the brain and thus the prefrontal cortex, where the neurological centers for clear attention and non-attachment are located. This means that the witness embodies the capacity for both clarity and compassion. Attention is the quality and quantity of focus the practitioner has in the fulcrum of her heart and third ventricle. Non-attachment is a disidentification from the effects of the autonomic nervous system, especially its speediness. Non-attachment is not becoming inert, overly passive, or disinterested. From the practitioner's point of view, this means that she can observe the physiological response emerging in her own or in the client's experience without losing the capacity to be still. The witness attunes with the to and fro of conscious attention, out to the horizon and back, at the tempo of Primary Respiration, as she observes the strong polarity being held in the client's fluid body.

The practitioner needs the skill of clear differentiation—knowing what she is identified with the autonomic nervous system especially and where her identification is located in or out of her soma, in order to bear witness to the pain and suffering of the client. The practitioner asks: "Am I identified with my role as a practitioner, am I identified with the client and his trauma, or am I identified with my own history of shock and trauma?" The practitioner-cum-witness must find which role she is identified with by attending to her sensorium and cycling back to a witness perspective. It is quite normal for the identification to automatically shift during a treatment. The skill is in recognizing how and when that happens, being able to nonverbally name or acknowledge that space, then gently shifting attention back to the role of biodynamic practitioner-witness.

The motivation of the witness is to become clear through a stillpoint and compassionate through the movement of Primary Respiration heart to heart. Ultimately, this is the desire to have the client being free from his pain and suffering and to have the client experience happiness and know its causes. Clarity and compassion are the true and necessary polarities of the client-therapist relationship.

Safe Space Is Sacred Space

The witness creates sacred space through the invocation of a deep stillpoint. This skill helps transform the chaos of trauma to the order and love inherent within sacred space. The practitioner is on the scent of the sacred. When trauma uncouples, sacred space automatically permeates the client and reestablishes a midline of stillness. Dissociation is just a molecule away from the divine! The effects of dissociation are the divine trying to get our attention. The brain stores the trauma in the same place that each of us has the potential to perceive the divine. The practitioner vacillates between feeling like a fool, not knowing how to proceed, and then a sacred fool when the stillpoint arrives. Sacred space has an organizing midline with resources of safety and trust. Thus, safety and trust are the first resourcing priorities in a healing relationship (Herman, 1997).

Safety and trust are engendered in the therapeutic relationship when the practitioner does not prematurely invoke the client's trauma issues. The practitioner recognizes the importance of establishing and maintaining therapeutic boundaries. She is holding a correct fluid distance out to the horizon and back to watch the therapeutic relationship unfold under the priorities established by Primary Respiration. By now, the reader might begin to have an idea of how the witness is an integral part of the creation of sacred space. One could say that the still witness is the embodiment of sacred space. Sacred space is a quality of the witness. The biodynamic practitioner is a shaman for a short period of time during each session. I will elaborate on this theme in detail in Section V, Mythology and Healing. Maintaining and recognizing sacred space is a basic function and responsibility of the biodynamic practitioner. The witness in this context is associated with the numinous connection to the divine, as opposed to the ego self, according to Ken Wilber (Wilber, 2000). Thus, the still witness as a Buddha or a Christ is continually self-regulating and self-organizing, constantly freeing herself from her neurotic mind and her own shock affects by periodically seeing them clearly and compassionately. Is this state possible to achieve? Can the practitioner embody these qualities and do they help facilitate healing? I believe that one is only ever in the process of becoming such a possibility. It is a fluid process and not static. It is truly the preexisting condition located in our mind and soma. That is one of the reasons that I believe biodynamic craniosacral therapy is therapist-centered therapy.

Safety has three aspects (Bloom, 1997). First, it is a perception of the reliability and trustworthiness of restorative life forces in the fluid body and soma. Second, it is the reliability of one's social environment and trust in the natural world.

Finally, it is one's personal connection to the divine or the numinous experience. Shock and trauma shatter the capacity to feel safe and this is imprinted in the fluid body and managed by its life forces from the moment the egg differentiates. Ultimately, this causes deep imprinting of annihilation and death anxiety, which are the embryo's constant companions. What is important now is to state a principle in traditional trauma resolution work: *physiology precedes meaning.*

Therapeutically, a trauma resolution expert must first help a client come into an appropriate relationship with his shock and trauma physiology and its related coupling to incoherent behaviors, intrusive sensations, numbing, freezing, nightmares, and other affects. Biodynamically, however, metabolism precedes physiology. The meaning is in the metabolism of the fluid fields of the embryo, as discussed in detail in Chapter 28 on metabolic fields. In biodynamic craniosacral therapy, all shock affects are reframed as a fundamental part of the ignition process, allowed to be accessed in present time, and held in a sacred container of Primary Respiration and stillness. Fluid shock uncouples from the speed in which it occurred or still exists and automatically shifts into a more appropriate relationship with Primary Respiration, which is the mind of the fluid body. Trapped heat in the fluid body is now able to permeate the soma. The release and distribution of heat from the inertial fulcrum is a key to understanding the life force, the heart and movement of the blood, both in the embryo, the adult, and the therapeutic relationship. This allows meaning to emerge as a midline experience in the fullness of time in the client's perception rather than the practitioner's time frame. Meaning, spiritual or otherwise, is an emergent property of sacred space and of the midline.

Self-Regulation and Attunement

The practitioner must be able to observe the cycling of the autonomic nervous system (ANS) in the early phases of treatment. When the practitioner sees activation, she waits for the activation to settle. She must not move in and engage or challenge the activation. The practitioner needs to get a sense of the activation and settling cycle (also called the freeze-thaw cycle) in the client before a biodynamic therapeutic process can begin with Primary Respiration. It takes at least three sessions for the practitioner to get a sense of the client's autonomic nervous system and whether it can achieve a wholistic shift to being moved by Primary Respiration. Otherwise, how can the practitioner know the client's capacity for self-regulation? Primary Respiration must direct each session.

Self-regulation is the ability of the autonomic nervous system to experience regular cycling of excitation and withdrawal, free from shock affect. This is linked to emotional development in the corticolimbic system during infancy. Self-regulation comes in two varieties. The first is *dependent* self-regulation, which occurs when two or more people interact and are able mutually to settle themselves in the relationship. *Autonomous* self-regulation, or auto-regulation, is a function of settling that occurs when a person is alone. Recent research regarding attachment processes between infants and their primary caregivers has made it obvious that many people do not learn to self-regulate emotionally and, consequently, become chronically activated autonomically while in relationship or when alone.

This inability to self-regulate the sympathetic nervous system with the parasympathetic system causes many downstream problems psychologically, physically, and spiritually, as will be detailed in Section III, Infants and Children. It is often spoken of in our culture as an addiction to excitement or speed and a variety of compulsive behaviors. It takes the form of a craving for overstimulation or withdrawal into a comatose state around a television, for example. These are learned neurological adaptations being regulated in the corticolimbic system (emotional brain) from a misattuned, ambivalent, or insecure attachment between infants and their primary caregivers, as also discussed in Volume One. The solution is slowing down and settling into the tempo of Primary Respiration and regular access to the stillpoint.

Self-regulation is modulated by the resonance established between the brains of the caregiver and the infant. It is no different in the client-therapist relationship. Someone must slow down to begin the therapeutic relationship and that responsibility is the practitioner's. The practitioner becomes consciously attuned to her own needs and then the client's needs for slowness and stillness throughout a biodynamic session.

Naming and Reflecting

When the client's autonomic nervous system becomes activated during a biodynamic session, it is important to verbally name any perceptions that relate to the autonomic nervous system, such as shortness of breath, shaking, heart pounding, trembling, tight abdomen, or feelings of anger or sadness. The practitioner must actively coach the client to say verbally when he notices any sensation that gets his attention or is producing discomfort. The practitioner also has the responsibility of verbally naming her own personal perceptual process when it is appropriate, during the early stages of biodynamic work. It could be as simple as saying, "I'm noticing a stillpoint fill the room." The practitioner must avoid self-indulgence, and it is very important that the practitioner reveal her

106 ▪ BIODYNAMIC CRANIOSACRAL THERAPY

own perceptions in a way that the client does not feel responsible for them. It's a question of attunement to affect and feeling. The practitioner must be attuned to the client's therapeutic process via the perception of Primary Respiration in order for self-revelation to be appropriate and therapeutically efficacious. The more attention the practitioner has on Primary Respiration, the less she will need to reveal anything about her perception.

When the client can also name his perceptions as an active witness, it helps to integrate the brain across hemispheres and develop self-regulation. The practitioner does not necessarily need to process what the client says, but, rather, needs to be an accurate mirror, reflecting the client's experience. This can be done with a simple acknowledgment like "Thank you" or "Good, you're having some strong sensation in your legs right now." I remember an old expression in psychotherapy: "If you can name it, you can tame it." Sometimes simply making a sound like *hmm* or *oh* is enough. Later in this section of the book I provide detail on verbal dialogue.

The reason that the practitioner may need to reveal her own perceptions is because often shock is a recapitulation or repetition of a developmental trauma that originated prenatally or perinatally. Most important, the *core shock,* the original experience that is the center of all the others held by the client, probably occurred when the client was *preverbal* and in an egg, zygote, or embryonic state. It is not necessary for a client to consciously and verbally access core shock material or even nonverbal states of activation from fight-or-flight to overwhelm, hyperarousal, and dissociation. Primary Respiration does not hold shock and trauma and in this way automatically uncouples the client from it very slowly. That is why one important antidote for helping to resolve preverbal shock is for each person in the therapeutic relationship, including the practitioner, to become conscious of Primary Respiration. Primary Respiration mitigates strong affect and reframes the core shock as an initiatory experience, which I will discuss in Section V, Mythology and Healing.

"No"

The client has the right to say no to anything. "No" is a complete sentence. An old expression from the self-esteem movement in the 1980s fits here: "What part of *no* don't you understand?" Always accept a no. This is a great act of client empowerment.

Also watch for a no nonverbally—expressed by the client's body movement and posture, vocal tone or lack thereof, arm and leg gesturing, and facial expression. Infants and children are experts at saying no with gesture. The soma can say no a thousand different ways.

Confidentiality

The client needs to be informed that everything he says, as well as everything that occurs in the treatment, is confidential. If the practitioner must keep notes of the session in a client's chart, then the notes should be very matter-of-fact (describing this hand position or that technique, for example). Avoid any written interpretation of the process that was evoked. Do not document or summarize any discussion that occurred during the treatment. Such documentation is not even within the scope of practice of most biodynamic craniosacral therapists. (See Appendix A.)

Pendulation

When a client begins to access shock and trauma material, it is important for the practitioner to remind the client of his available resources. Peter Levine calls this *pendulation*. It is also called *bridging*. When a client is activated or in hyper-arousal, the practitioner creates a gentle context of awareness of present time, verbally suggesting that the client slow down his physiological processes, which may include consciously slowing down thoracic respiration. The practitioner can then begin to acknowledge and attend to the sensations and physiological states that are arising in the client. This gracefully facilitates an ability to anchor the client's reaction in present time.

If a client is experiencing hyperarousal, the practitioner might coach the client that it is possible to slow down and notice the sound of the practitioner's voice or to focus on the color of the walls of the office, which activates his inner witness. This helps the pendulum swing back to the present moment (left hemisphere) and reduces the inertial pull of the trauma in the right hemisphere and soma. This can also be done verbally by saying something like "That is what happened back then and this is now" or "Back then it was very hard to breathe, but you can breathe right now." Levine said that whenever there is a trauma, there is also a counter movement of health to organize the life force of the soma. In biodynamic craniosacral therapy terms, there is a stillpoint located in center of the trauma and a fluctuation of movement in the fluid body toward the trauma, followed by a phase of equivalent movement of the fluid body away from the trauma. In biodynamic terms these movements in the fluid body are called lateral fluctuations (and are discussed in later chapters in this section).

It is the role of the practitioner to hold and contain the client between the two poles of the automatic shifting stillpoint in the trauma, whether it is inside or outside the client's soma. Yes, some of these stillpoints centering trauma in the fluid body are outside the skin of the soma. The fluctuating stillpoint is oriented to a midline. Staying within the tempo of Primary Respiration is the trail or bridge between the two. Pendulating between the stillpoint and the fluc-tuating fluid movement of Primary Respiration uncouples the trauma naturally. Simultaneously, by way of resonance, the practitioner helps the client pendulate between the inertia held in the right hemisphere and the therapeutic resources of the left hemisphere. The practitioner helps the client move back and forth across the bridge of the corpus collosum, the anterior commissure, and the posterior commissure surrounding the third ventricle of the brain. This is accomplished by attunement to the movement of Primary Respiration out to the horizon and back and up and down the midline of the soma.

In trauma, sensation in the soma becomes undifferentiated from the emo-tions, behaviors, memories, images, and affect. This causes a loss of coherence between these parts of the self. The practitioner helps to form a bridge of coher-ence for the client and gets the parts to talk to one another via Primary Respira-tion. This includes the skill of reflective dialogue. When the client says that he cannot feel his legs right now, the practitioner might say, "I wonder what part of your body you are sensing?" Then she might ask him to visualize using his legs, like running on the beach or out in nature, or, more preferable, coach the client to disappear the structure in his legs and imagine that the legs are filled with living ocean water and help him feel the tide moving through the legs. When one part of the self is not working too well, another part will be operational. These parts are preexisting in the self, according to Richard Schwartz (Schwartz, 1987). Each part is its own metabolic field, so to speak, and considered a whole unto itself. The unified self as the enduring perception of Primary Respiration goes underground in trauma and the protective parts of the self become apparent as shaping in the fluid body and ignition in the autonomic nervous system of the soma. Integration of the parts is not the goal but, rather, communication, harmony, balance, and self-regulation of the parts are the goals. Just as in the metabolic fields of the embryo, the parts of the self or its affects are already in relationship to one another in their own way.

There really is no such thing as a unified personality anyway—only the interchange between Primary Respiration and its fulcrum of stillness. "Parts is parts," as the old fried-chicken commercial said. Each part needs to be taken seriously because the boundaries between them from trauma are considerable. Without this dissociation and fragmentation, the client cannot access the feeling realization of a fluid body under the guidance of Primary Respiration and thus transform fragmentation into its natural instinctual state.

Slowing Down as a Resource

Slowing the therapeutic process is based upon the neurological model presented throughout this text and Volume One. The right hemisphere, as I've said, stores shock and trauma memories and it is very fast acting. The left hemisphere is slow acting and has decreased metabolic activity from shock and trauma. Shock and trauma cause the brain and soma to speed up because of the high volume of excitatory neurochemicals throughout the system and the evolutionary demand to move quickly to avoid death. This triggers the fight-or-flight response initially and it happens rapidly, well below conscious awareness. When stress hormones become chronically activated because of shock and trauma, feelings of confusion resulting from a disconnected left hemisphere occur constantly. This creates a fertile ground to become sensitized to experiencing overwhelm more frequently.

Telling the client something like "Let's slow down and take a breath" is especially helpful if the client perceives he is losing control of his breathing. The practitioner simply places a hand on the client's lower rib cage around the costal arch and coaches him to slow his breathing or to take longer, easier breaths. Slowing the process can also mean taking a break during the treatment, or getting a drink of water and just waiting for the client to take two or three breaths. This allows the nervous system to settle and integrate. Removing the practitioner's hands from a client is equally as therapeutic and healing as having them on the client. This level of attunement to approach and withdrawal of the hands is an exquisite biodynamic skill.

Another important aspect of slowing down is the ability of the practitioner to synchronize and sustain attention on Primary Respiration. This is the natural tempo of sentient behavior and an effect of an unencumbered autonomic nervous system. It moves freely from the horizon to the midline of the soma and back in rhythmic periods of fifty seconds. It does not hold trauma, yet it heals trauma. It does not change in relationship to autonomic nervous system activation, yet it can regulate the autonomics at the level of the fluid body. It sees autonomic activation as a normal ignition process. It is undiminished as it passes through the soma, giving normal shape and form to the fluid body through the activity of the metabolic fields of the embryo in the adult. This is the essential factor in healing trauma and that is the capacity of the practitioner to be in the tempo of Primary Respiration and accessing the life forces of the fluid body of the client to his ability to respond to the directions of Primary Respiration.

Titration

In a biodynamic craniosacral therapy practice, where it would not be unusual for the touch to be continuous for 10–15 minutes, the function of titration involves the quality of buoyancy of the hand contact on the client, as well as the ability of the practitioner to move her attention to the horizon with Primary Respiration. Thus, the function of titration is linked to the practitioner's witness skills and her ability to go to the horizon with Primary Respiration or into the earth and ocean with Primary Respiration or make contact heart to heart with a spiritual principle in the tempo of Primary Respiration.

Titration is further facilitated by a perceptual shift in the practitioner from rational thinking to meditative thinking, or, as Carl Jung said, "from reality thinking to dream thinking." It is within the meditative mind that the practitioner enters a space of unknowing or a clearing of the fixation to cognition and rational thought. This is followed by the arising of discriminating awareness and skillful means, which are two critical components of clarity and compassion. It is the awakening of an instinctual healing intelligence. These are the tools of the meditative mind and bridge the practitioner into the world of shamanism, which is trans-sensory experience. This is the ecstatic experience of dissociation and fragmentation.

Stillness

The embryo loves stillness because that is how it orients its development, first to fluid stillness and then to tissue stillness. This means that first there is an orientation to stillness inside the embryo and later in development to a stillness outside the embryo. Then the fulcrum of the stillness is able to automatically shift in and out of the body throughout the lifespan.

The brain loves stillness. Ask any baby. In biodynamic craniosacral therapy, the forces of creation arise from the Dynamic Stillness living at the horizon of the embryo or the natural world of the adult. Whenever the soma experiences shock and trauma, parts of the fluid body revert back to its basic nature, which is stillness. It is in this state of stillness that the forces of creation reside and trauma is held until Primary Respiration restarts the fluid body in right relationship to the midline of the soma. The practitioner waits for points of balanced stillness to occur in the therapeutic process, just as they did in the embryo. She sits in that silence and stillness, expanding her witness consciousness to include the therapeutic dyad, the office space, and the visible and invisible space outside the office walls and in to nature. This could be called waiting for the whole to connect with the totality. It is yet another quality of the ability to be a still witness free of conceptualizations and dualities.

A stillpoint is a localized quieting of either the tissues, membranes, fluid compartments, the fluid body, or a systemic quieting of them all together at once. The practitioner is waiting for a systemic stillpoint. The systemic stillpoint may expand to fill the room and the space outside to the horizon. Dr. Sutherland said that this kind of stillpoint is a most precious event. Within most stillpoints, the fluid body is able to shift automatically and reorient to the original midline of the embryo either in the spine, the heart, the third ventricle, or the umbilicus. A stillpoint may also be a window or threshold into deeper states of stillness. Thus stillpoints are hugely therapeutic and a central distinguishing feature of the biodynamic process of health and healing.

Intention

When a practitioner gets involved with trauma resolution work, it is exceedingly important to know what the client's intention is for the session. It must be clearly stated by the client and accurately reflected back to him by the practitioner, prior to beginning a session. The practitioner is obligated to inform the client if she does not feel that she can align with the client's intention (see Appendix A). Thus, the intention is negotiable. Let's say that a client wants his life and his relationships to improve. While that is a good intention, it is quite large. So the practitioner might say, "Well, that's a lot more than we might be able to do in this session. Why don't we see if there's something more specific we could work with in this session"?

Having a clearly stated and realistic intention at the beginning gives the practitioner a reference point that can be accessed anytime during the session with the client. The practitioner can remind the client of his intention or point out if the intention needs to be modified or amended during the session. Such an intention allows the therapeutic interaction with shock and trauma to stay in present time through verbal checking at various points in the session, if necessary. It is an essential organizational tool for the practitioner, especially since deeply held trauma can be contagious in a way that causes the practitioner to lose her identification in the session. I might also ask the client: "How would you know if you achieved your intention? What would that feel like in your body?"

Ignition

Relating to trauma at any level is considered to be a biodynamic ignition process. The essential skill in such a relationship is for the practitioner to maintain a sense of the stillness at the core of her midline. Witness consciousness is of the utmost importance when working with held trauma in the client's soma and fluid body. Because trauma can resonate with the practitioner, the practitioner must be able to witness her own process and that of the client with non-attachment and equanimity. The client has lost the ability to orient to the stillness or the sleeve of Primary Respiration around the stillness. This is sometimes called soul death or a heart in shutdown. Dr. Becker said, "The treatment does not begin until the will of the patient yields to the will of Primary Respiration."

The will of the patient is coupled to the autonomic nervous system (ANS) and its capacity to achieve equilibrium after a change process. When the ANS settles it may be possible to go through the process of a wholistic shift, since the wholistic shift is one of several interfaces between the soma and the therapeutic processes of the fluid body. Since the level of disturbance in the autonomic nervous systems of many clients is profound, it may not be possible to experience the wholistic shift. This is why in the final evaluation the practitioner can only rely upon the tide of Primary Respiration and its fulcrum of stillness.

The healing priorities of Primary Respiration are only known by themselves. It is up to the practitioner to synchronize with these priorities without grossly or even subtly interfering with Primary Respiration by overly focusing on fluid body imprinting. Primary Respiration is the mind and brain of the fluid body, as I have mentioned frequently. Let Primary Respiration guide you to the primary site in the fluid body.

Love

I frequently say the word *love* nonverbally as I am treating a client. I'll make up a sentence with the word love in it and use it as a mantra, such as "I am loved, you are loved, we are loved." This has a powerful influence on a client's well-being. I breathe love in between my heart and the client's heart at the rate of Primary Respiration. Make love real as a felt sense of warmth and heat rather than a concept. Try a little love in your next session.

CHAPTER 13

Going to the Void

Disassociation from the mundane world marks the entrance to the bio-dynamic therapeutic relationship. It is crossing a threshold into a very different world of experience. That is the world of shamanic healing where the presence of a benevolent intelligence as a force of nature is perceived by the practitioner to enter the office and participate in the physical contact with the client. James Jealous calls this the "other pair of hands" (Jealous, 1998) and Dr. Sutherland (Sutherland, 1998, 2002) called it the presence of the "Other."

The stillpoint, which is defined by Dr. Becker as the starting point for a session, must alternatively be viewed as a dissociative experience in which a gate to extra-sensory perception or subtle perception is opened. I noticed this quite by accident when I was teaching a cranial class some years ago and doing a demonstration of a cranial handhold. I suddenly noticed that I subtly fixed my gaze on an object in the room. In this case I was simply gazing at a student's shoe and spacing out in order to become still. I was actually putting myself into a light trance, and I was startled by this discovery because I became aware that I had always been doing it. I could not wait to get back to my office and see if this is what I did with my clients. Sure enough, I was always putting myself into a light trance and continue to do so before and even during a session.

Now I teach that every session begins with the practitioner establishing a stillpoint in herself, just as Dr. Becker taught. The practitioner must enter the world of spirit and leave the world of the mundane behind. The following is a practice that I teach that establishes a stillpoint as a beginning phase of a session. I call it *resting in the void.*

Resting in the Void

This is a meditation I do as I am preparing to make contact with the client. I like to do this as often as I need to during the session in order to establish a deeper and more profound stillpoint in the session.

Establish a comfortable seated position in preparation for making contact with the client. With your eyes open or closed, get in touch with the quality of your thoracic exhalation. Just notice the exhalation of air from your lungs with a little bit more attention than the inhale. This is not a manipulation of the diaphragm or a breathing technique. It is simply an observation of biological breathing with a slight focus on exhalation and noticing the small gap or stillpoint at the end of the exhalation before the next breath automatically comes in. There is a small biological stillpoint at the end of exhalation and helps to settle the mind by placing attention on that single moment of transitional stillness that is constantly repeated thousands of times each day.

Gradually, begin to disappear all the structure of your body, just as we did in Chapter 4, while guiding the client through much the same process. Start with all the bones, from the top of the head down to the bottom of the feet. Then disappear all the muscles of the body, starting from the top of the head down to the bottom of the feet. Then disappear all of the organs of the body, starting with the brain all the way down to the pelvic floor.

Now disappear all the fluid in your body and even your skin, so that your body actually no longer exists. Visualize empty space where you are sitting. Imagine that this was the time several seconds before your egg differentiated and that first cell of your body came into being. This happened when your mother was a five-week-old embryo herself. Imagine that your mother was a five-week-old embryo barely the size of a lentil and there was a moment of nonexistence. You did not in any way physically exist. Your egg that differentiated and then was fertilized by a single sperm from your father, and then developed into your body as it is now, first became something from nothing. Be that nothing. Take yourself back to that time through your life and then your mother's whole life and her time in her mother's womb. Take yourself back to that void when you have no body, but yet you were a potential contained in your mother's tiny womb within the womb of your grandmother and her womb being contained within the womb of the Great Mother Earth and Ocean.

Now disappear all of your personal belongings as though they never existed as well. If you are married and have a family, disappear them for the time being. Your nonexistence and their nonexistence are possible because none of it is present several seconds before the egg you developed from was brought into being when your mother herself was an embryo. Imagine your complete nonexistence as the state of stillness and space between every atom of your body extending out to the horizon and beyond. While contemplating this possibility, maintain contact with thoracic exhalation regularly. The empty space that you are has a reciprocal movement that is invisible. The respiratory diaphragm is a great wave-making machine in the ocean of empty space.

Now disappear the client. Imagine his body does not even exist. Imagine the time several seconds before the egg that the client developed from actually came into being. Make sure to disappear his body, his clothes, his problems, his symptoms, his family, even his car. Every single part of the client does not exist. This state of nonexistence present several seconds before his egg differentiated is carried forward as the Dynamic Stillness in the space between every atom of his body. Space is stillness. His empty space and your empty space intermingle. All is void and dreamlike.

Pay attention to your thoughts in your nonexistent body. Imagine that your thoughts also do not exist because of the way they arise from nowhere and dissipate and go nowhere. Just as with your body and personal possessions, the client's body and personal possessions, your thoughts also have no valid existence regardless of how spiritual or pornographic they are. They are all the same and do not exist. They are a mirage or a dream. Keep going to the void if your thoughts get hold of you and feel real.

Now listen to the silence in the room. Listen to the sound of the stillpoint in the room and see if it extends out into nature. Be facing a window in your office if possible and fix your gaze on a tree or a cloud and let yourself disappear into the tree and the cloud. Every part of nature out the window is a stillpoint also and does not exist either. Go into the cloud and into the tree and feel the stillpoint. Completely allow yourself to rest in this stillpoint until Primary Respiration really gets your attention. Repeat this sequence as necessary in order to establish the deep stillpoint that Dr. Sutherland spoke so fervently about. This is a deliberate and precise exercise in dissociating from the things of the world and contemporary society. Go to the void to create sacred space.

Postscript: A team of astronomers from the University of Minnesota recently discovered an expanse of 6 billion trillion miles of emptiness in the universe (Chown, 2007). The cosmic blank spot has no stars, no galaxies, no black holes, and no mysterious dark matter. It was called an atypical void and bigger than scientists could ever imagine. Go to the void.

CHAPTER 14

The Containment Principle

The process of personal integration is one of containment, not of elimination. … To integrate is to contain comfortably both ends of the spectrum of change. For example, we will become authentic in our self-presentation and at the same time we will still occasionally dissemble. Integration is not total anything; it is simply a rearranging of the proportions of life. Now we are more open and less guarded but both styles still appear in our overall behavior. (Richie, 1996, p. 89)

A core principle in biodynamic craniosacral therapy is *containment*. The practitioner silently holds the client with nonverbal and occasional verbal contact in order for deeply held imprinting to automatically shift under the direction of Primary Respiration. When deep shock imprinting can be accessed slowly and the client held in her totality with the love of Primary Respiration in the heart of the practitioner, then trauma can be slowly examined, understood, repatterned, and differentiated in the therapeutic relationship. The trauma can go into a state of suspension and be moved by Primary Respiration. Thus, Primary Respiration becomes the container that holds the client in her wholeness.

Containment is the basis of self-regulation. This means that when gradients of disproportion and density in the fluid body are contacted, the practitioner is free from any intention to release a particular charge, tone, or shape. Instead, the intention is to restore the relationship of the fluid body to the tidal body of Primary Respiration. In this way the midline of the fluid body can transmute the sensation of the life force in the fluid body as healthy and resourcing rather than stagnate and fractured, as one osteopath names it. This calls forth the client's lost ability to self-regulate her autonomic nervous system. Primary Respiration and its fulcrum of stillness manage the container for a healing process to be revealed. In other words, therapeutic contact with the client's Primary Respiratory System is done in small, incremental, manageable units at the tempo of Primary

Respiration. This allows the whole nervous system to integrate and heal compressed experience at its own pace. Frozen and dissociated densities of experience held in the fluid body are allowed to permeate, spread, circulate, fluctuate, and disengage frequently without the rapid discharge or tissue unwinding commonly employed in many release-based cathartic therapies. The client is given the correct amount of resistance from the practitioner to fortify the container of self-regulation for internal transmutation, but not too much so as to merely dissipate the emotional charge without effective transmutation and self-regulation.

Since this containment principle is especially suited for working with dissociation, verbal skills are frequently needed. The initial focus of the verbal interaction is to establish an orientation to present time. When a client is in an activated autonomic state, I might mention how I enjoy looking at the color of the client's shirt or repeat what she said to make sure I heard her accurately. What I am attempting to do is accurately reflect or mirror for the client what's happening for her now, so that she feels heard and held in safety. It is the left hemisphere that monitors present time, uses language, and tries to make sense of the external world of which I, as the practitioner, am a part. Some clients with shock affect are living in the right hemisphere, with a diminished connection to the left. Thus, the practitioner plays the role of the client's left hemisphere, until a time when the client is able to integrate both hemispheres herself. On the other hand, some clients with shock affect have so suppressed the memory of intense emotion in the right hemisphere that they use their left hemisphere exclusively and quite effectively by developing the skills of thinking and cognition. Here the practitioner might focus on the right-hemisphere skills, involving the client in choosing comfortable hand positions and soliciting the comfort and ease of the client verbally from time to time.

Containment also involves a set of nonverbal skills. The practitioner forms a receptive container for the client in his heart. The practitioner *holds* the totality of the client's past, present, and future together in the present moment. I like to teach my students to breathe in the client's pain and suffering directly into their heart and breathe out loving kindness and compassion to the client at the tempo of Primary Respiration with a bright color, especially red. It is much like a spiritual blood transfusion. The practitioner holds the container nonverbally, thus guarding it and protecting it in the stillness of his heart. This function of protection is an act of contemplation that includes maintaining an awareness of the midline of the practitioner and the client and the office space. The practitioner mediates the boundaries of the outside world with the inside world of the healing relationship.

Then the practitioner begins to immerse himself in thinking about the story of the client's shock dynamics. The practitioner holds the client's history non-verbally in his thoughts by repeating and elaborating the client's story with a felt sense of the story in the heart. This contemplation occurs before, during, and after the treatment. This creates a healing resonance between the conjunct nervous systems of the client and the practitioner. These are contemplative skills and are the foundation of healing in the containment principle.

The client must be given permission to *not* dive into the trauma memories or to relive them. What is known from clinical data is that the activation of the entire trauma schema may in fact retraumatize the client (van der Kolk, 1996). It is important to avoid inviting clients into prematurely revealing their trauma memories. On the other hand, some clients will leap to divulge their entire history. Perhaps they feel it is necessary because they have seen thirty other health care providers and believe that the practitioner wants them to do so. In this case, it is important to stop or slow down the story. Simple verbal interventions like, "Wow, that's a lot of information; let's slow this down and see what's important," followed by an explanation of the importance of titration and pacing are very effective. Therefore, it is important to only work with small pieces of the trauma at one time and in one session. Perhaps that one small piece needs to be worked exclusively over multiple sessions following the priorities of Primary Respiration.

This is an aspect of the containment model. First, the outer layer of trauma needs to be held in relationship until it is integrated with appropriate resources and across the hemispheres of the brain and systemically through the life forces of the fluid body. The client already lives at the center of her shock and needs to be shown the doorway out of it, back to the edge of the experience where she can actually pay attention without activation and self-regulate on her own. It is the edge of experience where the witness is reborn and transmutation takes place. The edge is a fundamental resource where the client can take control and witness her experience. This requires that the competently trained practitioner be willing to work with only small pieces of the trauma schema in any given session. Doing so helps to rebuild the proper sequencing of events that may be missing in the client's dilemma and also helps to avoid states of overwhelm. As I've said, trauma typically decreases metabolic activity in the left hemisphere. Along with monitoring present time, the left hemisphere is the logician of the brain and seeks order through the sequencing of life events. It requires discipline to avoid irritating the client's autonomic nervous system, which is what some release-based cathartic therapies tend to do. If a client starts to remember another part of the trauma schema, I will say: "Why don't we wait until the next session to work on that? I think you have enough on your plate right now," or "We have all the time in the world. Let's let this piece settle before we go on." It is time to resynchronize with Primary Respiration.

Only one layer of shock and trauma is elaborated and related with at any given time and with deliberate slowness. Biodynamic craniosacral therapy is slow therapy. The practitioner must move slowly to integrate the left hemisphere with the right, and the brain with the body and viscera. Touch and boundaries are constantly renegotiated, in order to avoid retraumatization of the client. The practitioner becomes a skilled observer of all the affects and nuances of activation at the edge of the client's nervous system and the fluid continuum of the body. It is the skill of staying at the edge that allows the client to self-regulate and helps her to develop an unbiased witness in the brain and heart, which is forgotten in trauma. The practitioner is merely listening to the client's story, as it is told through the fluids. At the same time the practitioner is listening to the inherent health of Primary Respiration as it moves the disturbance in the fluids, comes down to its fulcrum in the stillness, and automatically shifts the trauma of its choice. This builds the life forces in the fluid body, reconnects the two hemispheres of the brain, and creates a felt sense of wholeness in the soma of the client. The practitioner merely witnesses the activity of Primary Respiration and does not have to direct it.

In this regard, it is important for the practitioner to be able to evaluate how ready or prepared a client is to move through her shock and trauma issues. Criteria to look at include:

- The client's capacity for fluid awareness. Can her attention be directed to the inside ocean or outside in the sea around her?

- The client's capacity for containment (the inner ability to down-regulate strong emotions).

- The client's ability to maintain boundaries by not moving prematurely into deeper issues without the direction of Primary Respiration.

- The embryonic age from which the client is functioning. In other words, what stage of morphology represents the compression the client is holding?

- The conscious availability of the client's witness self. Has she formed a relationship between the situation and an internal, unbiased observer or stillpoint?

- The client's capacity for seeing irony and laughing at herself. Does the client have a sense of humor? Otherwise, it is a lot of hard work for the practitioner.

The containment principle was a value system used in pre-modern cultures for much the same purpose that a biodynamic craniosacral practitioner would incorporate it today. Shamanic healers recognized the need for the wild forces of adolescence and infantile narcissism to be harnessed, so chaos would not take over their society (such as what is occurring now in different parts of the world). The entire last section of this book is dedicated to shamanic healing. Containment of these wild forces occurred through an initiatory process that required a ritual container—a sacred space with an organizing midline—where power was rerouted back to its spiritual origin. This caused a symbolic reconception into a right relationship with the human, divine, and natural worlds. The container was held by a ritual leader who provided the participant with a rigorous initiation of how to channel and transmute the devastation of disease, anxiety, depression, and so forth. Much of contemporary shock and trauma is desacralized and devoid of a spiritual ground. In traditional cultures, the person had a premature initiatory experience of the raw power (misused) of the world and therefore it was uncontained. Thus the practitioner must build and manage a container with the skills mentioned to transmute and sacralize the client's experience.

There are several qualities necessary for the contemporary practitioner to develop in the skill of containment. The first of these is a *witness consciousness,* mentioned in a previous chapter. This is the ability to attune consciously to autonomic nervous system cycles of activation and settling, while being non-attached and nonjudgmental. How does one relate to unregulated states in the autonomic nervous system with equanimity? Developing a witness self allows fight-or-flight physiology to transform itself into useful therapeutic outcomes such as better self-regulation of emotions and greater empathy for one's personal dilemma. The witness looks at the larger pattern in the fabric of life without interpretation. The witness watches from the midline of stillness. Habitual physical and or emotional patterns are given enough space to naturally settle without collapse or exacerbation of its charge. This gives the brain and soma the ability to retain the potency of the energy, transform it, and use it to communicate with the other parts of the self that are lost in the affect of shock and trauma. This allows more dynamic choices in life.

Attunement is an important quality of the witness self. The therapist's attention is placed alternately on his own and the client's physical feelings, sensations, thoughts, memories, images, and body patterns buoyantly, like seaweed floating on the ocean or a feather on the breath of God. This type of attunement is extremely light and delicate, and moves slowly, at the rate of Primary Respiration back and forth between practitioner and client. Attunement also involves the ability to stay in present time. Staying in present time is an essential skill for healing. There is a little Timex watch in the left side of the prefrontal cortex and it definitely stops ticking in trauma. It is a function of the left hemisphere of the brain that is short-circuited during trauma and shock. Attunement is related to sequencing, another faculty of the left hemisphere. Traumatic stress interferes with the slow pacing of experience necessary for left hemisphere integration of the entire sequence of events that the client is accessing in the right hemisphere. Typically, shock and trauma leave big gaps in a person's memory, and these may need to be filled in for the client to make meaning of her experience. Proper containment in a session allows the client to attune to the sequence of events one at a time and put them back into the correct configuration as though completing a jigsaw puzzle.

Often a client will report gaps in her memory of traumatic events. Yet these gaps are imprinted in the nonverbal, sensory memory of the right hemisphere and the soma as a whole. They are below conscious awareness, and the job of the practitioner is to attune to his own sensory experience and alternate attention back to the client through occasional verbal interaction. If a client is experiencing an emotion, I must decide if I should say something or not. Frequently I do not. If I do, I may ask: "What is the sensation of the emotion you are having?" and "Where is it located in your body now?" Permission to contact the client at the beginning of the session must also be verbally negotiated. "Are you comfortable if I make contact right now?" is an example of something I would say to the client. Even removing your hands at the end of the session requires some verbal permission. "Is this a good time to remove my hands?" is something I frequently say to clients. Together, the verbal interaction, slowing the sequence of events, and focusing attention in present time represent some of the attunement skills that are necessary to contain and then reinhabit both hemispheres of the brain for self-regulation to occur.

The more life force a client can appropriately contain in her fluid body and soma, the more she is able to access freedom, self-regulation, and creativity as a natural instinctual process. This is attunement to the natural world. This allows life to unfold its original embryonic pattern and restores the lost freedom of a continuous unfolding of the human heart. This principle of containment requires the practitioner to develop another important skill, which is to hold both the trauma history and the forgotten but preexisting health of the client simultaneously. This is called the *holding function* in biodynamic craniosacral therapy. It requires the practitioner to expand his own container to hold the polarities of the client's pain and suffering as well as the client's intrinsic capacity and potential for health and healing through Primary Respiration.

Holding the client's totality and attunement to the polarities of life and death that are continually dancing in the client are crucial when contacting disorganized states in the client's nervous system such as non-normal dissociation. Equally important biodynamic containment skills are attunement to the horizon and back and establishing a stillpoint in the office. These skills also lead to more effective self-regulation and differentiation. Gradually, the client begins to build coherence between these qualities of containment inherent in her own nervous system and can disengage from the soma into the life forces of the fluid body. This is a reassociation to fluid sense, fluid image and fluid shape as the fundamental resource, which is the core of the biodynamic geography. It is fluid sensation that is at the heart of all feelings, emotions, and perception in the soma. Sensations are islands of experience mediated by the fluid compartments of the soma. As fluid experience they are designed to flow and move, to swell and recede. They are the soma's primary language. Fluid sensations are the link relating physical states of being, posture, and gesture to the psyche and to the divine. They are the voice of the Breath of Life. It is the responsibility of the practitioner to maintain regular contact and awareness of his own sensations as part of the holding function of the therapeutic container. This includes cueing the client to tune into the fluids in her body, as discussed in the first section of this book. I will often suggest images like a river, a lake, or the ocean for clients to contemplate. This greatly facilitates the practitioner's ability to synchronize with Primary Respiration in the client. It is important to help the client get out of her nervous system so it can be supported and resourced by the fluids from which it came into being.

Formerly, the practitioner maintained the role of the ritual leader to bring order and spiritual integration to the culture. This gave society the ability to maintain stewardship of the earth benevolently and justly. Ultimately, that is also the goal of containment in biodynamic craniosacral therapy—to bring order to the body-mind system, to come into a right relationship with the natural world within the loving container of Primary Respiration, and to form a loving and ordered relationship with the numinous experience of life via an organizing midline.

Finally, it must be said that this is the most important aspect of the containment model. It is the midline. The container must have a sacred midline for the forces of the divine to manifest their inherent order and love in the client.

The forces of healing and the creation of wholeness via Primary Respiration and stillness become available at every moment in a person's life in a safe container. This is the container of a still heart.

To review, there are six basic components of the containment model:

- The capacity of the therapist to hold strong polarities present in the therapeutic relationship

- The capacity to create sacred space, defined as having an organizing midline of stillness

- The ability to witness the trauma story with equanimity

- The skill to stay in the present time

- The recognition of a stillpoint and its value

- The capacity of the therapist to sense his or her heart and body

CHAPTER 15

The Fluid Body, Soma, and the Brain

Longitudinal Fluctuation

The fluid body permeates the soma, breathing the physical body as a condensation of the tidal body. This ignites the longitudinal fluctuation of the fluid body from the coccyx up to the brain. Two basic qualities describe this directional flow. First, it has a fluid drive, and second, it has lateral fluctuations. The inner resources of the unified fluid field contain a bioelectric magnetic (BEM) force and a drive or potency carried in and around the cerebrospinal fluid. Dr. Sutherland called it the "direct current." It moves precisely up from the coccyx for 12–15 seconds and when it intersects with Sutherland's fulcrum it cascades out and around the body for another 12–15 seconds before coalescing again at the coccyx. This cascade creates a kind of outer skin for the fluid body. It is like a permeable membrane 10–15 inches off of the skin and completely surrounding the physical body.

The fluid midline with its longitudinal fluctuation is exceedingly important because they ignite the embodying function of mesoderm in the third week of embryonic development. As the embryo turns in relationship to its connecting stalk (at its caudal end), the fluid pressure in the amniotic cavity increases in a longitudinal direction on a caudal-to-cranial axis. The amnion begins a central spiraling movement along this fluid axis. This creates a kind of rip current, which is a strong flow. This vertical flow rises from the cloacal membrane (future anus) and travels up and through the plate of the ectoderm. It is this rip current that initiates the arising of the primitive streak and notochord. Mesoderm floods the space between the ectoderm and endoderm, creating the lateral canals that will eventually form the heart. The future matrix for the musculoskeletal system now forms the middle of the embryo and will give rise to the connective tissue structures of blood, bone, ligaments, tendons, and muscles.

Thus the fluid drive of the longitudinal fluctuation is of critical importance in embryonic growth, development, health, and healing.

Lateral Fluctuations

The vertical fluid drive of the longitudinal fluctuation transduces itself into a horizontal movement called lateral fluctuations. This is the second aspect of the longitudinal fluctuation. The embryonic laws of the fluids, as stated by Erich Blechschmidt and Raymond Gasser (Blechschmidt and Gasser, 1978), clearly say that fluids move vertically and perpendicular to limiting membranes. This is sensed as a horizontal movement perpendicular to the longitudinal fluctuation, anywhere from the coccyx up to the top of the head but especially in the cranium. In the palpation of the lateral fluctuations, the fluids may appear chaotic or speedy, due to traumatic experiences.

The dilemma of contemporary clients is a diminishment of their longitudinal fluctuation, which effects compensations in the lateral movements. Rapid or irregular lateral fluctuations are a systems response for the loss of whole-body orientation. The lack of orientation and vitality within the fluid drive may develop into metabolic problems in the subcompartments of the soma such as the blood and lymph. Inflammatory neuro-immune chemicals are now a major cause of many illnesses because the immune system is overactive and a part of the fluid body has become very toxic with chronic inflammatory processes. Speed is the underlying problem.

Aberrant lateral fluctuations within the cranium may arise as a figure-eight motion, fast single vectors of movement, rapid reciprocal oscillations in the fluid body, or other expressions of a system seeking balance. The practitioner's intervention, however, is initially the same. It is through an orientation to stillness that the therapeutic process can be initiated. Whenever the practitioner senses fast movement, he moves his perception away from it and locates a stillpoint somewhere outside the body, within the treatment room or out in nature. Often, the practitioner may sense the cessation or deceleration of movement in the fluid body as a state of balanced stillness becomes manifest. This frequently means that the center of an inertial fulcrum has been found and this particular stillness ignites the felt experience of the therapeutic force of Primary Respiration. The resolution of inertial or traumatic fulcrums, then, is the result of Primary Respiration expressing itself as the fluid body and related tissue and physiological systems return to a state of balanced stillness. Potency within the tide of Primary Respiration automatically shifts the held compensation back into a right relationship with the midline.

Stillpointing the Fluid Body

There are two ways in which a biodynamic craniosacral practitioner can attend to the stress held within the fluid body in a way that makes possible transmutation rather than traumatic reenactment. The first lies in working with the stillness and its relationship with the longitudinal fluctuation of the fluid body. When trauma occurs, it creates inertial phenomena—a decrease in normal movement, tissue-fluid density, or improper heat distribution in both the fluid and physical body. Just prior to the trauma, the fluid body briefly experiences a systemic stillpoint. At the center of the trauma, stillness also functions to organize the chaos of the traumatic event. Heat is trapped in the inertial fulcrum. Thus both types of stillness are present in the fluid body holding condensations of stress.

Orienting to the presence of this systemic stillness around the client's body is the second key in relating with trauma in biodynamic craniosacral therapy. Thus the practitioner orients to both a systemic stillpoint in the fluid body and, since the fluid body extends beyond the skin of the soma, the practitioner also orients to a stillpoint outside the soma. This is done by the practitioner gently placing both hands under the lower thoracic and upper lumbar vertebrae. The area around this junction in the spine is the fulcrum for the entire fluid body. It may automatically shift down to the second and third lumbar vertebra, in which case the practitioner lowers his hands to that area. The practitioner waits for the reciprocal tension potency (RTP) of the fluid body to stillpoint and notices whether it occurs at the end of its inhalation phase or exhalation phase. This is called a fluid body CV4 (exhalation) or EV4 (inhalation). The RTP usually inhales for thirty seconds and exhales for thirty seconds. Concurrently, heat is usually released from the inertial fulcrum and may likely be perceived in the practitioner's own fluid body and soma.

Therapeutic Focus

While gently cradling the client's cranium, it is important that the practitioner evaluate the motions of the following tissue structures and therapeutic rates:

- The transverse widening and narrowing of the cerebellum within the slow rate of the fluid body

- The transverse widening and narrowing of the tentorium within the slow rate of the fluid body

- The transverse widening and narrowing of the lateral angles of the occiput within the slow rate of the fluid body

- The intraosseous motion of the occiput (intraosseous motion of each bone is a fundamental perceptual skill in biodynamics) within the slow rate of the fluid body

- The shape and form of the fourth ventricle in relationship to the brain stem and cerebellum

- The perceived quality of fluid drive (vertical) versus the reciprocal tension potency (horizontal RTP) or lateral fluctuations in the fourth ventricle

- The capacity of the RTP to stillpoint in the fourth ventricle

- The transverse widening and narrowing of Primary Respiration across the cranium

The CV4 or EV4 is a preference toward a direction-of-ease, either toward inhalation or exhalation at 1–3 cycles per minute (CPM) in the fluid body. The tempo of the practitioner's physical contact and state of mind is ideally always within Primary Respiration or stillness. A CV4 (exhalation stillpoint) clarifies and strengthens the midline of the fluid body. An EV4 (inhalation stillpoint) helps distribute the RTP away from the midline and throughout the fluid body.

When oriented to stillness and Primary Respiration, the biodynamic practitioner supports the amplitude of the longitudinal fluctuation and full lateral expression, as well as the balance of the fluid body as it interfaces with both the nervous system and connective tissues of the soma. By settling into stillness and synchronizing with the therapeutic force of Primary Respiration, the practitioner is able to distance himself from the erratic and compensatory function of the Cranial Rhythmic Impulses—these quicker rhythms are linked to stress levels in the autonomic nervous system (McPartland, 1997). In this way, clients remain resourced and the fluid body can automatically shift in stillness and at the tempo of Primary Respiration.

While the nature of the Cranial Rhythmic Impulses is compensatory, the longitudinal fluctuation and its expression of the RTP systemically are some of the deep formative forces in the fluid fields of the embryo. These aspects of the fluid body infuse every cell in the body with heat, which is the felt sense of self-healing and self-correction as the heat permeates and warms the body with a sense of animation, grace, and at times, awe. They are all aspects of the body's innate self-healing system. Therefore, when a practitioner encounters inertial states in the client's fluid body and soma, there are at least two healing vectors that can be tracked. One is through synchronizing with stillness. The other is through Primary Respiration. The starting place is rarely in the activity of the fluid body until the movement of the whole via Primary Respiration has been established and a stillpoint has been located and can be referenced. This allows the heat distribution function of the RTP to not burn out. In this sense, Primary Respiration acts as a catalytic converter for the heat to be maintained at a temperature and speed that can be integrated throughout the soma.

The Soma

I would like to talk about the soft tissue of the soma since many biodynamic practitioners are trained in soft tissue therapy. The myofascial system of the soma unwinds as a secondary process. It reorganizes itself metabolically to the movement of the whole, which is Primary Respiration. Tissues and their cells are in a constant process of transmutation—changing from one state to another. The tissues of the body are in a process of continual metabolic renewal. Death and rebirth happen every second within the soma. The chains of amino acids, which make up the protein structure of fascia, are always breaking off, rebinding, and reconnecting with other chains. The body is in a nonstop process of adapting to an infinite variety of stresses from both inside and out. It is constantly reshaping itself dynamically and creatively under the catalytic function of Primary Respiration and the fluid body.

Synchronization with the movement of the whole, followed by the reestablishment of the longitudinal fluctuation in the fluid body, precedes the decompression of the mechanism of trauma in the myofascial system. This is an appropriate sequence for treatment. The client can then be skillfully guided back to an embodied sense of her midline. The client must have both personal and metabolic resources operative in her life for trauma to be transmuted biodynamically. Proper diet, nutrition, and elimination must be considered in all chronic conditions because of inflammatory processes in the immune system, intestinal tract, blood, and lymph. The tissues may need to remember an accident back to the beginning, or they may not. How do we know? What is known is the critical importance of turning off inflammatory conditions that are interfering with the normal function of the fluid body.

The biodynamic practitioner listens to the client's midline of stillness and the movement of the whole—Primary Respiration—for direction in supporting the client's healing process. This is the catalyst that will help put out the fire of inflammation. This must occur in an environment free of preconceptions on the part of the practitioner about what the client needs, especially how to "fix" her. The client must be stabilized first with stillness and such things as metabolic dietary support as needed and guided by an appropriate health care provider. Fixing simply is not possible. The fluid body needs the space to slow and shift under the directions of its own connection to the Intelligence of Primary Respiration. Decreasing inflammatory processes allows the fluid body to slow down. Then perhaps a midline of stillness can be reestablished.

It is crucial to start a therapeutic relationship with stillness and wait for the fluid body to invite the practitioner to witness its function; otherwise, the practitioner may induce what one osteopath calls a false fulcrum. If that happens, the practitioner is following his own projection into and through the client. The client's body is instinctually reacting to the practitioner's input, much like an immune system response to a pathogen. Both cause irritation within a client's system. The client may unconsciously withdraw or become retraumatized, which to the unskilled practitioner appears as a state of relaxation or an emotional release. Actually, it is a euphoric dissociative state of shock affect where true healing is thwarted. During these non-normal dissociative states, what seems like a stillpoint is actually a deep state of being withdrawn from the world, which is a preverbal defensive strategy. The seeming stillpoint is flat and numb without dynamism and clarity. It usually feels like the effect of a recreational drug which can also be anesthesia imprinting from birth or surgery. A false fulcrum is often precipitated by a practitioner's contact that is too quick or heavy and full of mechanistic intentions.

What the client's soma may be saying is, *Get away from me!* When the practitioner has a projection around the client's process, such as "What this system really needs is …" or "I have the tools and techniques to fix this," or worse, "I can heal you," that projection will easily go into the client and diminish the freedom and possibility of Primary Respiration. The practitioner ends up tracking his own thoughts and actions within the client. The client's body reflects the practitioner's fixations. It is antithetical to healing. Healing shock and trauma requires the practitioner to remain as a still witness and synchronize with Primary Respiration in himself rather than excavating to find the trauma in the client. The client already lives in the trauma. Healing occurs when the stillness of the fluid body and its relationship with Primary Respiration are accessed and the fluid body is allowed to automatically shift and balance the whole body-mind continuum. It is an inside-out process.

Neurology of Trauma

Within any accident or trauma, no matter how slight, the fight-or-flight physiology of the sympathetic nervous system is activated. The degree of activation-arousal and internalization-withdrawal generate a somatic ignition in an attempt to reach equilibrium.

This process may be linked to several genetic and neuro-endocrine-immune factors, such as the following.

- The autonomic set point in the hypothalamic-pituitary-adrenal (HPA) axis, the hypothalamic-pituitary-thyroid axis, and the hypothalamic-pituitary-gonadal axis that are established pre- and perinatally, as a function of the ability of the mother to help co-metabolize the anxiety and frustration of the embryo, fetus, and child. Likewise, the child metabolizes the mother's stress state through the attachment and bonding process (Schore, 1994).

- Genetic factors that predetermine states of arousal. Prenatal stress states imprint genetic expression, especially around protection and defense for life.

- Immune system regulation that is either speeded up or depressed, causing chronic inflammatory responses systemically in the body. Excessive cortisol production from chronic stress is toxic to the brain and body and causes the immune system to generate inflammatory processes because it thinks the body is about to be overcome with bacteria and it wants to be ready to fight the invasion, which has already arrived and is locked in place.

- Chronic inflammatory processes that cause high-threshold pain receptors (nociceptors) to mutate into low-threshold receptors, which then create pain symptoms everywhere in the body, even in areas of weak links with minimal stimulus.

- The irony of life. Frequently practitioners do not have enough respect for the vicissitudes of life and the seeming randomness of misfortune. It is simply not possible to know what the client is holding and whether it even had a beginning or will have an end. Appreciating the irony of life generates deep compassion.

Trauma fixates at all levels of the brain and is right lateralized, especially in the brain stem, corticolimbic system, the midbrain, and orbitofrontal cortex (Schore, 2001b). The corticolimbic system is the emotional brain and it contains the amygdala (the fear center), the hypothalamus (responsible for fighting,

fleeing, fornicating, and feeding), the locus ceruleus in the reticular formation of the brain stem (which secretes the chief neurochemicals driving the
sympathetic system), and the orbitofrontal cortex (responsible for emotional
self-regulation and "reading" the context of physical touch as either nurturing
or not). These are all co-regulators of the autonomic nervous system. The locus
ceruleus has been linked strongly to the neurobiology of shock and trauma
(Perry and Pollard, 1998). The human central nervous system, however, is a
unit of function. It must be viewed as a part of a whole.

Trauma is stored in the right hemisphere (please refer to Volume One for
a discussion of the right hemisphere) and the fluid body systemically. It is a
simultaneous event across body platforms, so to speak. Trauma short-circuits
the orbitofrontal cortex (thinking brain), from the limbic midbrain (emotional
brain), cuts off access to the left hemisphere, and overstimulates the brain stem
(action brain). It compresses the midline of the fluid body. Trauma produces
shock affects, such as flooding emotions, withdrawal from reality, and stress-
induced analgesia, which is linked to non-normal dissociation (van der Kolk,
1996). These are all biodynamic ignitions that are stabilizing the system and
under the guidance of Primary Respiration and stillness.

The orbitofrontal cortex is where conscious self-regulation of emotions
occurs, as well as organized conscious responses to stress and pain. The orbitofrontal cortex is where we pay attention to reality. These conscious responses
are often lost in shock trauma. The inner world of hyperarousal, withdrawal,
fragmentation, and non-normal dissociation replaces them. Reality becomes
greatly distorted. These are adaptive and quite useful organismic strategies that
are preexisting in the body. Hyperarousal, non-normal dissociation, and sensory
intrusion like sudden pain indicate core relationships in the body-mind that are
fragmented or coupled to past trauma acting in the present time. Likewise, the
fluid body is also fragmented or, as one osteopath has said, fractured. This is
why the practitioner must know how to orient to a stillpoint and synchronize
with Primary Respiration.

Impact Trauma

It is quite well known that stress patterns in the myofascia of the body crystal-
lize along lines of stress (Feitis and Schultz, 1997). The fluid gel of the fascia
dehydrates and contracts within seconds following an impact. An automobile
accident that causes a whiplash will imprint in the autonomic nervous system
of the soft tissue, the right hemisphere of the brain, and in the fluid body from

the trajectory and velocity of the accident. However, other life elements may be crystallized in the accident as well. These other life elements—such as impending divorce, loss of employment, or even seemingly less important events like being able to balance a checkbook—may be more central to the physical resolution of the accident than the traumatic tissue pattern or the fluid body condensations.

Years ago, I worked with a client who was a passenger in a tractor-trailer truck that overturned on an icy road and flipped over and over as it slid down a steep embankment. During the course of her treatment, her body insisted on recapitulating the tumbling that occurred while she was in the cab of the truck. This took 15–20 minutes yet never occurred again in subsequent sessions. At one point during this session, she rolled off of the treatment table onto the floor and kept going until she stopped in the same position she had occupied on the floor of the cab. Through our work together I learned the importance of assisting the client to slow down whatever movement her body was making and to actively resist moving in habituated and perseverative patterns, to stay within the tempo of Primary Respiration, and to keep the client oriented in present time. Fortunately for this particular client, her movements were an uncomplicated automatic shifting process (her husband was the driver and uninjured, and they were completely in love with each other and their work). Very few are this simple.

Genuine Change or Not?

Is automatic shifting genuine or nongenuine? The biggest challenge for biodynamic practitioners is to discriminate between an automatic shifting that is genuine and one that is not. As stated previously, a client may react to the work by establishing a false fulcrum in her body that the unwary practitioner thinks is genuine therapeutic process. Synchronizing with Primary Respiration is one way to know if the trauma is being contained. If the practitioner continues to be drawn into the same story line with similar fluid and tissue movement, the practitioner may actually be touching a deeply held belief system, or a developmental issue.

This may also be an indication that it is not the right time for the client's story line to be advanced. It is imperative that the focus of the practitioner remain on the stillpoint and Primary Respiration. Physical and emotional symptoms may be the surface features of a developmental crisis that is necessary for the client to be experiencing. As Dr. Becker once said, "Leave my primary lesion alone." They are important to the maturation and growth processes of all human beings. These crises typically occur during the lifespan as a way to realign ourselves with the divine plan in the fullness of time. All the practitioner can do is wait, watch, and wonder at the unfolding of life process.

Automatic shifting may not occur until more awareness is brought to a pattern by slowing down the therapeutic expression within the tempo of Primary Respiration. This gradually uncouples the trauma and allows both the trauma and the embryonic forces in the adult to automatically shift to a more normal midline relationship. Chronic stress or trauma shapes the body around inertial fulcrums from other preexisting patterns, like transparent overlays in an anatomy book. Each trauma in life in some way is a recapitulation of an earlier one.

These historical threads are intimately connected within the systemic relationships and emergent shapes held within the fascia and surrounding fluid matrix of the fluid body. The nervous system contributes its time-line perspectives of held memory and context held in the right hemisphere of the brain. The immune system contributes an inflammatory process designed to get rid of the foreign invader. Family, culture, and society contribute beliefs and attitudes that are often antithetical to an individual's healing process and promote fragmentation. A client may have to distance herself from family, friends, and the familiarity of context in order to actualize her healing potential.

CHAPTER 16

Somatic Ignition Skills

In this day and age, it is an unfortunate fact that almost everyone has experienced some degree of trauma. To restate the preliminary guideline for working in a therapeutic setting involving traumatic history, it is imperative that the practitioner orient to the stillness of a client's fluid body by synchronizing with Primary Respiration. Ideally, the first three sessions of biodynamic craniosacral therapy involve an assessment of the client's autonomic nervous system. This is the essence of somatic ignition described in Volume One and throughout this section of Volume Two. The practitioner develops the skill to observe how the client resources herself in the context of the excitation of the sympathetic system and the settling activity of the parasympathetic system. Without knowing this preexisting somatic ignition process in the client's soma, the practitioner may continue to leave false fulcrums in the client's soma and fluid body.

By adhering to these somatic ignition assessment skills, the client's autonomic nervous system can be expected to respond to the priorities of Primary Respiration and a deepening level of trust and safety can be established with the client. What follows is an elaboration of a set of principles or natural laws that define somatic ignition in the Primary Respiratory System as it relates to held inertia in the brain, soma, and fluid body.

Visualizing the Client Three-Dimensionally

I begin each session by settling into stillness, waiting for a felt sense of Primary Respiration to arise in and or around my body. I do this by orienting to the three-dimensional surface of the skin of my own soma. This may lead me to a body-sense of Primary Respiration moving up and down the middle of my spine, breathing back and forth to the horizon. I will occasionally look at the second hand of the clock in my office and time Primary Respiration to make sure it has two phases of fifty seconds each.

Since Primary Respiration is part of a three-dimensional matrix or "sea around us," practitioners must be able to visualize the surface of the client's body three-dimensionally. This includes the part of the client's body that is unseen and lying on the surface of the treatment table. I like to imagine the client inside a bubble or sphere of the fluid body. The idea is to visualize the whole and total surface of the body from some vantage point in the practitioner's imagination, and then to visualize the entire inner space of the client's body as clear, living, moving water. This opens the spatial intelligence of the right hemisphere of the practitioner to be able to sense Primary Respiration. Sometimes when I am specifically working around the cranium I visualize the client's occiput and the original movement of neural cells that formed the head moving at the tempo of Primary Respiration in the fluid body from posterior to anterior.

Allowing Micro Movement

During the middle phase of a biodynamic session, the autonomic nervous system may begin to thaw. This may appear as phases of shaking, jerking, and/or trembling (sympathetic) followed by phases of settling and stilling (parasympathetic). Note the frequency of these phases. Do not impede this motion but allow the movement, especially if the client is in a deep state of relaxation. It may be helpful to verbally acknowledge such spontaneous movement if the client is alert. In most cases, however, I verbally discourage larger motions because these motions are actually very superficial and require a much slower tempo in order to deepen the therapeutic process. Unless the practitioner senses micro movement in relationship to phases of stillness, he will miss the subtleties of the automatic shifting in the fluid body and soma.

The practitioner's hands may sense small oscillations and vibrations on the surface of the skin as the fluid body begins to change shape and affect the soma. The practice of evenly suspending attention between the horizon and self is a necessary and developed skill. Such kinesthetic perception is facilitated by the slow-acting nerve receptors in the palms of the practitioner's hands coupled with the ability to be calm and still within the practitioner's own body and mind. Small perturbations of the fluids are points of ignition and shape changing that must be accommodated and not interfered with. It is an allowing and slowing process rather than an active tissue guiding process.

The client's body may begin to make large or quick motions. The practitioner verbally suggests that the client inhibit the motion and uses his hands to inhibit the motion with the intention to slow it down. Very often it is the hyperarousal of the autonomic nervous system that is so damaging to the brain and body and slowing down the motion allows for resonance to occur across the right hemi-sphere of both the client and the practitioner. This allows the self-organizing of the fluid body to occur within the tempo and direction of Primary Respiration. It allows for self-regulation of emotions to be reestablished in the prefrontal cortex of the client. This helps complete the freeze-thaw cycle of immobilization in the autonomic nervous system, which is thwarted in shock and trauma.

Slowing down the motion of an automatic shifting process in the fluid body and soma at the tempo of Primary Respiration allows for the longitudinal fluctuation of the fluid body to be reestablished and deepens the uncoupling of the event from its origin. Slowing a client's process acts as a type of insurance policy against retraumatizing the client. It is an invitation rather than a demand placed on the client's fluid body and soma. This is a critical skill with children as well. Just as Italy's "slow food" movement has spawned numerous worldwide organizations dedicated to slowness, so too biodynamic practice is part of this international shift in the consciousness of slowing and stilling.

Scanning the Body

The practitioner frequently scans the surface of the client's body for areas of auto-nomic arousal. All such activity of the autonomic nervous system is considered to be an ignition. In these instances ignition refers to the neurological activa-tion and intensity that is arising unconsciously through synchronization within Primary Respiration. This was referred to as somatic ignition in Volume One.

These areas give the practitioner clues about the state of the client's ANS. The practitioner may observe one or more of the following.

• The eyes are direct indicators of limbic system activation—the practitioner might see the eyes glazing (exophthalmia, a bug-eyed look) or fixating on an object in the office. This may be an indication of numbing and fragmentation, which may be transient, or part of the client resourcing herself in a normal dissociation, like staring at an object in the office or on the wall or ceiling.

• The face and parts of the body may flush red or turn white or grey. The prac-titioner is alert to visible skin color changes, especially around the face.

• The jaw and mouth may clench or tremble.

• The head may turn slowly from side to side.

• The neck and atlanto-occipital joint may tense into flexion.

• The head may begin to rotate from side to side, either slowly or quickly.

- The upper thoracic cavity may flex on one side or the other as the client's shoulder and upper arm lifts off the table and relaxes back down.

- Sweating (sudomotor response) may be observed on the forehead of the client, around the face, under the axilla, or up and down the spine. This aspect of somatic ignition is common and much deeper than crying.

- The respiratory diaphragm registers all autonomic activation as a part of somatic ignition called the startle reflex and needs to be observed, along with the movement and position of the rib cage. Is the chest getting depressed or lifted up? Is breathing quiet or rapid? If rapid, the client is usually alert so the practitioner can place a hand gently over the diaphragm and verbally coach the client to breath more slowly.

- Sleep apnea is not unusual when a client goes into a deep relaxation. The chest will heave up and down without taking any air into the lungs and then the client will gasp for a breath, which usually awakens her. I have seen some clients have episodes of apnea for more than a minute before taking a breath. This is the way a fetus breathes fluid and the way a person dies when the lungs fill up with fluids. It is a very deep ignition.

- The abdomen and pelvis are areas of vibration or flaccidness when the autonomic nervous system starts to ignite. This is usually due to blood being shunted from the viscera to the extremities for fight or flight.

- The most typical indicator of the ignition of the autonomic fight-or-flight mechanism beginning to thaw is when the lower extremities shake or tremble. Shaking and trembling when occurring consciously need to be encouraged with deliberate slowness and then connected through the whole body by verbally asking the client to allow the sensations to move and expand to other areas of the body and ideally toward the core. The practitioner may need to ask the client the name of the body part closest to the vibration that is not moving; for example: "Can you tell me where the vibration is not happening?" or "Can you connect those areas?"

If the client is in a deep relaxation, the practitioner remains still and keeps his hands in place until the autonomics have finished cycling. The phase of thawing within the somatic ignition process known as fight-or-flight activates the midline function of the fluid body as well as the release of heat. It often causes tissue releases and frees the fluid body to breathe with reciprocal tension potency. Aberrant lateral fluctuations can diminish and the longitudinal fluctuation can reassert itself as a strong life-sustaining midline.

- Sometimes, however, the extremities will be still while the whole area in the front of the client's spine trembles and vibrates. I often ask my client to allow the deep trembling in the core of the body to move freely and gently up to the surface of the skin. Let the submarine come to the surface. Then I suggest to the client to find an area of the body where the vibration is missing and allow vibration to move there in small increments or body part by body part. This empowers the client and gives her control of the body. This lets the whole fluid body automatically shift from the experience of fragmentation and recouples to Primary Respiration breathing back and forth to the horizon in rhythmic periods of fifty seconds.

- These events of the sympathetic nervous system may cause a parasympathetic vagal reflex such as nausea, headache, arching the spine in extension, and quick, whiplike motions of the spine that appear much like a seizure.

I rarely see all of these different somatic expressions, the more I work with Primary Respiration. These responses, usually resulting from preverbal imprinting, can be contained, uncoupled, and reintegrated into the wholeness of the tidal body and fluid body with Primary Respiration. The reintegration process rarely requires such strong somatic responses. It is here where biodynamic practice by focusing on the slow movement in the fluid body and tidal body can actually allow the central nervous system to decompress with order and organization inherent in the relationship of Primary Respiration to stillness. For those times when the autonomic nervous system of the client needs to express itself more fully, the biodynamic practitioner can rest in his own perception of Primary Respiration and Stillness.

These are all important functions, however, of the autonomic nervous system that allows the soma to ignite and automatically shift its fulcrum to a deeper integration with the fluid body and tidal body. All three bodies must have the opportunity via such ignition to reestablish a functioning midline between them. The practitioner supports the comfort and ease of the client at all times.

Tissue Work

Some practitioners have specialized training in tissue work. The only time to intend mechanical pressure into the tissues is when the practitioner's instinct is drawn to the membrane system, and even then it is incremental and used only for brief moments. I like to use what I call the rule of three. Since I practiced Rolfing for many years, if my instincts tell me to approach the tissues during a biodynamic craniosacral therapy session, I ignore it twice until it comes through loud and clear a third time. It requires the delicate skill of switching between the metabolic fields of the embryo and the tissue fields. The fluid fields were the first to congeal in development and the tissue fields were last. Not every practitioner may wish to work within a spectrum that spans both metabolic formation and levels of tissue density. Making the bridge between these formations requires additional study. Biomechanical pressure into the tissues is only used to experiment with tissue barriers that impede the fluid body. It is only done in the middle of a session rather than at the beginning or end. Then the practitioner listens to the response in the fluid body (the early metabolic fields) while staying in the tempo of Primary Respiration.

By definition the fluid body will go still when pressure is applied to its tissue condensations. Consequently, the practitioner must be able to wait for the fluid body to reinitiate its movement. When perception is on the fascia of the body, it may begin to automatically shift the tissue fulcrum and advance the story line in that metabolic field. The fascia is actually very thick fluid. The fluid body responds to stillness and Primary Respiration. This is the preexisting condition in the embryo. Muscles and bones were the last structures to form in the embryo.

The best advice I can offer is for the practitioner to schedule separate sessions for tissue work if compelled to work in the soft tissue. In this case I would switch to biodynamic craniosacral therapy at the end of such a session to decompress the nervous system and reestablish the link to Primary Respiration. This builds a bridge across a spectrum of touch and intervention.

Therapeutic Tips

Here are some therapeutic tips if somatic ignition surfaces with a client in a session: Keep the eyes open—be attentive, playful, and studious. Avoid techniques and protocols except rarely as a way to initiate a conversation and then only briefly in the middle phase of a session. Work with subtlety and deliberate slowness. What heals is the practitioner's stillness and slow, conscious tempo of Primary Respiration. Stillness evokes presence that is a function of poise and dignity being embodied. Presence implies silence, stillness, and being in present time, which is the heart of biodynamic craniosacral therapy. Along with presence comes listening. Biodynamic craniosacral practitioners are listening for the priorities of Primary Respiration to manifest. There is a buoyant accommodation that practitioners' hands make in response to any fluid movement. Rather than taking up slack, like reeling in a fish that has just been caught, the hands create a sense of space and lightness, becoming transparent or even disappearing from sensory perception. This opens the deeper intentions of the midline to manifest.

Listening and Observation Skills

Eye contact and mental concentration on a client's speech and reflecting it back to the client are critical elements in developing trust and safety in a therapeutic relationship. These two elements feed and nurture the client. They nourish others sometimes without ever having to say a word—just a nod of the head or a sound of acknowledgment is usually enough. When words are used they are based on personal curiosity much more so than therapeutic demeanor or technique. The key element in observation skills is monitoring the internal self-talk of the practitioner, letting the mind rest occasionally in a stillpoint, and extending the senses out to the horizon via Primary Respiration to include the whole environment. Accurate observation and reflection is crucial. There is a need to develop resonance with clients—eyes to eyes, breath to breath, body to body with hand contact, body with feelings, and so on. This develops resonance in the biodynamic attunement. Healing is based on self-awareness, self-discovery, and cooperation that is generated by this resonance.

It is better to err on the side of gentleness. We live in a very aggressive society. The health care system is aggressive in its approach to treating disease, pain, suffering, and death (Illich, 1976). Without awareness of the stillpoint and its exchange with Primary Respiration, subtle cues from clients are missed through lack of attunement. The client may be retraumatized. Rather than facilitating integration and reeducation, the practitioner becomes part of the system of negative reinforcement and aggression. Non-normal dissociation is unable to transform into normal dissociation, or a slowed-down perception of the world.

This gentle normal dissociation of personal sensing and body awareness is crucial to reawakening the whole fluid sensorium from what Thomas Hanna (Hanna, 1988) calls sensory amnesia. Biodynamic practitioners must approach themselves and the client with profound gentleness by placing one's self on the bottom of the ocean. The biodynamic practitioner is indeed a submariner. It is more a witnessing of a gentle unfolding process that goes on within the practitioner and client as the beauty of the undersea life swims by. I grew up watching the Jacques Cousteau television specials about undersea life and was transfixed by them. The practitioner is a guide like Jacques Cousteau, one who has taken the journey below and knows the uneven terrain of aquatic life. There is a willingness to explore that which is uncharted or unknown. Modern parlance calls it risk-taking, but it is much deeper than that. It means letting the lungs breathe fluid just as they did for nine months in the womb and just as they will as we die.

Feelings, emotions, and bodily sensations are foreign, discarded as an *epiphe-nomenon,* something outside of meaning and unimportant in the healing process according to biomedicine. The soma is not such a machine; it is a sentient ocean. A soma cannot be understood only from studying its parts, through anatomy and physiology, or through its cells, atoms, viruses, and bacteria. Biodynamics is the study of the perception of a heart-to-heart connection. The soma is a living fluid—the therapeutic relationship is a connection of ocean to ocean, blood to blood, and heart to heart.

Resolution and Healing

In helping a client to heal trauma held in the fluid body with a biodynamic craniosacral approach, the point is to access the stillness and to observe how this forms a relationship to the client's longitudinal fluctuation and Primary Respiration. One of the keys is to sense stillness in the fluid body. It is imperative for the practitioner to change his own perception by expanding and extending his senses out to the horizon and synchronize with the stillness of nature. Then the healing process becomes instinctual.

Any system of healing will be correct when it follows the morphological laws of the embryonic development. The embryo grows and develops cavities first (visceral, thoracic, and cranial) around fluid fulcrums formed by organized fluid forces and membrane boundary interaction. The cavities are then connected via a circulatory system and finally the scaffolding of the musculoskeletal system that it all hangs on is built. This dynamic, whole fluid field then folds and unfolds throughout life. It is a biodynamic fluid process. The adult body contains that original embryonic matrix, or blueprint for health and healing, within the tempo of Primary Respiration. The body heals itself by these natural laws. The original-ity of the embryo may be hidden or dormant, but it is nonetheless present. All trauma processes are embryonic processes.. Ignition describes the therapeutic process of biodynamic craniosacral therapy.

Practitioners deepen their relationship with healing when they realize they cannot heal their clients and that it all starts at home in the practitioner's own body and mind, healing himself through stillness and silence and self-regulating his emotions. Then the soma can begin the road to recovering the deep resources of Primary Respiration. When the equation of practitioner and client becomes equal as one embryo to another, growth and differentiation can arise naturally and spontaneously. A practitioner who works with his own personal issues psychologically and spiritually becomes grounded in the process of his own illness and limitations. This will reflect directly to the client, and the client's original embryonic Intelligence of Primary Respiration will respond.

When practitioners can become comfortable with *not knowing,* then the self-correcting Intelligence of the Primary Respiratory System will reveal itself. This requires faith, respect, and sacrifice. It is not an Old Testament sacrifice but rather a sacrifice of self-aggression. Biodynamic craniosacral therapy affords practitioners a golden opportunity to have the health of the embryo be revealed rather than disease. As one of my first osteopathic teachers once said, "Cranial work is a way of life."

CHAPTER 17

Verbal Skills:
Principles and Practice

I would like to review the various principles I have discussed throughout this section on relating to trauma. Then I would like to present several sample dialogues from my clinical experience. The intention is to give the biodynamic practitioner an example of skills I have learned over the years in my training in psychology. My hope is for biodynamic practitioners to relate appropriately and sincerely with clients and not be therapeutically "clever" in relating to a client's dilemma.

Safety

The first requirement in a therapeutic relationship is to establish safety. One way is to verbally solicit the comfort and ease of the client. The practitioner asks the client: "Are you comfortable?" or "Are you comfortable where my hands are?" or "Could my hands be in a better place?" The client also needs to be informed that she has the power to stop the session, take a pause, or make a request of any kind for her personal comfort. The practitioner is expected to educate the client on when to take a pause, if necessary.

Mirroring

When the client tells her story, the practitioner occasionally repeats back to the client what is being said. It does not have to be verbatim, but rather a reflection that lets the client know she is being heard. The client must know she is being heard for healing to happen. This is a simple acknowledgment and is a skill of paying attention. Attention is a deliberate way of listening to the emerging process in the client.

Synchronizing

The practitioner encourages the client to synchronize her attention with fluid sensations, fluid images, and fluid shapes in her body. Conversation around emotions is redirected to the sensory and fluid strata of the client's experience. The practitioner might ask: "What's the shape of that?" or "Where is the sensation of that located in your body?"

It is not in the scope of practice of a biodynamic craniosacral practitioner to get involved in the content of a client's story line. When the sensate is unavailable, the practitioner helps the client synchronize with where the client's attention is located. This is the sentient rather than the sensate in biodynamic craniosacral therapy.

Attunement

Attachment literature shows that the autonomic nervous system in many people has become uncoupled from its natural homeostatic cycling of states of sympathetic activation followed by states of parasympathetic settling. In fact, the sympathetic and parasympathetic nervous systems have become uncoupled in many clients and are both overactive at the same time. Attunement involves the development of a witness consciousness. This means that a practitioner is observing his own cycles of activation and settling very slowly. Such attunement creates a resonance with the client and enables the autonomic nervous system to recover its coupled reciprocal function.

Curiosity

The practitioner avoids therapeutic cleverness, generalizations, and aphorisms. The practitioner helps the client explore her arising states with open-ended questions and even small talk as a way of creating integration across hemispheres. Everything is considered ordinary. I often precede a question with the words, "I wonder,..." The practitioner tracks his own internal state of attention and possible projections onto the client. This means that the practitioner is allowed to self-disclose his own state of mind, emotions, or sensory experience. This should not intrude upon the client's experience or create a demand for emotional attention from the client.

Verbal skills in biodynamic craniosacral therapy are exploration skills. The use of language is open-ended and nondirective. Please remember that if a client is asleep or in a deep state of relaxation, she should not be verbally interrupted. A cranial treatment is 80–90 percent nonverbal. The little verbal work done in a session is used primarily to integrate the client's left hemisphere to the right and to help the client become conscious of the total fluid continuum of the body from which the nervous system was born. From time to time, however, the client may experience emotions before, during, or after a session. As a teacher of mine once said regarding emotional process work, "Seek not, forbid not." It is really about curiosity and play rather than therapeutic cleverness. Please avoid poking around in someone's emotional body.

Sample Dialogue

When a client exhibits a state of sympathetic overactivation or hyperarousal, the practitioner may ask, for example, "What's the sensation of the cushion you're sitting on?" Or the practitioner may ask the client to place her attention on other people in the room, or "I wonder, what does it feel like when you see other people in the room?"

Other questions or observations by the practitioner to bring the client's attention to the fluid continuum might include the following. These examples show a sequence of focusing the client's attention.

"Are you aware of any sensations in your body that tell you that you are okay?"

"Where's the openness in your body right now?"

"Where is the space in your body located right now?"

"Where are you?"

"What's happening with your body right now?"

"Where are things soft and easy?"

"Is there something that needs to happen with the leg?" (if it is shaking)

"Can you imagine that happening?" (the opposite of the process being observed, such as relaxation)

"Let yourself prepare to do that."

"What does your whole body need to do?"

"Slowly let your legs do that."

"Something is trying to clear here."

"Is that arm trying to do anything?"

"Can you stay with that intention?" (a slow exploration of movement or sound)

"Can you imagine that you are going to do it?"

"Can you prepare to do that?"

"Let yourself do it, but do it slowly so all the energy comes through."

"Ah, that's interesting."

"Something is arising that's important."

"Are you in touch with resources in your body right now?"

On the other hand, when the parasympathetic nervous system is overactive, the client will appear withdrawn. When you are working with a spaced-out client ask her, "Where are you right now?" If a client says she is not in her body, get precise about the location of her attention and support it. Conscious dissociation is a resource. Work with the process of coming and going from the body with Primary Respiration. Start an inquiry into what is happening inside the body and what is happening outside the body. Uncouple any emotional charge by slowing down the process. You could ask the client, "Can you stay with the sensation under the emotion and let it move?" or "Is there a fluid image or shape you can access right now?"

"What's possible here?"

"How much space is there around you right now?"

"I wonder what this is about?"

"Are you in contact with the ocean of support?"

"Can you sense your fingers or toes right now?"

Staying at the Edge

You must give the client permission to *not* jump off the deep end into her trauma: "Can you stay at the edge of your discomfort and not dive into it?" Clients already live there and need a lifeline out of the quicksand.

You could say: "This is an old process your system is trying to complete. Be slow now because it takes time to put this all together" or "This is your nervous system discharging and it is very normal" or "Can you sense the trembling in your (name a body part)?" The rule of thumb is to slow it down.

Staying in the Present

When there is something new, you do not have to de-skill yourself. Keep in verbal contact with your client. Don't become the client's process. Appreciate the process and engage the adult. Some focusing questions:

"Are you present?"

"Is your adult here?"

"What do you need to do now?"

"What's next?"

"Can we wait here?" (a good cue either verbally or with your hands)

"What's happening now?"

"What's the space around you like?"

"How do you sense yourself in that space?"

Containment

Your voice creates containment. Think of stillpoints and EV4s. It occasionally helps to meet something with resistance in order to slow a movement down and create the possibility of a stillpoint, but only with pacing and titration.

"What is the space around you like?"

"Are you alone?"

"What's the sense of where you are?"

It's not just pain and anguish that we touch into, but there's the possibility for happiness, spiritual awareness, and relaxation. Can we actually rest in the space between all the atoms and molecules in the body? This space is filled with the Dynamic Stillness. Help make the relationship with the adult more concrete and still: "How is it to be here?" Go slowly one step at a time and maintain an orientation to the present.

"What tells you that you are okay with your body?"

"What feels okay?"

"What sensations tell you that you are okay?"

"Can you contact a place of safety in your body?"

"Is there an image of a place, thing, or activity that is a resource for you?"

"What tells you that you feel good?"

"What's familiar after all of that?"

"What's different now?"

"What's happening now?"

"And how is that for you?"

"Just let the wave come through."

"Take the time to acknowledge what is happening."

"Why don't you take a minute to greet what you're feeling now."

"Take the time to acknowledge that there is something important there."

"Make space between what you're experiencing and the adult in you."

"How is that for you now?"

Nonverbal Dialogue

You are not doing something to release something. You are conversing with it in relative stillness. You are in collaboration with it. "Now where is the natural instinct to heal?" is the question to ask your own fluid body. The answer is given as a systemic movement or localized shaping in your own fluid body that is already in nonverbal dialogue with the client's fluid body. All that is required is to maintain awareness of your own tidal body and fluid body as the client shapes it through the relational field of the fluid. Anytime you engage tissue, you engage history, so stay with the fluids. Start another nonverbal conversation about space. "And then what?" is a question to ask with your hands while the client's fluid body is automatically shifting. It may help to advance the story line. Don't fixate on one particular aspect of the fluid body if it speeds up, but keep offering "Let's take a pause" or "Let's get still for a moment." or "Be still and know." These nonverbal phrases are offered as a type of prayer with a respect and reverence first suggested by Dr. Sutherland. This prayer is offered while having your hands in buoyant contact with the client.

This concludes the section on relating to trauma from a biodynamic perspective. I highly recommend specialized training in trauma resolution if a biodynamic practitioner is interested in helping a client in that way.

SECTION III

...

Infants and Children

CHAPTER 18

Attachment, Affect Regulation, and the Developing Right Brain: Linking Developmental Neuroscience to Pediatrics

Allan N. Schore, PhD

We are in the midst of an exciting period for clinical practitioners, one in which the connections between the basic and applied sciences are being more tightly forged. A powerful engine driving this progression of knowledge is the recent remarkable advance in biotechnology, especially imaging technologies. Noninvasive studies of organ systems have increased substantially our understanding of the biologic processes that underlie various diseases of the body. At the same time, neuroimaging research of both psychological functions and psychiatric conditions has generated more complex models of the normal and abnormal operations of the human mind. Another catalyst of the continuing dramatic increase in information is the rapid expansion of collaborative interdisciplinary research. Of particular relevance to pediatrics, this same time period has seen an explosion of infant research that integrates neurobiological studies of brain development and psychological studies of emotional, social, and cognitive development. Developmental studies, which span a spectrum of scientific and medical disciplines, now are serving as a convergence point for complex models of structure and function, brain, mind, and body.

A paradigm shift is occurring in the basic sciences that underlie pediatrics. Research in developmental biology and physiology now strongly supports a model of the "developmental origins of health and disease" (Gluckman and Adler, 2004[3]). Although the role of early expressed genetic factors is an essential focus of current study, it has become clear that genes do not specify behavior absolutely; prenatal and postnatal environmental factors play a critical role in these developmental origins. The social environment, particularly the one created together by the mother and infant, directly affects gene-environment interactions, and, thereby has long-enduring effects. The newer interdisciplinary models, therefore, detail the mechanisms by which "mother nature meets mother nurture" (Crabbe and Phillips, 2003). Complementing this conception of the nature-nurture problem, studies in neuroscience indicate that development represents an experiential shaping of genetic potential, and that early experiences with the social environment are critical to the maturation of brain tissue. Thus, nature's potential can be realized only as it is facilitated by nurture (Chicchetti and Tucker, 1994).

In parallel advances in developmental psychology and child psychiatry, attachment theory, initially proposed over thirty-five years ago by John Bowlby (Bowlby, 1969) as a conception of the mother-infant relationship, has now become the dominant model of human social-emotional development available to researchers and clinicians over a broad array of disciplines. In his attempt to integrate psychology and psychiatry with behavioral biology, Bowlby speculated that the attachment system, an evolutionary mechanism common to both humans and animals, ultimately would be located in specific areas of the brain. Updated models of attachment theory that emphasize both emotional and social functions and neurobiological structures now are interfacing with developmental neuroscience and generating a large body of interdisciplinary studies.

This recent information on the developmental origins of health and disease can be translated directly into clinical practice. It has both expanded the amount of factual knowledge and altered the theoretical constructs that model the diagnoses and treatments of a variety of psychological and physical disorders of childhood. These advances are, in turn, directly relevant to pediatricians' interest in the normal and abnormal functions of the developing child's mind and body. The common ground of the expanding body of knowledge in the developmental sciences, therefore, can strengthen the ties of pediatrics to the allied fields that border it: developmental neurology, child psychiatry, and developmental psychology.

This ongoing paradigm shift in the basic and applied sciences is expressed in three converging themes. The first arises from the wealth of neurobiological data that became available in the last decade, the "decade of the brain." These findings strongly support the idea that the most powerful conception of development may come from a deeper understanding of the brain's own self-organizing operations. Currently, there is an intense focus upon the human brain growth spurt, which begins in the last trimester of pregnancy and continues to 18–24 months of age. Myelinization of the brain is so rapid and extensive at this time that the brain takes on an "adultlike" appearance by the end of the first postnatal year

(Paus, et al., 2001). Neuroscientists are concluding that the accelerated growth of brain structure during critical periods of infancy is dependent on experience and influenced by "social forces." Neuropsychiatrists refer to "the social construction of the human brain," and posit that the cellular architecture of the cerebral cortex is sculpted by input from the social environment embedded in the early attachment relationships. These data suggest that "the self-organization of the developing brain occurs in the context of a relationship with another self, another brain" (Schore, 1996).

Furthermore, we now are aware that "the brain" is actually a system of two brains, each of which has very different structural and functional properties. Of particular interest to the developmental sciences is the early maturing right brain, which undergoes a growth spurt in the first two years, before the verbal left, and is dominant in the first three years after birth (Chiron, et al., 1997). This growth is not encoded totally in the genome, but it is shaped indelibly by the emotional communications within attachment transactions. Because the right hemisphere is dominant for the emotional and corporeal self (Devinsky, 2000), the social experience-dependent maturation of the right brain in human infancy is equated with the early development of the self (Schore, 1994). The early development of the brain-mind-body, the origin of the self, therefore, is a reflection of the development of the right brain and its unique functions.

The second theme emerges from transformations within the psychiatric and psychological sciences. All subdisciplines within psychology, from developmental through abnormal, are shifting their focus from cognition to emotion. Research suggests that the attainment of an attachment bond of emotional communication and the maturation of affect represent the key events in infancy more so than does the development of complex cognitions. Models have moved from Piagetian theories of cognitive development to psychobiological models of social-emotional development. Clinical psychology and psychiatry are moving from cognition to emotion as the central force in psychopathology and psychotherapy. This emphasis on emotion is also reflected in: (1) the emergence of affective neuroscience and its focus on the specializations of the right hemisphere for processing affective states, and (2) psychiatry's current interest in the emotion-processing limbic system, the brain system that derives subjective information in terms of emotional feelings that guide behavior and functions to allow the individual to adapt to a rapidly changing environment and organize new learning.

The third theme revolves around the critical concept of self-regulation. The process of development itself is believed to represent a progression of stages in which adaptive self-regulatory structures and functions enable new interactions between the individual and the social environment. It is now established that emotions are the highest-order direct expressions of bioregulation in complex organisms, that the maturation of the neural mechanisms involved in self-regulation is experience-dependent, and that these critical affective experiences are embedded in the attachment relationship.

In other words, attachment relationships are essential because they facilitate the development of the brain's self-regulatory mechanism. Studies reveal that these essential self-regulatory structures are located in the right (and not left) brain (Schore, 2003a). Consensus now indicates that attachment can be defined as the dyadic regulation of emotion, that the attainment of the self-regulation of affect is a major developmental achievement, and that normal development represents the enhancement of self-regulation.

I now use the perspective of regulation theory (Schore, 1994, 2003a, 2003b) to discuss and interpret recent studies on attachment, affect regulation, and the development of the right brain. These advances in understanding the neurobiology of attachment are now being incorporated into clinical models of the development of childhood mental health and mental illness, areas that that are directly relevant to pediatrics. The mission statement of the American Academy of Pediatrics states its commitment to "the attainment of optimal physical, mental, and social health for all infants, children, adolescents, and young adults" (www.cispimmunize.org/mission.html).[4]

Interactive Affect Regulation as a Fundamental Mechanism of Attachment Dynamics

The primary goals for the infant during the first postnatal year are the creation of an attachment bond of emotional communication with the primary caregiver and the development of self-regulation. From birth onward, infants use their expanding coping capacities to interact with the social environment. In the earliest proto-attachment experiences, infants use their maturing motor and developing sensory capacities, especially smell, taste, and touch, to interact with the social environment (Van Toller and Kendal-Reed, 1995; Weller and Feldman, 2003). At around eight weeks of age, there is a dramatic progression of social and emotional capacities. Within episodes of mutual gaze, the caretaker (usually the mother) and infant engage in nonconscious and spontaneous facial, vocal, and gestural communications. Such highly arousing, affect-laden, face-to-face interactions allow the infant to be exposed to high levels of social and cognitive information.

In face-to-face emotional transactions the mother makes herself contingent, easily predictable, and manipulatable by the infant. To regulate the high positive arousal, the dyad synchronizes the intensity of their affective behavior within split seconds. These episodes of "affect synchrony" occur in the first expression of social play, and generate increasing levels of joy and excitement. In these interactions, both partners match states and simultaneously adjust their social attention, stimulation, and accelerating arousal to each other's responses. According to Lester, Hoffman, and Brazelton, "synchrony develops as a consequence of each partner's learning the rhythmic structure of the other and modifying his or her behavior to fit that structure" (Lester, Hoffman, and Brazelton, 1985). In such moments the empathic caregiver's sensory stimulation coincides with the infant's endogenous rhythms, allowing the mother to appraise the nonverbal expressions of her infant's internal arousal and psychobiological states, regulate them, and then communicate them back to the infant.

In this process of "contingent responsivity," the tempo of their engagement, disengagement and reengagement is coordinated. The more the empathic mother tunes her activity level to the infant during periods of social engagement, the more she allows him to recover quietly in periods of disengagement. The more she attends to the child's reinitiating cues for reengagement, the more synchronized becomes their interaction. Thus, the caregiver facilitates the infant's information processing by adjusting the mode, amount, variability, and timing of the onset and offset of stimulation to the infant's unique, temperamentally determined integrative capacities. These interactively regulated, synchronized interactions promote the infant's regulatory capacities and are fundamental to his or her healthy affective development.

In such interactions the mother must be attuned not so much to the child's overt behavior as to the reflections of the rhythms of his or her internal state, enabling the dyad to create "mutual regulatory systems of arousal." To regulate the infant's arousal, she must be able to regulate her own arousal state. The capacity of the infant to experience increasing levels of positive arousal states is amplified and externally regulated by the primary caregiver and depends on her capacity to engage in an interactive communication of emotions that generates feelings in herself and her child. Maternal sensitivity, therefore, acts as an external organizer of the infant's biobehavioral regulation.

Research also shows frequent moments of misattunement in the dyad, or ruptures of the attachment bond. In early development, an adult provides much of the modulation of infant states, especially after a state disruption or a transition between states, and this intervention allows for the development of self-regulation. The key to this beneficial interaction is the caregiver's capacity to monitor and regulate her own (especially negative) affect. In this essential regulatory pattern of "rupture and repair," the attuned "good-enough" caregiver who induces a stress response in her infant through a misattunement remedies the situation and helps her infant regulate his or her negative affect via her participation in "interactive repair." The process of reexperiencing positive affect following negative experience allows the child to learn that negative affect can be tolerated and that relational stress can be regulated. Infant resilience emerges from an interactive context in which the child and parent together transition from positive to negative and back to positive affect. The adaptive regulatory capacity of resilience in the face of stress is an ultimate indicator of secure attachment and optimal mental health.

Affect synchrony that creates states of positive arousal and interactive repair that modulates states of negative arousal are the fundamental building blocks of attachment and its associated emotions. These arousal-regulating transactions, which continue throughout the first year, underlie the formation of an attachment bond of emotion regulation between the infant and primary caregiver. Indeed, psychobiological attunement and the interactive mutual entrainment of physiologic rhythms are fundamental processes that mediate attachment, and thus throughout the lifespan attachment is a primary mechanism for the regulation of biologic synchronicity within and between organisms.

These data clearly suggest that affect regulation is not just the reduction of affective intensity or the dampening of negative emotion. Affect regulation involves an intensification of positive emotion, a condition necessary for more complex self-organization. The attuned mother of the securely attached child not only minimizes the infant's negative states through comforting transactions but also maximizes his positive affective states in interactive play. Regulated affective interactions with a familiar, predictable primary caregiver create not only a sense of safety, but also a curiosity that fuels the child's exploration of novel socioemotional and physical environments. This ability is a marker of adaptive infant mental health.

Interpersonal Neurobiology of Right Brain-to-Right Brain Attachment Communications

Learning how to communicate emotional states is an essential developmental process. Because these communications are nonverbal and subjective, it was believed that their underlying mechanisms were unavailable to experimental analysis. However, studies in developmental psychobiology have offered important contributions to this problem, revealing that during optimal moments of bodily based affective communications, the adult's and infant's individual homeostatic systems are linked together in a superordinate organization that allows for mutual regulation of vital endocrine, autonomic, and central nervous systems of both mother and infant by elements of their interaction with each other.

Basic developmental neurobiological research findings are consonant with the psychological models of early mother-infant communication described in the preceding section. Coordinated visual eye-to-eye messages, auditory vocalizations, and tactile and body gestures serve as channels of communicative signals that induce instant emotional effects: the positive feelings of excitement and pleasure build within the intersubjective field created by the dyad. According to Trevarthen (Trevarthen, 1993), the intrinsic regulators of a child's brain growth are adapted specifically for coupling, by emotional communication, to the regulators of adult brains.

Attachment communications, therefore, are "built into the nervous system," inducing substantial changes in the developing brain. Which parts of the brain are affected by the interactive regulation embedded within various types of visual, auditory, and tactile communications? Keeping in mind that the brain actually represents two unique hemispheric processing systems, a substantial body of research indicates that the right hemisphere begins a critical period of maturation before the left. This hemisphere is more advanced than the left in surface features from about the twenty-fifth gestational week until the beginning of the second postnatal year, when the left hemisphere undergoes a growth spurt (Trevarthen, 1996). Neuroimaging studies demonstrate that the brain mass increases rapidly during the first two years after birth, normal adult appearance is seen at two years, and all major fiber tracts can be identified by age three years. Infants younger than two years of age show higher right than left hemispheric volumes (Matsuzawa, Matsui, and Konishi, 2001).

Several studies supports the principle that "the emotional experience of the infant develops through the sounds, images, and pictures that constitute much of an infant's early learning experience, and are disproportionately stored or processed in the right hemisphere during the formative stages of brain ontogeny" (Semrud-Clikeman and Hynd, 1990). The neurobiology of attachment, therefore, is an interpersonal neurobiology of right brain-to-right brain communications. Although the later developing left hemisphere mediates most language functions, the early developing right hemisphere is more important to the broader aspects of communication.

In support of this right brain-to-right brain communication model research indicates that at about eight weeks (onset of intense face-to-face communications), a critical period is initiated in the occipital cortex during which synaptic connections are modified by visual experience (Yamada, Sadato, Konishi, et al., 2000). Infants as young as two months of age show right hemispheric activation on positive emission tomography when exposed to a woman's face, and particular areas of the right hemisphere are timed to be in a plastic and receptive state at the very time when sensory information that emanates from faces is being attended to most intensely by the infant (Tzourio-Mazoyer, et al., 2002). During synchronized face-to-face transactions, patterns of information emanating from the caregiver's face, especially of low visual and auditory frequencies, are processed by the infant's right hemisphere. Studies demonstrate that the development of the capacity to process information from faces efficiently requires visual input to the right (and not left) hemisphere during infancy (Le Grand, et al., 2003).

Over the first year, emotional communications embedded within mutual gazing are etched into developing right lateralized networks that are specialized for assessing familiar faces and gaze direction and for processing visual and auditory emotional signals. The right cerebral cortex is dominant for the infant's processing of individual faces, recognition of maternal facial expressions, and response to the mother's voice. Similarly, the mother's mature right hemisphere is faster than the left in appraising emotional facial expressions; responding to the positive aspects of facial expressions, visual stimuli, touch, and smell; and assessing visual or auditory emotional signals.

Other studies reveal that the maternal response to an infant's cry, a fundamental attachment behavior, is accompanied by an activation of the mother's right brain. These data support the idea that engrams related to emotional voices are imprinted more strongly on the infant's early maturing, more active right hemisphere (Lorberbaum, Newman, and Horwitz, 2002). With respect to tactile communications, most women tend to cradle infants on the left side of the body. This left-cradling tendency facilitates the flow of maternal affective signals into the infant's left ear and eye and processing in the developing right hemisphere, and the ensuing infant's auditory and visual communications are then fed back to the center of emotional decoding in the mother's right hemisphere (Manning, Trivers, and Thornhill, 1997). Researchers conclude that this left-cradling context allows for maximal somatoaffective feedback within the dyad and that "the role of the right hemisphere is crucial in relation to the most precious needs of mothers and infants" (Sieratzki and Woll, 1996).

From a neurobiological perspective:

When the child is held and hugged, brain networks are activated and strengthened and firing spreads to associated networks; when the child is sung to, still other networks are strengthened to receive sounds and interpret them as song. The repeated appearance of the mother provides a fixation object as in imprinting. (Epstein, 2001)

The cortical and subcortical systems of the infant's right brain become tuned to dynamic self-organization upon perceiving certain patterns of exteroceptive social information, namely, the visual, auditory, and tactile stimuli emanating from the smiling, joyful, soothing, and calming face as well as the expressive body of a loving mother.

These imprinting experiences are "affectively burnt in" (Stuss and Alexander, 1999) developing limbic circuits in the infant's right brain, which are known to undergo extensive myelination in the first eighteen postnatal months. Thus, at a fundamental level, the mother functions as a regulator of the infant's socio-emotional environment, and her regulatory interactions play a critical role during the establishment and maintenance of developing emotion-processing limbic circuits. The spontaneous emotional communication that occurs within the attachment relationship has been described as "a conversation between limbic systems." Because the early maturing right hemisphere, which is deeply connected into the limbic system, is in a growth spurt at this time, attachment experiences specifically affect developing limbic and cortical areas of the right brain networks that are critical to self-regulation.

This research indicates that the mother functions in the short term as a regulator of the child's homeostatic alterations and in the long term influences the child's capacity to cope adaptively with the social-emotional environment (Ovtscharoff and Braun, 2001). Although the mother initially provides an external regulating mechanism for the infant's immature neurobiological processes, by the end of the first postnatal year, the infant becomes self-regulating through the maturation of internal regulatory mechanisms entrained to the mother's stimuli. Current psychobiological models refer to representations of the infant's affective dialogue with the mother, which can be accessed to regulate its affective state. Studies are detailing how even subtle affect-regulating transactions alter activity levels permanently in the child's maturing brain. During the last ten years, many studies have documented the enduring impact of maternal visual, vocal, and tactile emotional stimuli on the infant's brain development, and on resulting emotional, social, cognitive, and regulatory capacities in later life (Schore, 2003b). (A detailed discussion of the relevant anatomy and physiology of the brain is presented in the appendix to this article.)

Secure Attachment, Optimal Right Brain Maturation, and the Psychoneurobiological Origins of Mental Health

In optimal interpersonal environments, co-regulated emotional communications between the securely attached infant and the primary attachment object facilitate the self-organization and increased complexity of the infant's right brain. Following the child's attachment to the mother in the first year, the child forms another attachment in the second year to the father, allowing the child to have affect-attuning and arousal-regulating experiences with two different types of caregivers. As a result of this interaction with caregivers, the infant forms internal working models of attachment that are stored in right-lateralized nonverbal implicit-procedural memory. Security of attachment relates to a physiologic coding of an expectation that during times of stress homeostatic disruptions will be set right. These interactive representations encode strategies of affect regulation and contain coping mechanisms for maintaining basic regulation and positive affect in the face of environmental challenge. The infant's ability to develop more complex self-regulatory coping capacities, to regulate stressful alterations of psychobiological state either interactively or autonomously, emerges out of its experiences with the social environment.

In all later interpersonal functioning, this right hemispheric representation of a working model of the attachment relationship, acting at levels beneath conscious awareness, is accessed to appraise, interpret, and regulate socioemotional information and guide future action in both familiar and novel interpersonal environments. For the rest of the lifespan, the right hemisphere that has been imprinted and organized by early relational experiences, is dominant for the nonconscious reception, expression, communication, and regulation of emotion, essential functions for creating and maintaining social relationships, especially intimate ones (Borod, Cicero, Obler, et al., 1998; Blonder, Bowers, and Heilman, 1991; Dimberg and Petterson, 2000; George, Parekh, Rosinsky, et al., 1996). Studies suggest that attachment psychobiology and right brain neuropsychology represent the substrate of three other capacities that are critical to human interactions: trust, empathy, and moral development (Perry, et al., 2001; Shamay-Tsoory, et al., 2003; Winston, et al., 2002).

Indeed, the right brain is dominant for the regulation of fundamental physiologic, endocrinologic, immunologic, and cardiovascular functions, thereby controlling vital functions that support survival and enable the organism to cope actively and passively with stress. A growing body of data underscores a strong association between alterations in maternal-infant interactions, early programming of the hypothalamic-pituitary-adrenal axis, pre- and postnatal critical periods of brain development, and adult health and disease (Matthews, 2002). This work is paralleled by studies linking attachment, stress, and childhood attachment (Maunder and Hunter, 2001; Schmidt, et al., 2002) with adult cortisol and cardiovascular function (Luecken, 1998) and research showing the right hemisphere plays a unique role for pain sensitivity and negative affect (Pauli,

Wiedemann, and Nickola, 1999). Assets or limitations of right brain survival functions, thus, affect not just on "psychological" but also essential "psychobiological" capacities of coping with both emotional disturbance and physical disease. These regulatory capacities, significantly influenced by optimal attachment experiences, are critical indices of adaptive physical and mental health.

In addition to self-regulation, the right hemisphere is specialized for generating self-awareness and self-recognition, and for the processing of "self-related material" (Decety and Chaminade, 2003; Keenan, et al., 2001). Devinsky (Devinsky, 2000) posits an evolutionary role of the right hemisphere in the following adaptive functions: maintaining a coherent, continuous, and unified sense of self; identifying a corporeal image of self and its relation to the environment; distinguishing self from nonself; recognizing familiar members of a species as well as other familiar organisms, items, and places; recalling autobiographical information; appraising environmental reality; and emotionally understanding and reacting to bodily and environmental stimuli. All of these critical adaptive functions are present by the second postnatal year (the end of the right brain growth spurt), and all are essential components of the earliest manifestation of mental health.

According to the unpublished manuscript of the Infant Mental Health Task Force of Zero to Three, National Center for Infant, Toddlers and Families:

> Infant mental health is the developing capacity of the child from birth to three years to experience, regulate, and express emotions; form close interpersonal relationships; and explore the environment and learn. …
> Infant mental health is synonymous with healthy social and emotional development.

The earliest expression of mental health reflects the adaptive or maladaptive functioning of the right brain, the neurobiological locus of the emotional self (Schore, 2000, 2001a).

Although the right brain reorganizes later in life and retains plasticity, conditions affecting its initial stages of evolution have an enormous impact on its subsequent development. The postnatal maturation of limbic-autonomic circuits is influenced significantly by the primary caregiver's provision and regulation of social-emotional experiences within the attachment relationship. Neuroscience now reveals that at the most fundamental level, regulated attachment experiences facilitate the brain's major regulatory systems, located in the right brain. However, studies also show that unrepaired and chronic stressful dysregulating interactions within the early social environment lay the groundwork for an insecure attachment, right brain dysfunction, limbic-autonomic deficits, and the development of a predisposition to later psychiatric and psychosomatic disorders.

The principle that early disruption of the mother-infant attachment relationship has a negative impact on brain plasticity and predisposes to later psychopathology is well established (Schore, 1994; Caldjii, et al., 1998; Cirulli, Berry, and Alleva, 2002; Graham, et al., 1999; Schore, 2001b, 2002; Siegel, 1999).[5] Helmcke and associates concluded:

> Positive (formation of emotional attachment) or negative (e.g., maternal separation or loss) emotional experience may carve a permanent trace into a still developing neuronal network of immature synaptic connections, and thereby can extend or limit the functional capacity of the brain during later stages of life. (Helmeke, et al., 2001)

The increasing appreciation of the profound and indelible impact of early interpersonal relationships on the psychological, physiologic, and neurobiological trajectory of the self over all stages of life substantially alters our view of human infancy. In the middle of the last century, the pediatrician-psychoanalyst Donald Winnicott asserted that there is no infant without the mother (Winnicott, 1960). This developmental psychological conception is mirrored in the previously mentioned developmental neurobiological principle that "the self-organization of the developing brain occurs in the context of a relationship with another self, another brain" (Schore, 1996). This other brain is the right brain of the primary caregiver, the mother. Although controversies have existed in the past, a large and consistent body of developmental neuroscience research across both human and animal species confirms the central role of the early relationship with the mother in the neurobehavioral development and, therefore, future social-emotional and stress-regulation capacities of the developing individual (Carter, 1998; Sieratzki and Woll, 1996; Ovtscharoff and Braun, 2001; Cirulli, Berry, and Alleva, 2002; Caldjii, et al., 1998; Fleming, O'Day, and Kraemer, 1999; Gunnar and Donzella, 2002; Meaney, 2001; Menard, Champagne, and Meaney, 2004; Nitschke, et al., 2004; Weaver, Cervoni, and Champagne, 2004).

There is an intense interest in neuroscience in the enduring impact of early "enriched experience" on brain development in the first eighteen postnatal months and in the applications of this knowledge to child development. These studies indicate that enriched experiences "are especially effective early in life and they set the basis for later use and maintenance of the brain and of ability" (Rosenzweig and Bennett, 1996). In the past, an "enriched environment" has been defined narrowly as a complex physical environment, and the reputed impact of early exposure was on cognitive development. It now is clear that for optimal brain development, the infant also needs to interact with an enriched social environment. The spectrum of regulated affective transactions within a psychobiologically attuned mother-infant attachment relationship defines an enriched environment more correctly—one that has a long-term impact on emotional development and the essential capacity of self-regulation.

In accord with these conceptualizations, a very recent National Institute of Child and Human Development study on the mother-child relationship and affect dysregulation concluded, "Self-regulation in infancy is best conceptualized as a quality of the infant-caregiver relationship, rather than a characteristic of the infant alon." (NICHD, 2004). The authors cited a large body of data that:

> emphasize the importance of the child's relationship with the primary caregiver as central to understanding the developmental processes leading from early affective arousal and attention control to later functioning. … Children's inability to control negative affect in early interactions with their caregivers may forecast continuing difficulties with affective regulation across multiple contexts.

Psychobiological markers that assess attachment relationships, regulation of affect, the right brain, and infant mental health need to be included in the diagnostic armamentarium of the practicing pediatrician. This information allows the clinician to understand the system of nonverbal communication and interactive regulation that lies at the core of the mother-infant relationship. To assess the social and emotional capacities of the nonverbal infant and the status of the nonverbal communications within the attachment dyad, the pediatrician must use clinical skills that involve her or his subjective right brain as well as objective left brain. The principles of regulation theory that apply to the mother-infant relationship also apply to the clinician-patient relationship (Schore, 1994, 2003a). According to Adler (Adler, 2002), the art of the doctor-patient relationship, which involves the physician's empathy and the capacity for responsive listening, "entails establishing the same kind of person-to-person attunement that is essential to the development of the newborn" (Schore, 1994). Psychobiological markers that assess attachment relationships, regulation of affect, the right brain, and infant mental health need to be included in the diagnostic armamentarium of the practicing pediatrician. (See the table in Figure 18.1 for a schematic of clinical observations of affect regulation and right brain development.)

Summary

Recent interdisciplinary data on attachment, affect regulation, and the right brain can be applied directly to clinically relevant models of the earliest manifestations of normal and abnormal social and emotional development. Adaptive infant mental health, an outcome of optimal attachment experiences, can be defined as the earliest expression of efficient and resilient right brain strategies for regulating both negative and positive affective states and for coping with novelty and stress, especially interpersonal stress (Schore, 2001a). The formation of an increasingly complex right brain system for communicating emotion allows the developing individual to switch internal, bodily based affective states in response to perceived changes in the external social environment via autoregulation or interactive regulation, thus maintaining a cohesive sense of self in both autonomous or interconnected contexts.

On the other hand, maladaptive infant mental health is manifest in a poor right brain capacity to enter into emotional communications with others, prolonged frequent and intense episodes of affect dysregulation, a fragile self system, and an inability to adapt to demands of the dynamically changing social environment in a timely manner (Schore, 2001b). The former is a resilience factor for coping with the psychobiological stressors inherent in social interactions; the latter is a risk factor for interruptions of developmental processes and a vulnerability to the coping deficits that define a predisposition to later-forming psychopathology. These conceptions directly relate to what the American Academy of Pediatrics terms "the attainment of optimal physical, mental, and social health for all infants" and thereby the primordial expression of health in "children, adolescents, and young adults."

Appendix: Anatomy and Physiology of Cerebral Functioning in Attachment and Affect Regulation

In his initial outline of attachment theory, Bowlby hypothesized that a succession of increasingly complex regulatory systems involving the limbic system and brain arousal areas mediate attachment processes. The neuroscience literature now refers to the "rostral limbic system," a hierarchical sequence of interconnected limbic areas in amygdala, anterior cingulate, insula, and orbital cortex, and a "circuit of emotion regulation" consisting of amygdala, anterior cingulate, and orbital frontal cortex. Based upon the principle of caudal-to-rostral brain development, I have offered a model of the early experience-dependent maturation of the limbic system and proposed a sequence of regulatory systems that are imprinted by more complex attachment communications and evolve over the first two years of human infancy (Schore, 2001a, 2003b). The optimal formation of these brain areas essential to the child's emotional development depends on the interactive regulation embedded within the attachment communications of the mother-infant relationship.

At birth only the amygdala, a primitive subcortical limbic regulatory system that appraises crude information about external stimuli and modulates autonomic and arousal systems, is online. The right amygdala processes olfactory stimuli within the mother-perinatal infant relationship, and mediates the infant's recognition of the mother's scent as well as the mother's recognition of the neonate through olfactory cues. At eight weeks, a critical period for the development of the anterior cingulate commences, allowing this system to regulate play and separation behaviors, laughing and crying vocalizations, face representations, and the modulation of autonomic activity. The first year also is a critical period of experience-dependent maturation of the right insula, a structure within the temporal lobes that is involved essentially in the subjective awareness of inner body feelings and emotionality, and the right parietal cortex, a posterior cortical area involved in the representation of the physical self and the ability to distinguish self from others.

By the last quarter of the first postnatal year, the orbital (ventromedial) areas of the frontal lobes enter a critical period of growth which continues through the middle of the second year. The orbitofrontal cortex, the hierarchical apex of the limbic system, acts at the highest level of control of behavior, especially in relation to emotion, and is identical to Bowlby's control system of attachment. I have suggested that in mutual gaze transactions, the mother is downloading programs from her limbic system into the child's developing limbic system. A very recent fMRI study by Nitschke and colleagues of mothers viewing a photograph of their own infant shows maximal brain activation in the mother's orbitofrontal cortex, especially on the right side (Nitschke, et al., 2004). These authors conclude that this cortex plays a critical role in the representation of attachment-related positive affect, as described by Bowlby, that it linearly tracks the intensity of positive emotions underlying maternal attachment, and that individual variations in orbitofrontal activation to infant stimuli reflect an important dimension of maternal attachment.

Other studies demonstrate that the right prefrontolimbic areas play a primary role in the appraisal of biologically meaningful exteroceptive and interoceptive self-related information and in the integration of internal physiologic states with salient environmental cues, processes central to the attachment mechanism.

This right cerebral hemisphere is critically involved in regulating the hypothalamic-pituitary-adrenal (HPA) axis and in activating physiologic stress responses (Wittling, 1997). More than any other area of the human prefrontal lobes, the right orbitofrontal cortex, which plays an executive control function for the entire right brain, is linked most directly to the brain's stress regulatory system (Sullivan and Gratton, 2002). Recall, the regulation of stressors in social relationships, modifies prefrontal maturation, and in this manner a secure attachment facilitates the transfer of regulatory capacities from caregiver to infant. Lyons and colleagues state, "Theories of human development suggest that stressful experiences in social relationships modify prefrontal maturation" (Schore, 1996) and demonstrate that conditions that affect early maternal variability in infancy produce "significant differences in right but not left adult prefrontal volumes, with experience-dependent asymmetric variation most clearly expressed in ventral medial cortex measured in vivo by magnetic resonance imaging" (Lyons, et al., 2002). Thus, on a fundamental level, the attachment relationship between the child and primary caregiver is formative because it promotes the development of the brain's major self-regulatory mechanisms.

More specifically, the attachment relationship mediates the dyadic regulation of both positive and negative emotion via the maternal interactive regulation of the infant's postnatally developing autonomic nervous system (ANS). Optimally regulated communications embedded in secure attachment experiences imprint the connections between the postnatally maturing central nervous system limbic system that processes and regulates social-emotional stimuli and the ANS that generates the somatic aspects of emotion. A growing body of work reveals that the right hemisphere is deeply connected into the ANS and that it, more so than the left, controls both sympathetic and parasympathetic responses (Spence, Shapiro, and Zaidel, 1996). The hypothalamus, the head ganglion of the ANS, is right lateralized, and the hypothalamic nuclei are considerably larger on the right side of the human brain. This hemisphere is dominant for the production of corticotrophin-releasing factor and the glucocorticoid cortisol, the neurohormones that mediate stress coping responses. Convincing evidence shows that the infant's relationship with the mother regulates the development of the HPA axis (Gunnar and Donzella, 2002), that neonatal social behavior associated with the HPA axis increases right hemisphere dominance, (Tang, et al., 2003), and that perinatal distress leads to a blunting of the stress response in the right (and not left) prefrontal cortex that is manifest in adulthood (Brake, Sullivan, and Gratton, 2000).[6]

Figure 18.1. Schore's model of affect regulation and right brain development

	INFANT CONTEXT	**MOTHER CONTEXT**	**INTERACTIVE CONTEXT RIGHT BRAIN TO RIGHT BRAIN**
RIGHT BRAIN COMMUNICATION PROCESSES			
VISUAL/ FACIAL			
REGULATED RESPONSE	Orients, explores, gazes at face of mother and others; seeks eye contact. Displays bright, wide-eyed facial expressions. Uses a wide range of affective expressions. Resting quiet-alert state of pleasant facial expressions.	Responds (attunes) to infant's cues with variety of affectively expressive facial expressions (eye contact, smiling, pleasant facial expressions).	Dyadic visual-affective arousal regulation. Each member of dyad focuses gaze upon the other, engaging in mutual eye contact; smiling, bright facial expressions. Interpersonal resonance amplifies positive states in both.
STRESS RESPONSE	During relational stress, transiently avoids orienting, exploring, or gazing at mother's face or engaging in eye contact.	Flat, absent, fear-inducing, or incongruent facial expressions (laughing when infant is distressed).	One breaks off mutual gaze and/or eye contact. Dyad transiently out of sync (misattuned); acute dyadic stress. Absence or avoidance of eye contact by either mother or infant may be a significant indicator requiring further investigation.
VOCAL TONE AND RHYTHM			
REGULATED RESPONSE	Turns toward mother's voice. Uses inviting or playful tone in response (cooing, babbling).	Vocalizes soothing responses with varied tones and rhythms. Modulates tones and rhythms of voice to infant's psychobiological state.	Dyadic auditory-affective arousal regulation. Both match or imitate the other's vocal tones and rhythms.
STRESS RESPONSE	During relational stress, transiently turns away from mother's voice. Uses distressed tone (crying) in response or is nonresponsive.	Uses discordant, harsh, loud, or unmodulated tone and rhythm of voice or does not use vocalizations in response to infant's emotional communication. Does not vocalize or mirror (match) infant's vocalizations.	One uses discordant tone while the other is silent, or both use distressed or discordant tones. Nonresponsivity or turning away from mother's voice may be a significant indicator requiring further investigation.
GESTURAL/ POSTURAL			
REGULATED RESPONSE	Moves limbs and body evenly and fluidly; relaxed posture; reaches and turns toward other or novel social stimulus.	Approaches to soothe, manipulate, or maneuver infant gently and cautiously. Responds to and interprets social bodily based gestures.	In intimate physical context, dyad's rhythmic matching allows bodies to cradle or mold into each other. In social referencing late in first year, gestures become purposeful and synchronized, promoting intersubjective engagement.

STRESS RESPONSE	In socially stressed contexts, moves limbs unevenly and/or frantically. Fails to reach out; averts head, turns body away, stiffens, or arches body to mother's touch.	Approaches infant too quickly or responds to infant in threatening or fearful manner. Handles infant awkwardly or roughly. Misinterprets infant's gestures or does not attempt to soothe, respond, or interpret gestures and body movements.	Infant continues or increases distressed gestures and postures and is unresponsive to mother's efforts. Mother increases rough or awkward gestures and postures. Mother continues to misinterpret infant's gestures and body movements. Dyad becomes frustrated or ceases/fails to attempt to soothe and comfort interactively.
RIGHT BRAIN AFFECT PROCESSING			
POSITIVE AFFECT PROCESSING			
REGULATED RESPONSE	High, positive, arousal. Enjoyment-joy, interest-excitement. Vitality expressed freely.	Happy demeanor; responsive to, supportive of, and matching of infant's affect and positive arousal.	Mutual delight. Mother or infant leads affective interaction while other follows. Non-overwhelming and turn-taking behaviors. Dyadic amplification of positive arousal in relational play.
STRESS RESPONSE	Hyperaroused (overstimulated) or hypoaroused (understimulated).	Incongruent happy demeanor to infant's distressed cues or sad demeanor to infant's positive cues. Continues to fail to create regulated, positive arousal stimuli for infant. Low frequency of play behavior.	Mismatched (misattuned) arousal states. One or both hyperaroused (overstimulated) or one is in positive arousal state while the other is hypoaroused (understimulted) or hyperaroused (overstimulated). Overwhelmed dyad.
REGULATED RESPONSE	Fussy, moody affect expressed freely. Resilience.	Able to tolerate and express sadness, anger, fear in self and infant while seeking to interact appropriately. Participates in interactive repair.	Mutual attuning to disquieting stimuli or condition.
STRESS RESPONSE	Withdraws or is nonresponsive or becomes agitated, frustrated, or fearful when experiencing sensations of distress (dysregulated states). Increasing intensity and duration of either state precludes infant's quick response to soothing attempts and return to regulated state.	Unable to tolerate own negative feelings and responds inappropriately (expresses anger, irritation, or frustration or withdraws and is nonresponsive toward infant). Poor capacity for interactive repair.	Mutual frustration. Mother cannot or does not soothe infant and repair negative affect; dyad remains in distressed state.

RIGHT BRAIN REGULATION			
INTERACTIVE REGULATION	Expresses and recognizes affective facial expressions, vocalizations, and gestures. Infant seeks out mother to co-regulate inner state of being.	Responds with arousal or regulating facial expressions, vocalizations, and gestures. Mother seeks to affect infant's inner state of being.	Each member of dyad contingently responds to other's facial expressions, vocalizations, and gestures (right brain-to-right brain) Mother and infant interactively seek attunement. Frequent episodes of interactive play.
AUTO-REGULATION	Self-soothing behaviors (sucks finger or pacifier, rocks body, holds soft object). Self-created solutions for regulating inner state of being.	Self-calming behaviors (deep breaths, self-talk). Mother lets infant struggle with distress briefly and then regulates (assists in autoregulation).	Each member of dyad remains calm in presence of the other. Each regulates own state of being autonomously.
RIGHT BRAIN DYSREGULATION			
INTERACTIVE DYSREGULATION	Averts gaze, becomes agitated by sounds and gestures. Startles to parent. Habitually disconnects from mother's attempts to co-regulate while inner state escalates. Sense of safety threatened by interaction.	Frequent angry, hostile, facial expressions, harsh tone and uneven rhythms, threatening gestures. Does not look at infant or shows unresponsive "dead face." Repeatedly fails to respond to infant's affective struggle despite infant's escalating inner distress.	Mutual arousal dysregulation. Each individually or dyadically ignores cues of other; dyad fails to collaborate in regulating infant's inner need state. Inconsolable infant may lead to mother's negative feelings toward him/her and diminish mother's confidence in her being a "good enough" mother.
AUTO-DYSREGULATION	Crying, arching, flailing, and vomiting; or blank stare, limp, motionless. Infant repeatedly fails to self-regulate inner state, becoming overwhelmed, eventually exhausted and withdrawn. Dissociates to maternal stimuli. Chronic sense of threat or lack of sense of safety.	Irritable, threatening, intrusive, and rough or flat affect; unresponsive. Disregards infant's ability to autoregulate by quieting or stimulating self. Dissociates to infant's stimuli.	Both agitated or withdrawn in presence of other. Both fail to allow infant to enlarge capacity to self-regulate affect. No relational or intersubjective context.

CHAPTER 19

Birth Ignition Skills, Part 1

The Stillpoint

What is an infant? No one quite knows the inner experience of an infant or even what an infant truly is because of a mass of cultural confusion. This comes from many disciplines in the scientific or psychological communities competing for the discovery of the infant's experience. For example, some in the scientific community say that infants do not experience physical pain yet the pre- and perinatal psychology community says that they do. Both have evidence to support their claims, and children who are ill and their practitioners are caught in the middle of the debate, not to mention the challenges faced by parents. Thus, from the biodynamic craniosacral therapy point of view, the use of manual therapy in a pediatric practice must find a common ground, or, as one osteopath says, a meeting place, where the infant as client and the practitioner can meet halfway, so to speak. The recognition and perception of the movement of wholeness in the practitioner, which is the perception of the outside presence of Primary Respiration, is a starting point in a relationship. This is the tempo in which an infant is to be greeted at the beginning, middle, and end of a session. Primary Respiration is the sense of unconditional love that so frequently permeates the treatment room when in the presence of a child who is chronically ill, experiencing developmental issues, or traumatized from birth.

There is another meeting place that must be found as the practitioner settles into the field of the infant-mother dyad. That meeting place is a fulcrum of deep stillness in between these two wholes of practitioner and mother-child. The practitioner has the responsibility of entering the fulcrum of stillness and waiting there until the infant or child can join her in the stillness. The stillness is the health spoken of in osteopathy. Biodynamic work with children, especially with newborn babies, spontaneously proceeds from this meeting place where two wholes breathing at the tempo of Primary Respiration come together and rest in a stillpoint. It is a stillpoint that automatically shifts from the horizon to the treatment room.

The meeting place is actually the shared heart between the mother-child dyad and the practitioner. It is as though the therapeutic relationship is an extended cardiovascular system with the center point being the actual heart in between the two people. Embryologically, it can be observed that the pericardium of the heart first develops directly in front of the face and neck of the embryo and then is brought into the interior of the embryo. It is this image of the shared heart space that is actually in front of our very face and neck that is the meeting place. The heart primordium is a fluid-filled space, empty of any structure. Initially, it is dynamically still and thus the meeting place is nothing other than the embryonic heart waiting to be ignited by the shared empathy and compassion of the mother-child dyad and the practitioner. The infant is so close to its conception that he still wears the actual face of creation. The face is a stillpoint in the developing heart and pericardium from which unconditional love moves. The heart of loving kindness and compassion is the meeting place. Is it any different when working with an adult?

Once the meeting place has been found by the practitioner and other considerations are held and contained, such as the infant's relationship with the mother, a sequence of biodynamic contemplations regarding the pre-conception, conception, gestation, and birth process can be observed in the therapeutic relationship. The mother is usually physically present with her child and so she is included in the still meeting place by the practitioner. It is not so much a triad (therapist-infant-mother) as it is two metabolic fields interacting. The mother-child is a coupled metabolic field and the practitioner is an autonomous metabolic field. Therefore the practitioner is in relationship with the mother-infant dyad as a metabolic field that is usually under stress and must have the freedom to self-regulate within a slow tempo and a stillpoint.

Subsequent birth ignition skills in a biodynamic approach to working with infants and children are focused on the stillpoint as the starting point, so to speak. Ignition of the first breath follows and the first gaze and first touch are covered in the next chapter. Birth ignition requires knowledge of what one osteopath calls rebalancing skills. These skills apply to adult clients and especially infants and children. Regarding children, they are based on a biodynamic understanding of the complex metabolic and physiological transition that an infant makes before, during, and after birth, discussed in Volume One. They are also based on understanding the relationship of the birth process to the dynamic morphology of the embryo. In other words, birth is a recapitulation of embryonic development. It is therefore out of sequence to work on an infant's cranium in the initial phases of session work for several reasons. First is the sequence of the timing of the development of the endoderm in the embryo. After birth the endoderm derivatives relate to the suck-swallow-breathe reflex, compression in the fluid body, and their interrelationships. These are the first clinical considerations when treating an infant or a child that I will discuss.

The second consideration when treating infants is that the developing brain is being guided by the mother. In this context the mother needs to be treated and have her stress levels reduced. This reflexes directly into the infant's brain. Regarding cranial molding and sutural overlapping from a vaginal birth, it must be remembered that mothers naturally stroke their babies all over their body and especially the head. It has been observed in other cultures that the way a mother strokes her baby's head gradually relieves cranial molding and normalizes the shape of the infant's cranium, even in some severe cases of plagiocephaly. I rarely meet an infant who accepts my touch on its head. This is the mother's job and I frequently teach mothers how to gently stroke their baby's head.

What follows is a simplified nonlinear sequence of biodynamic explorations with the infant while being held by its mother or the child crawling on the floor in the presence of the mother or father or other family members. This exploration is also done with adults who need rebalancing.

1. Orienting to a stillpoint outside the infant's body, in the room, or out in space is of paramount importance.

2. Synchronizing with Primary Respiration in the mother and her baby. When contact is appropriate, I like to work with both the mother and her baby while she is holding him. I place my hand on the mother's back and the other hand over her hand as it cradles her baby. Then I wait to sense Primary Respiration breathing between my two hands. I coach the mother when I sense Primary Respiration changing directions and see if she can perceive it along with me.

3. Orienting to a stillpoint in the fluid body, either in back of the umbilicus (L2–L3) or at the abdominal-thoracic junction (the floating ribs). This is sometimes called an EV4 of the Reciprocal Tension Potency (RTP) of the fluid body manifesting as a horizontal and three-dimensional movement perpendicular to its midline of the longitudinal fluctuation. This is accomplished by approaching the baby from the side or, alternatively with adults, by sitting at the head of the client with both hands under the scapulae. This is called a scapular EV4.

4. Orienting to a stillpoint on the long axis between the fourth ventricle and the lumbar cistern. All phases of a vaginal birth cause compression on the

long axis of the body and the fluid body, especially the birth lie side. The fluid body tends to naturally stillpoint in the fourth ventricle as a result of a vaginal birth. The stillpoint may automatically shift between the third ventricle and the lumbar cistern, depending on the nature of the birth such as a C-section. It may automatically shift outside of the infant's body depending on the amount of trauma associated with the birth. Gentle contact with the occiput and low back allows the long-axis birth stillpoint, if accessible in the body, to manifest even in some C-section babies. This is a critical ignition for the spinal nerves, the cerebrospinal fluid (CSF), the brain, and the fluid body in general.

5. Subsequent evaluation of children involves the biodynamics of what is called the "first breath" in osteopathy. Facilitating a biodynamic first breath is accomplished by synchronizing primary inhalation with secondary inhalation, first in the practitioner and then with the client. This requires classroom training and the ability to attend to Primary Respiration through its five-step conception-ignition cycle of synchronization, augmentation, spark, permeation, and disengagement. Once the practitioner has a clear perception of a personal relationship with the outside and inside presence of Primary Respiration in relationship to secondary respiration in herself first, she can pendulate to sensing the client's Primary Respiration. She listens for the last several seconds of primary exhalation as it is decelerating and entering its phase of augmentation. At that point, the practitioner asks the client (or observes in the infant and child the place where the secondary respiration changes) to take a deep, slow inhalation with the respiratory diaphragm. This augments the spark at the beginning of primary inhalation and reorients the body's physiology and metabolism to be permeated by the potency of Primary Respiration and for the body's physiological systems to disengage, which means to assume a normal relationship with the midline of stillness.

6. A phase of the session, or perhaps a marker for the end of a session, occurs when the practitioner is able to differentiate one of the following: three cycles of unchanging amplitude in the fluid body; two cycles of Primary Respiration going out to the horizon and back; or a stillpoint that expands from the center of the client-therapist dyad out to the horizon. Alternatively, the child gets up and moves away to take a break.

7. Biodynamic palpation skills involve the use of buoyant hands that are empty of tissue. This means developing the capacity to allow the tissue structure of the soma to become totally fluid on the inside of one's hands and body

as well as the same in the client in order to be immersed in the protoplasm while maintaining contact with the whole via Primary Respiration. The hands become transparent, living water with the thickness of liquid soap. Gradually the practitioner imagines the structure of her body and that of the client becoming a three-dimensional liquid and waits for his fluid body to be moved by Primary Respiration, much like a sea sponge or a piece of seaweed in the ocean. The practitioner attends to the ocean around and inside her body first, and then the seaweed. The priority is always the movement of the whole after orienting to a stillpoint. The use of metaphor and image is a way to contact the fluids.

8. The focused intention of biodynamic craniosacral therapy after the stillpoint is to maintain a systemic sense of the whole body and the sea around us. In other words, the practitioner senses and images her body three-dimensionally. It starts by sensing the total surface volume of the skin (see Volume One for an extended meditation on sensing the skin). The next step is maintaining an awareness of the whole body and the space around it as a fluid-filled egg shape and pendulating toward the client's whole body as an egg-shaped fluid ocean or sea sponge. Imagine the practitioner expanding her egg out three-dimensionally until it enfolds the client's body as a function of its expansion and contraction. The client is influenced by the practitioner's tide more than the hands. This requires a wide perceptual field, a mind of equanimity, and a heart-centered stillpoint that is the fulcrum the egg breathes around.

9. The stillpoint and Primary Respiration are dynamically related to one another. They both originate from the horizon and inform the midline of the body. They are supposed to change places with one another during a session as a function of the practitioner's perception. This is the basic rhythm of a biodynamic craniosacral therapy session. The perception of this rhythm guides the session as the constant background beat in case functional and biomechanical skills might need to be employed with a particular child.

10. The skin develops in utero as the floor of the ocean of the yolk sac then the chorion and finally the amniotic fluid. The skin of the embryo separates the outside ocean of the yolk sac from the inside ocean of the amnion in the early embryo, and then it reverses itself and the skin gets turned inside out. The majority of the internal embryo is 98 percent protoplasm. Therefore when sensing the skin of the client, it must be imaged and palpated as a kind of diaphragm between the ocean outside and the ocean inside the body. It is this diaphragm that automatically shifts with Primary Respiration. Imagine

that the skin is actually a membrane sandwiched between the longitudinal fluctuation of the fluid body inside the soma and the outer edge of the fluid body approximately 12–15 inches off of the soma. This skin diaphragm is synchronized with the respiratory diaphragm during the first breath and then is used to sense the mother's autonomic nervous system, heart, and respiratory diaphragm while being held.

11. Concurrent with these biodynamic considerations is the attachment and bonding process between the caregiver (mother) and her child. Parenting skills, especially the CALMS method (Contey and Takikawa, 2007), are recommended. CALMS stands for the following sequence: C = Check in with yourself, A = Allow a breath, L = Listen to your baby, M = Make contact and mirror the baby's feelings, and S = Soothe your baby. As a practitioner comes into relationship with an infant and mother, she must be able to assess any attachment stress between them. This CALMS method is a very simple way to assess the mother-infant dyad. Frequently, the baby is the identified patient in a therapeutic situation but in reality the mother's stress levels are being metabolized by the infant and consequently the focus of work needs to be on relieving maternal stress. I always work on the mother separately because I have seen it over and over that this will improve the baby's symptoms in many cases of noncomplex trauma.

12. The next part in an evaluation sequence would involve orthopedic considerations and facilitation of the suck-swallow-breathe reflex in the infant. This is especially needed to free up the heart in relationship to pulmonary circulation, the mesenteries in relationship to bowel movements, and umbilical affect for digestion and absorption of nutrition. The celiac, superior, and inferior mesenteric arteries must be free to move since the endoderm is oriented to them. These arteries are directly anterior to the spine and form the middle or fulcrum for the whole fluid body. I gently place my hand under a baby's floating ribs and lumbar spine and sense the RTP until it stillpoints as outlined in number 2 above.

13. Finally (but not by any means the last consideration), the practitioner tends to the cranial base and the embryological aspects of the viscerocranium (face). The intention is to normalize motion in the fluid body of the face and this includes the top of the cranial base via the sphenoid bone. Precise knowledge of the embryological development of the face must be known, especially its horizontal orientation in growth and development. The development of the face is responsible for organizing the whole head. One of the reasons for this is that the face derives chiefly from endoderm, which

again relates to the suck-swallow-breathe reflex. In addition, precise knowledge of the anatomical development after birth of the cranial base over the first six years of life must be known before approaching an infant's head. The cranial bones are not fixed to the dura mater after birth as they are in the adult. The perinatal development of the cranial base is related to the social nervous system that I will discuss in a later chapter. Consequently, the cranial base is related to emotional expression. Biodynamic work with infants and children is sequenced from the belly, to the heart, and finally to the face and calvarium rather than the vault and never during the opening few sessions. Even with moderate to severe cranial trauma from birth, the biomechanical practitioner would always consider the sacrum first. It is the same in biodynamic practice.

Conclusion

I consciously avoid teaching the four stages of birth in the early stages of any biodynamic craniosacral therapy foundation training. This is partly because it leads the new student into a very mechanical representation of a complex nonlinear process and into the domain of tissue imprinting (conjunct sites and pathways, etc.) of the birth process, especially the cranium of the infant. I look at birth embryologically first and, from this point of view, understand birth as a recapitulation of embryonic development. I believe the infant is trying to tell his story of creation that started nine months ago more than the more immediate experience of birth, because they are both the same to the infant.

So in the sense that birth is initiated by a mechanical flexion motion of the infant's cranium engaging the maternal pelvis and then going into a phase of extension, one could say it is the opposite or the reverse of the morphological fluid process of embryonic development. I mean to say that the last stage of the morphological development of the embryo is flexion-extension (folding-unfolding) and that motion somehow initiates the beginning of the birth process. Then the infant must twist himself out of the birth canal. Late-stage embryos twist like a Sufi dancer as well. Can this also be considered a preexercising of a later birth function? Then after considerable compression throughout the whole birth process, the head is born and decompresses. This is clearly similar to the compression-decompression of the first two weeks of development postfertilization. So the infant comes out in the reverse order of its embryonic development, such that upon birth the newborn is a newly conceived human being. At all times we could learn to touch our clients and infant clients as though we are touching an embryo. Is that possible and what type of sensitivity would that require?

The baby is starting over again in a new phase of development just as being conceived was a new phase of development and hardly the beginning of a "new life." All stages of birth involve a recapitulation of embryonic morphology. The first week postfertilization is about tremendous compressional forces, soon to be reexperienced nine months later, as I mentioned above. That is why the focus in a session is on the stillpoint found at the middle place of all the compression-decompression, twisting, and flexion-extension, and often that middle place is located at a considerable distance outside the body. After establishing the meeting place, the practitioner synchronizes with Primary Respiration in the mother and her baby and then facilitates decompression in the fluid body via the stillpoint, rather than decompression in the tissue fields and cranium. It is a matter of discovering the correct sequence for the application of biomechanical work. Biodynamic craniosacral therapy is an honoring of the metabolic physical forces of creation (biokinetics). The infant, therefore, is closer to its creation than ever before and is the visible symbol of the invisible movement and manifestation of creation and incarnation. The meeting place is therefore the space of creation and is sacred.

Initially, the main event biodynamically in treating children is evaluating the endoderm derivatives, as I said above. It is not so much that the endoderm gets compressed during birth and is part of the recapitulation process. It is more that the purpose of the compressional forces of birth is to initialize the endoderm derivatives with the ignition of potency for suck-swallow-breathe, emotional development, and pulmonary circulation to begin. Furthermore, the endoderm is the *first* differentiation to occur in the central body of the embryo at the end of the first week and beginning of the second week. It is the endoderm that is responsible for a very core perception of our internal reality. It is now sometimes called the "gut brain" (Gershon, 1998). The endoderm initially differentiates as the first fluid cavity outside the embryo and then continues its differentiation inside the body wall of the embryo as a tube. The organizing midline of the gut tube occupies the body location of the acupuncture meridian of the conception vessel in Traditional Chinese Medicine, from the pubic symphasis up to the glabella of the frontal bone. It is not the conception vessel per se, but rather the same line in that space, as the skin in the anterior surface of the embryo is the last to close and form the definitive container of the soma.

Clinically, when working with children and infants, the endoderm derivatives are the most easily accessible from both the front and back of the child, and the infant is usually more receptive to having a practitioner come into relationship with the endoderm derivatives first, rather than the cranium or nervous system (both of which are primarily mom's job, not the practitioner's). It is the mother's job to stroke her baby's head and smooth out the infant's cranium, not mine, as I said above.

Finally, that leaves us with the mesoderm derivatives—the main ones being the heart and blood. Well, this means that the heart and blood are intimately connected to the endoderm derivatives and closer to the fluid body and more important biodynamically as the communication system between ectoderm derivatives and endoderm derivatives. An infant is expected to take his first breath within five minutes after leaving the aquatic breathing environment that has nurtured him for nine months. But the heart itself takes a year to transition after birth, to grow into a relationship with pulmonary circulation. One must consider that the infant needs up to six years to successfully transition physiologically from the aquatic breathing environment to an air breathing environment.

Now, if we look at the endoderm embryonically, we see that it is the endoderm that is inducing the brain and cranium as well as parts of the cardiovascular system. It is rather simple to extrapolate these embryonic realities, and add that understanding into clinical pediatric practice. Biodynamic craniosacral therapy with infants and children is indeed a somewhat different approach, but it is an authentic and clinically appropriate way of relating to infants and children in this day and age of infant trauma. It is the demand of our time to examine our developmental models and begin to see the infant as an embryo and the adult as an embryo. Then we must ask ourselves this important question: What is an embryo?

CHAPTER 20

Birth Ignition Skills, Part 2

The First Touch—The First Gaze

I would like to take some time explaining the next phase of birth ignition more deeply. Birth ignition is the biodynamic and biomechanical process of transitioning from inside the womb to outside the womb. In the previous chapter I focused on the stillpoint, the first breath, and other therapeutic concerns. The first breath is that literal moment when the infant has been birthed from the mother's womb and takes his first oxygenated breath. This transition is very brief and initially occurs within minutes of being born or brain damage may happen. I have worked with many children who have such challenges. For the previous nine months, the prenate has been breathing fluid and within moments of being born, must accomplish an incredibly sophisticated physiological transition from aquatic breathing to air breathing. Chapter 26 in Volume One covers this transition in detail.

The most important principle of birth ignition, however, is not only the physiological aspects, but also the psychospiritual dynamics of this huge transition. At the very least, birth ignition necessarily includes the entire time of pregnancy, labor, and delivery, and the first two years of life outside the womb. It is a sequence of developmental transitions that spans at least three years rather than the first breath, which is one of many transition points that contain risks for death or trauma. Following the first breath in an uncomplicated birth, it is natural and instinctual for the newborn baby to be placed on the mother's abdomen skin to skin and given the opportunity for self-attachment and bonding to the mother and her breast and to settle after this stressful transition.

The infant ideally is able to move up from the mother's abdomen to a resting position over her heart in alignment with one of her breasts. Infants and mothers are particularly oriented to feeding from the left breast and it seems that this is in association with a closer proximity to the mother's heart so the infant can maintain a felt sense of the movement of the mother's heart just as he did in the womb. Through the galvanic skin response the infant is also resonating with the mother's autonomic nervous system and movement of the respiratory diaphragm as well as the heart. This skin-to-skin contact tells the infant the inner emotional state of the mother and whether the infant needs to modify his physiology unconsciously. This positioning also facilitates neurological reflexes in the right hemisphere of both the mother and her infant that are critical for learning self-regulation of emotions. As a matter of fact, the first two years of perinatal neurological development are focused on the learning of emotional self-regulation while in relationship with the caregiver. Please refer to Volume One for an in-depth discussion of self-regulation and the two chapters in this section on the biodynamics of self-regulation.

It would not be unusual at all for the infant to need some assistance in learning how to suck, swallow, and breathe all at the same time from the mother's breast. Each infant's transition involves a degree of life-death intensity and even moments of overwhelm in order to get out of the womb. Such stress during birth has the potential to delay normal self-attachment and bonding, especially if coupled to medical interventions. The system is very forgiving and some researchers believe that a mother and her infant have up to six months to self-attach and breastfeed without harmful consequences for the baby. Other researchers have said that it is never too late in a person's life to receive love and heal the past, even if one was bottle fed or experienced attachment trauma. But for all babies, it is a natural instinct to nurse immediately and some may take longer than others to settle and become still. The key words here are *settling* and *stilling*. This is a dramatic change in tempo from the hours of labor and delivery that preceded the self-attachment and bonding process. It is interesting to note that the German word for breastfeeding is *stillen,* which means to become still and be in a settled place and relatively free of stress in order to nurture the infant through the breast.

Self-attachment is also an endocrine role reversal, so to speak, as the hormone oxytocin at the beginning of labor helps to speed it up and now that breastfeeding has begun, oxytocin is associated now with a slow tempo and a pervasive feeling of warmth, nurturing, and love that is distributed through the body via the heart and cardiovascular system. Dr. Michel Odent (Odent, 1999), a French researcher, has called oxytocin "the hormone of love."

Research has shown that the infant's naked body should ideally have complete skin-to-skin contact (SSC) with the mother's bare skin over her heart. This facilitates thermal regulation and the lowering of stress hormones in both the mother's and the infant's body from the recent birth (Bergman, Linley, and

Fawcus, 2004). In addition, it may take up to a year for the liver, heart, and pulmonary system to complete their structural transition from prenatal arteries and veins to postnatal ligaments and full pulmonary circulation. This includes proper closure of the foramen ovale between the right and left atrium of the heart and the full opening of the pulmonary artery from the heart to the lungs. It is my contention that the position of the infant's body over the mother's heart for prolonged periods of time contributes to the proper closure of the foramen ovale. It also allows the mother to stroke her infant's head with loving kindness. I call this the *first touch*. This is a natural instinct that mothers have to caress their baby with absolute loving kindness. It also has the effect of decompressing the infant's cranial molding (sutural overlapping and asymmetrical head shape from a vaginal delivery). In fact, the natural instinct of the mother is to stroke every inch of her baby's body! This is part of nature's welcome party for the newborn.

Those were some of the physiological and structural considerations regarding the self-attachment and bonding sequence. There is, however, another event that occurs around the first touch that I call the *first gaze*. As the infant settles into an embodied experience of being nurtured and held, the mother likewise begins to settle from the enormously hard work she has just accomplished. At that moment of settling and stilling, it has been frequently reported that a mother looks at her baby calmly for the first time and enters a portal into a pervasive and embodied sense of unconditional love for her infant as the infant also radiates pure love for the mother.

There is a radiance and a warmth that emanates from the mother as she looks deeply at her baby. Likewise, the infant gets to gaze, sense, and express love to the mother. This radiance and flow between the mother and her child flows from the first gaze. It is unconditional love. At last the mother can see the first visible manifestation of creation that up until now has been hidden in her womb and known only through its movements, its size, and weight, and perhaps an invisible communication or dream between the two of them. Even an ultrasound is the most unaesthetic picture of an unborn baby that could be seen. Now with the first gaze, creation is viewed in all of its glory. It is creation as close as it can be to its point of origin nine months previously.

Unconditional love is ignited after birth as a dynamic relationship between the mother and her child. Love gestated for nine months now becomes embodied. Unconditional love from the infant to the mother is reflected back to the infant and imprinted through the skin of the baby, the cardiovascular system of the baby, the autonomic nervous system of the baby, the central nervous system of the baby, and so forth. All systems of the body, including the fluid body itself, receive a massive influx of unconditional love that breathes not only back and forth between the mother and child, but fills the room. Thus unconditional love becomes the ground of being of the newborn baby and the proper field of growth for all future development. It is the felt sense of the emotional grace of Primary Respiration.

Clinical Exercise: The First Touch—The First Gaze

In this particular exploration, we will be working in triads. There will be the position of client, the position of caregiver, and the position of the therapist. The client will be lying supine on the table. The caregiver will sit at the side and be prepared to place her hands in the "pietà" position with one hand under the client-infant's shoulder blade and the other hand under the leg or knee, depending on the reach of that caregiver.

The location of the therapist is at a discreet distance away from the caregiving dyad and must be negotiated with the dyad in terms of a comfortable distance that is respectful and unobtrusive, visually and energetically. The first phase of the exercise is the phase of settling and stilling without physical contact. All three members of the triad are seeking the meeting place of a stillpoint spoken of in the last chapter. The meeting place is that common area outside of their three bodies where a stillpoint can be perceived by one or more members of the triad. It may take time to do so and there is very little verbal interaction to affirm that all three are located in the meeting place of the stillpoint. What is important, however, is that the caregiver has a sense of a stillpoint located somewhere inside or outside of her body.

I usually suggest to students that they begin by accessing a stillpoint either in their umbilical area, their pericardial area, or the area around their third ventricle. These are the three embryonic fulcrums of stillness mentioned in Section I on clinical practice. Then I ask the students to connect those fulcrums with the horizon, with nature, or with the earth and ocean below. By connecting one or more of the fulcrums with the outside world and its farthest edge, the student can then tune in to the slow tempo of Primary Respiration. The next step is synchronizing with Primary Respiration. Once Primary Respiration has been accessed, it will normally recede from the student's perception and be replaced with the perception of a more systemic or global stillpoint that permeates the inside and outside of the body of the student-practitioner. There is a rhythmic interchange of the stillness with Primary Respiration regularly in a session.

The next step involves the student in the role of caregiver negotiating permission to make contact with the client. This is the first touch—that first moment when the mother touches her newborn as though touching the face of God. This is the divine child in her eyes. The first touch is indeed a feather on the breath of God. This first touch establishes a context of touch as nurturing and loving in the infant's brain and heart. It establishes a baseline of nonconfusing physical contact to be established for a lifetime and thus allows the infant to develop clarity of perception when touched by other people later in life. If damaged, this context center of the brain will become irritated even from the loving touch of other people. Once this loving first touch has been established, the caregiver returns her personal perception to the stillpoint or the meeting place.

Here is a sequence of contemplations.

The first contemplation is that the caregiver is one whole, huge heart from head to foot, the client is the vascular system and all the blood, and the hands and arms of the caregiver represent the connecting stalk with the umbilical veins and arteries. Always the student-practitioner is encouraged to perceive the interchange between the stillpoint and Primary Respiration in himself first. Then this image is reversed. The client becomes the heart, and the caregiver the blood, and so forth. It is important for the practitioner to remember to stay within the tempo of Primary Respiration and its moving fulcrum of stillness.

At the next stage I suggest that the triad begin sensing where warmth and heat are located in their bodies. I may ask each of them to imagine that they are radiating heat from their heart to the heart of the other person in the tempo of Primary Respiration. The felt sense of love biodynamically from the first touch and the first gaze is heat. This is because a major development happening with the first touch and first gaze is physiological thermal regulation in the brain, heart, and whole body. Its perception as an adult may start in the hands, the spine, the face, or the chest and heart area of the practitioner. The practitioner focuses on the heat permeating his whole body. Many clients get warm and practitioners begin to break out in a sweat spontaneously during a session. This is the active combustion of the ignition system under the guidance of Primary Respiration. This is the heart of the therapeutic response in biodynamic craniosacral therapy. The heat tells you that you are permeated with love or being loved. It is the movement of the mystery.

The next important phase is that the caregiver actively imagines being the mother and the client his or her biological child. It has been said by many Buddhist teachers that even a man has been a mother in a past life. So if the student-practitioner is male, as I have indicated throughout this chapter, he should engender and imagine himself as mother at this particular time. The client on the table is the child. This is the phase of the exploration called the first gaze. This is an attempt to deepen the perception of Primary Respiration and stillness into its feeling tone of unconditional love.

The caregiver-mother now begins to contemplate unconditional love flowing between him and his child on the table as the color of blood. This is done in the tempo of Primary Respiration and I like to imagine that the blood has the viscosity of liquid soap as it flows from heart to heart. The child on the table is also contemplating this aspect of being held by the mother and all that that means to receive her blood as during pregnancy. The heart warms the blood through the power of unconditional love. The heat mixes with unconditional love and moves through the blood and circulates throughout the soma. The heat of love becomes the felt sense of the flow of grace within and between two people.

After several minutes, the roles are reversed. The dyad stays located in its same physical position and only mentally and emotionally changes positions. The child on the table is the mother lying on the table and the caregiver is the child who is holding the mother. The child now radiates unconditional love to her mother in the role reversal because this is the way it was at the beginning, or was supposed to be. All an infant knows how to do is shower mom with love and now this primal act is recapitulated between two adults under the supervision of Primary Respiration. These contemplations, when held in the context of Primary Respiration and stillness as the heat and grace of unconditional love, allow the student-practitioner to uncouple from the past and reorient memory to the preexisting state of unconditional love. Rather than grieving for the loss of something missing, it is discovered that it was there all along and simply forgotten. This is a heart-to-heart connection that requires some genuine emotion in the form of heat to reignite the torch of unconditional love.

What is the role of the third person in this triad? That person is actually the therapist. It is the job of the therapist to maintain contact with the outside presence of Primary Respiration and occasionally check in to the meeting place of the stillpoint. The therapist is witnessing a metabolic field between a mother and her child and places the caregiving dyad in a protective bubble. The therapist helps to hold the bubble for the expression of unconditional love by staying in touch with its midline. The therapist witnesses and holds that caregiving relationship with deep feeling and emotion as he also has the opportunity to uncouple from his own personal past and history, just as the other two people in the dyad are loving each other as a mother and newborn baby.

The therapist is placing himself in a stillpoint located somewhere outside the biosphere around the mother and her infant, as Dr. Becker called it. This is the outer edge of the chorionic cavity. It is not immediately located within the body of either the mother or the child, but is a dynamic state of circulating blood and stillness that can be felt in the room or perhaps somewhere all the way out to the horizon. It was during the second week postfertilization that the chorion became surrounded by stillpoints so the mother's blood could orient to her embryo. Imagine that the whole edge of the bubble of the mother-child dyad is all stillpoints. The chorion allows the embryo to orient to a place outside its body as it goes through enormous structural and functional processes for quite some time after conception and then after birth. Likewise the body of the mother takes up to two years to integrate her physiological changes after birth. So both the mother and her baby have a sanctuary to rest in when necessary outside of their bodies but in a place they both can share in private. The practitioner must support this sacred sanctuary as a type of holy chorion.

Conclusion

It has been said by Dr. Alan Schore that the client-therapist relationship is a direct analog of the mother-child relationship. The *first touch* and *first gaze* are important biodynamic contemplations that will bring to consciousness one's personal history of issues with unconditional love. It is an opportunity to uncouple gracefully from conditional love and without overactivation because of the ability to rest in the dynamic container of Primary Respiration and its fulcrum of stillness now located everywhere around the two. This is the great mother beyond biology. It is more like a great heart. It is an opportunity to shift one's allegiance from a personal history of heart wounding to the felt sense of Primary Respiration as unconditional love and the heat that flows from it. Whether people perceive that they did not receive unconditional love from their original caregiver is not a problem when it comes to Primary Respiration. The issue is whether we have the courage to uncouple from our history and let our infant body be gazed upon by the open heart of another person in the safety of stillness and silence.

CHAPTER 21

Biodynamics of Self-Regulation, Part 1: Projection, Dissociation, and Safety

The basic principle of biodynamic practice is that the client-practitioner relationship is a direct analog of the infant-mother attachment relationship. For those unfamiliar with attachment literature, please read the section on pediatric practice in Volume One (Shea, 2007) or Daniel Siegel's book *The Developing Mind: Toward a Neurobiology of Interpersonal Experience* (Siegel, 1999). To summarize: There are four styles of infant-mother attachment. Only one of them is considered to be a "secure" attachment and is likely to occur in 50 percent or less of the population. The remaining three styles of attachment are considered to be "insecure" and, therefore, damaging in varying degrees to the development of the infant's capacity to self-regulate emotions. One type of insecure attachment tends to interrupt the infant when she is trying to settle, another to ignore the infant's needs, and a third to generate chronic fear in the infant as the result of the parents' behavior.

Self-regulation of emotions is the primary function of an infant's brain. It is now considered to supersede sensory-motor development and cognitive development (Immordino-Yang and Damasio, 2007) throughout the lifespan. It involves the critically important making of a filter through which to view life psychologically, and respond to life behaviorally and physiologically into adulthood (Schore, 2001a). Evaluation and support of self-regulation, then, is a key to effective therapeutic outcomes in *any* system of therapy, especially biodynamic craniosacral therapy.

The style of attachment shapes the brain. The shaping process imprints the brain with emotional tendencies and beliefs about getting needs met and the way the world works that are carried through life as unconscious behaviors and working models of reality. The models are learned filters of experience over one's body and mind that change the perception of the environment (reality). Filters include internalized images and story lines (autobiography and mythology), since this is how the mind of a newborn baby and toddler works. Cognitive ability develops after infancy, as the child matures. Imprinted emotions are usually very strong emotions that cause substantial mental affliction. Such strong affliction results in the need to dissociate, project, and use transference to unload the unbearable internal pressure and conflict, all of which is largely below conscious awareness. This is what I call the cycle of affect from an insecure attachment. The place of repair in biodynamic craniosacral therapy is how the practitioner is attuned to stillness and Primary Respiration in himself first and the client second. This attunement mimics the attunement of a secure attachment and thus decompresses the corticolimbic system of the client and builds an internalized still witness, both of which are essential for self-regulation. The practitioner becomes an equal partner in the therapeutic process of reestablishing self-regulation.

Brain Mapping

Brain mapping has provided a wealth of new information on how the brain grows and develops. There are vertical-hierarchical models and horizontal-functional models. The hierarchical model of Paul MacLean (MacLean, 1973) is a great teaching model because of its simplicity. He divided the brain into three structural-functional components: the brain stem or action brain, the limbic system or emotional brain, and the cortex or thinking brain. The limbic system has been renamed the corticolimbic system and has components throughout MacLean's triune brain concept. Joseph Chilton Pearce (Pearce, 2004) points out that Schore's work indicates a fourth component to the hierarchical brain, which is the orbitofrontal cortex (OFC). The OFC has top-down regulatory control over the other three components via its capacity for witness consciousness. Additionally, by way of principle, the brain is fundamentally organized horizontally into two parts, a right hemisphere and a left hemisphere. While this is old information, the new paradigm states that the right hemisphere is dominant before and after birth and, therefore, forms the foundation of crucial lifelong self-regulatory functions. Figure 21.1 shows these different regions of the brain.

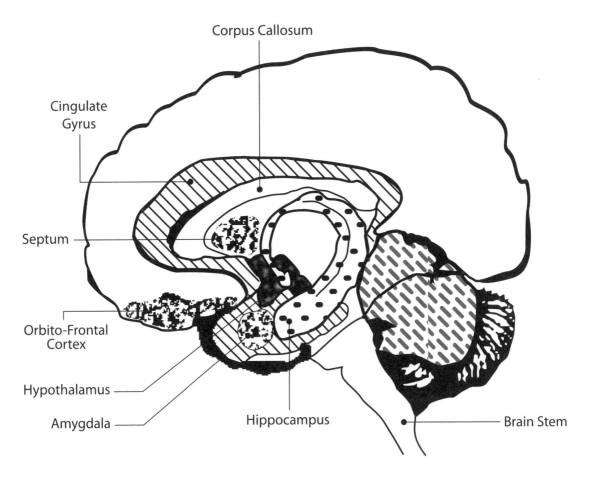

Figure 21.1. A cross-section of the human brain
showing the corticolimbic system

The left hemisphere is no longer considered to be the dominant hemisphere with its cognitive functioning. Rather, the right hemisphere is dominant, particularly in the first two years after birth, and consequently throughout the lifespan. It is this hemisphere that develops the capacity for self-regulation of emotions in the OFC, the primary goal of the brain during this period of development, through the experience of being in a relationship with a mother-person. In other words, interpersonal experience wires together the function of the right hemisphere from the brain stem through the limbic system and forward into the OFC from its first appearance at thirty-three days postfertilization. Because there are no cognitive functions in place during those first two years of life, the right hemisphere designs the basic wiring mechanism. The corticolimbic system is the predominant aspect of the right hemisphere. Its apex is in the prefrontal cortex or the OFC. This is the highest neurological center known for regulatory function in the human body. Its ability to differentiate during the first eighteen months after birth is dependent upon a cumulative set of experiences mediated neurologically between the infant's right hemisphere and the mother's right hemisphere.

Right-brain processes optimally involve empathy, managing strong emotions, social adjustment, mood control, drive and responsibility, the highest level of control of behavior, witness consciousness, image-generating picturing or "image-thinking," nonlinear cognition, spatial awareness, the capacity to sustain attention over time, and the capacity for complexity and chaos. In addition, the right hemisphere monitors the totality of our bodily sensations (interoception) and visceral functioning. Through the dorsal motor nucleus (DMNX) of the polyvagal system (the vagus nerve is the tenth cranial nerve), the right hemisphere monitors visceral functioning. All of this happens quite rapidly in the right hemisphere. Imagine that the right brain is constantly monitoring the totality of the inside of the body, all of its systems, every second of our waking life! This is an enormous job. So, there is a lot happening below our conscious awareness. The right brain has to filter all of this information and build a filter that is predictive of future events. Those filters that sort out relevance and context, especially emotionally, develop early in an embryo, continue with the fetus, and come to fruition in a newborn during the first two years after birth.

The OFC and its self-regulatory capacities are designed to stabilize moods and emotions and help the system rapidly recover from disruptive emotions and distress states in general. A mature OFC will move toward positive emotions and states. An immature OFC fails at such recovery processes and classically overreacts to minor stimulus. It is important to watch the stimulus-response system in a client. This provides a lot of information about the client's preverbal time of life. The OFC inhibits subcortical emotional processes such as overactivation of the hypothalamus and it is the regulator of arousal. It maintains responsibility for certain important controls over autonomic activity, especially if the OFC experiences a secure attachment. This is especially true in the right hemisphere of the brain. The right hemisphere and the right lateralized OFC are responsible for the primary processing of emotions and are typically considered to be unconscious. The right hemisphere, including the amygdala and cingulate gyrus, are therefore the regulator of projection in the first year of life and the OFC for transference phenomena linked to emotional information in the second year of life (Schore, 2003a). This system of auto-regulation manifests its structural organization and functional onset during toddlerhood 10–18 months after birth. Concurrently at that time, a system of compassion, empathy, and loving kindness is dawning in the infant as a complex relationship between the heart and the brain.

Emotional Effects

The basic working models of life or filters are caused by the formation of implicit memory from the imprinting of life experience via the attachment and bonding with a caregiver(s). Unconscious behaviors derived from insecure attachment processes with a parent usually result in the following affects later in life in response to stimuli: dissociation and/or withdrawal; projection of uncomfortable feelings and thoughts onto other people; activation and/or hyperarousal; and transference of strong emotions and blame onto other people. These four effects of relational stress start as an embryo and solidify during infancy. This imprinting or implicit memory is carried through adult life and acted out with no conscious recall of its etiology because it came from a preverbal time of life. The rule of thumb is that these responses may not necessarily match the life stimulus and are consequently difficult to self-regulate. They are the most fundamental impairments to experiencing love.

What I am going to focus on in this chapter are the first two effects, dissociation and projection. I will continue with the third and fourth, activation and transference, in the next chapter. I believe these four components of emotional responsiveness are more likely to be seen by biodynamic practitioners. The consequences of insecure attachment processes in childhood require a well-attuned therapeutic relationship in adulthood to heal. The practitioner provides the quality of attunement that was missing early in life. The principle of a well-attuned therapeutic relationship means that the biodynamic practitioner is able to differentiate his personal issues from the client's, to have a felt sense of stillness, outside and inside his body, and to access Primary Respiration outside and inside his body as the first priority in the therapeutic relationship. This builds autonomy in the relationship and begins to repair that function in the client through right brain-to-right brain resonance. Thus, I consider biodynamic craniosacral therapy to be a therapist-centered therapy. The practitioner must manage his own perception and fluid sensorium for the majority of time that he is in contact with a client. This may be 80–90 percent of the time allotted for a biodynamic session.

Dissociation

It is my contention, as a biodynamic practitioner for thirty-plus years, that a core side effect in body-centered therapies is the phenomenon of both normal and non-normal dissociation, as described in Section II, Relating with Trauma. I divide dissociation into two categories: normal and non-normal. I believe all practitioners, including myself, frequently co-induce both states of dissociation with the client. Both reveal themselves in numerous ways and must be respected as important friends in the healing process. I feel each is a valuable state if contained, but without biodynamic trauma skills non-normal dissociation is frequently mistaken for an effective therapeutic outcome by itself, since the client, at the time, no longer feels her symptom(s) or has them exacerbated. The former I call euphoric dissociation and the latter I call intrusive dissociation. Each becomes the starting point for a biodynamic therapeutic process rather than the end and must be normalized by the practitioner's ability to be a guide in the wilderness of strong affect with only stillness and Primary Respiration as light.

The exacerbation of physical symptoms as intrusive physical sensation requires extra care from the practitioner, thus mimicking an interactive repair by a mother-person. Often such intrusion is linked to the metabolic digestive system and immune system of the client. These systems, and others in the client's body, are managing chronic inflammatory processes that will have a probability of being exacerbated from craniosacral therapy, especially with biomechanical work. This means the client may need extra time after the session is over or need to return for "rebalancing." The practitioner must also consider referring the client to another health care provider who specializes in anti-inflammatory therapy. I believe the current epidemic of inflammatory body processes has its roots in early developmental stress and trauma and thus such side effects are normal results of the physical touch of any practitioner. Therefore, it is imperative that biodynamic craniosacral therapists develop the ability to modulate their physical touch to identify the effects of non-normal dissociation, especially chronic inflammatory conditions. The priority is for the practitioner to identify his own inflammation metabolically and psychologically. This has great value when the practitioner can identify his own irritation and allow it to be moved by Primary Respiration. This comes about through personal psychotherapy or clinical supervision, skilled self-regulation by receiving biodynamic sessions regularly, nonjudgmental self-observation, continuing biodynamic education in some form of the containment model of self-regulation, and, last but not least, a clean diet. All these help a person learn to love himself.

As part of a traumatic experience in the prenatal and perinatal time, powerful fight-or-flight physiology is generated later in the lifespan. Early imprinting in the fluid metabolism of the embryo is carried forward throughout life. Chronic dissociation and its inflammatory effects as well as the neurochemicals of fight-or-flight are toxic to the brain and body. The effects from non-normal dissociation include repeated sympathetic cycling, a tendency for emotional flooding, heat distribution problems, hypomobility, frozen states, susceptibility to inflammatory processes as mentioned, and fluid condensation. Non-normal dissociation generates these effects throughout the fluid body and soma. It is a systemic reaction experienced frequently as a fragmented state—a loss of three-dimensional awareness of the body. When these states are accessed with physical contact, the aberrant sensations, as well as the associated or coupled traumatic memory, may be evoked regardless of the quality of the contact. This usually begins unconsciously and then escalates to a point of conscious intrusion as the client's autonomic nervous system amplifies feelings and develops the perception of an emotional charge. The best remedy is for the practitioner to be in the tempo of Primary Respiration and able to access a stillpoint inside and outside of his body. This is the basis for a much deeper healing solution for the client.

Dissociation is normally a valuable resource in the developing organism. The embryo, fetus, and newborn are very fragile, using contraction and withdrawal as a first defense when threatened. Dissociation is also a normal sentient gesture. Sentience is the awareness and movement toward an outside source of stimulus and the awareness and movement toward an inside stimulus. Sentience is mediated by the fluid body and secondarily by the autonomic nervous system in the soma. The chronic rapid withdrawal and loss of flexibility of the movement of sentience (which prefers to move at the rate of Primary Respiration) between the inside and outside of the body is a pervasive expression of the need to defend (and also to self-soothe) in an infant. Thus in the speed, awareness is lost. Typically, non-normal dissociation involves undersomatization (loss of body perception) or oversomatization (excessive body perception). These states of implicit memory are preexisting from the preverbal time of life. These states can simply be evoked through the neutral light contact of the hands of a craniosacral therapy practitioner and especially more heavy-handed approaches. There are powerful affective states or imprints coupled to non-normal dissociation (terror, rage, hopelessness, death anxiety, and fear of annihilation) can cause the practitioner to resonate with the client both consciously and unconsciously. The practitioner needs to recognize these imprints both in the client and himself as part of the healing process called ignition in biodynamic craniosacral therapy. Dissociation is an ignition for conception to recur in the adult and requires Primary Respiration to regain sentient flexibility between the outside and inside of her body. Non-normal dissociation needs to be transmuted with the Dynamic Stillness.

The practitioner always orients to a deep stillpoint at the beginning of a session and sometimes for the whole session. The biodynamic practitioner then attunes to his own sense of Primary Respiration and lets the client resonate with his first. It is like the story of Hansel and Gretel following a trail of sweets deep into the woods. The wicked witch of non-normal dissociation is cured with Primary Respiration and its fulcrum of Dynamic Stillness.

Sentient attention is designed to breathe freely from inside to outside and outside to inside the body in rhythmic periods of fifty seconds in one direction and fifty seconds in another direction. It is not possible to be fully aware of embodiment at all times. The brain and body are not designed that way. Even the first visceral bodily functions of the embryo are projected outside her central body onto an external body. These functions are then incorporated back into the body when there is a structure for them. Structure and function is breathed in and out of the body in rhythmic periods of fifty seconds each. Furthermore, research has shown that awareness of the self (the unique person who is having these experiences) becomes embodied at different times during prenatal and perinatal existence (Wade, 1998). Therefore, it can be interpreted that embryos, fetuses, and infants teach us that we are naturally designed to move our attention and awareness flexibly within and out of our bodies, creating a balance between function first and structure second moving at the rate of Primary Respiration. It is all oriented to a stillpoint. Awareness of such still and slow functions would be therapeutically valuable and a start in understanding the power and relative value of dissociation and projection. Dissociation is merely the organism's attempt to slow us down. It must be honored as a biodynamic process. Clients must be taught to synchronize their attention with the inside and outside presence of Primary Respiration by the practitioner.

Projection

Projection is a biological and metabolic necessity in the human organism. This is what the embryo teaches us. The early embryo separates itself into a central and peripheral body. The central body becomes our soma many differentiations later. The peripheral body becomes our placenta many differentiations later, and not before it has performed many other functions that the central body cannot yet do. For instance, before we have an actual liver in the central body, the central body projects specific functions of the liver out to the lining of the peripheral body such as specific liver enzyme activity before the structure of the liver is present (Vogler, 1987). Many types of visceral functions are projected out to the peripheral body before there is a structure in the central body to host such functions. When the structure is built centrally, the embryo retrieves the externalized function and reclaims the projection, so to speak. What begins as a metabolic process in the embryo continues as a physiological process in the newborn. During the first year of life the newborn must project her love and needs into the mother to get them met and the love mirrored back. Gradually the physiological process of projection in the infant will become psychological projection processes in later stages of the lifespan. Projection, then, is a natural process, or at least it starts as a natural process.

Biodynamic practitioners must understand that negative or adaptive projection, which is the way we unconsciously place parts of ourselves (previously unmet needs or even new undiscovered developmental needs) into the mind and body of another person, is directly related to dissociation. Projection takes place between the two right hemispheres of the client and practitioner. The infant has basic developmental needs such as warmth, food, a dry diaper, and loving touch in the first year of life and beyond. A developmental need is also a psychological need. The infant has to get the mother to feel what she is feeling, sometimes very loudly and without words. The client or spouse with preverbal wounding has to get her partner or practitioner to feel what she is feeling without language as well. This is where projection comes into play, so to speak. The infant projects her needs unconsciously into the mother through sound, gesture, and emotion. It's kind of like a game of charades. It is received in the right hemisphere of the mother-practitioner and recreated as a neural network and total-body experience. The mother-person tends the garden of the autonomic nervous system of the infant-client until she can contain and auto-regulate her emotions by herself. Thus, the mood and the inner emotional tone of a client-infant are rapidly projected into the mother-practitioner's waiting brain and body. Rapidly means within milliseconds. The mother-practitioner receives it in the right hemisphere and recreates the information as a neural network and felt body state. By doing so, the caregiver metabolizes the content as a form of digestion, assimilates it, and mirrors back to the client-infant a nonreactive (empathetic) mature brain state. If the practitioner as mother has personal early emotional issues activated unconsciously, he will be challenged in the ability to separate personal issues from those of the client. The practitioner must monitor his body frequently during a session to auto-regulate his autonomic nervous system.

Parenting is not a perfect process. It depends on the quality of interactive repair by the mother after a break in the continuity of her relationship with her baby. Breaks in continuity are normal. The regularity of the interactive repair of the caregiver allows the infant to wire together or connect the highest centers of the brain for emotional self-regulation while in relationship and to auto-regulate eventually when alone. Regular repair through verbal apology and affection imprints the filters of implicit memory that life is good and repairable in the corticolimbic system. Self-regulation of emotions begins with the primitive amygdala coming on line in the third trimester of pregnancy and especially in the first months after birth. It continues with the OFC at 10–18 months, the subject of the next chapter. Depending on the mother's ability to accurately attune to her infant's needs is the degree to which the infant will split off such needs and use negative projection to get future needs met as a maladaptive form of self-regulation. Dissociation and projection are linked together in this way, because auto-regulation is thwarted at the level of the OFC and the infant learns to rely upon stress reactions coming from the hypothalamus, amygdala, and brain stem, which are well below conscious awareness. When they eventually come to awareness, it is through inflammatory processes and by then stress reactions are chronic.

G. Vanaerschot contended:

> The first level [of therapeutic relationship] refers to the bodily implicitly felt whole concerning a situation and originates in the interaction between person and situation or environment. … The interaction between body and situation gives rise to an implicit, bodily felt sense, which is preconceptual and undifferentiated. It is a knowing without words: a knowing that precedes words and from which words emerge. … The bodily feeling is implicit. (Vanaerschot, 1997, pp.142–143)

Thus, two of the most powerful states that a practitioner can experience with a client are dissociation and projection. Both are normal metabolic states when synchronized with Primary Respiration. Because an infant is so dependent upon her caregiver, especially in the first year of life, the basic nature of projection is particularly valuable and necessary. In a secure attachment "my self" as physiology is reflected back to me by a mature adult brain. The infant's right hemisphere and autonomic nervous system have been projected into the mother, who metabolizes them with her right brain and body. At that time of life "my self," as a psychophysiological being, is expressed through the body as a need for warmth, food, sustained skin contact, and loving emotional reflection from the caregiver. The projection can then be "owned" unconsciously (psychologically), because the *physiological* need is fulfilled. The amygdala is soothed and more parts of the OFC get "wired" together without the need for aberrant behavior later in life. I am not suggesting that well-attuned parenting is the complete panacea for a happy life, but it is a significant component.

The insecure attachment features the projection of "my self" into the caregiver but it is not returned or reflected accurately, and the infant's physical needs are only partially fulfilled or not fulfilled at all. She must then learn to manipulate her world unconsciously to get fed, have her diaper changed, be soothed, and receive love. A pattern is set into place that continues for a lifetime. In this pattern she uses other people to hold the split-off, partial selves or the unconnected, unbalanced OFC, partial selves in her psyche. She then chooses people to enable her lack of self-regulation. She has no conscious recall of the origin of these imprints and it is terrifyingly painful to change them. It is important to remember that the client will naturally choose someone strong enough to hold the projection. That someone may be a spouse or a psychotherapist or even a pet. Projecting the split-off inability to self-regulate (partial self) onto a strong person gives one an opportunity to recreate the original wounding and potentially heal it with love. The goal of this projection is to finally work through the wounding toward healing. If that doesn't work, she can fire the practitioner or, of course, get divorced.

A healthy fluid body must be created in the practitioner and in the client. This is done with stillness and Primary Respiration. We are driven to do this in order to reclaim and re-own adaptive emotional imprints and states of non-normal dissociation from embryonic wounding and insecure attachment stress and trauma. The soma (the inner experience of the body of the client) must be approached from the fluids outside the central nervous system for a chance to heal. A critical aspect of the healing is to develop a stillpoint in the soma by finding a self-existing stillpoint in the belly, heart, or third ventricle in the brain. These are the original embryonic fulcrums of growth and development. The originality and wholeness of the embryo are accessed rather than the aberrant imprinting. Healing happens through the fluid body and tidal body of Primary Respiration before it can do so through the soma in biodynamic craniosacral therapy. Meaning naturally arises in the fullness of time after the senses have been acknowledged. Because the therapeutic environment is organized by preverbal communication, the continuously attuned biodynamic practitioner must have a right-brain regulatory strategy that allows him to remain in a state of "regressive openness and receptivity." The essential step in creating a container in which an emotion-communicating reconnection can be experienced is the practitioner's ability, initially at a nonverbal level, to detect, recognize, monitor, and self-regulate autonomously the stressful alterations in his bodily state that are evoked by the client's transferential bodily communication (Rubin and Niemeier, 1992). The bodily state is preceded by the fluid body state that is preceded by the tidal body state of Primary Respiration. And it all starts with a stillpoint, which is the original state.

Non-normal dissociation dysregulates those parts of the right brain that monitor bodily sensation. I believe that non-normal dissociation actually places people directly in their fluid body and they have absolutely no reference point for that state or ability to describe it. It frequently causes a person to experience a state of being "beside herself" or outside her body—inside her body but fragmented, frozen and immobile, or intrusively inside her body with irregular and varying degrees of pain or numbness, including hypersensitivity in the autonomic nervous system. These are fluid body perceptions. This strong survival mechanism (filter) involves the sympathetic nervous system but especially an overregulated parasympathetic nervous system (PNS) of the soma; consequently, that is where therapeutic attention goes and rightly so. The autonomic nervous system must be stabilized for Primary Respiration to move the dysfunction in the fluid body first and then the soma. The PNS is the infant's self-soothing mechanism in an insecure attachment now that the fluid body cannot do that. This means that a person will carry this dissociation, self-soothing throughout life, and build it into larger, more complex defensive mechanisms, both physiological and psychological, such as addiction, aberrant behavior, or chronic relationship or employment failure. A person can continue to be soothed by failure because "someone else is doing it to me" (projection as a conspiracy theory). Biodynamically, there is a complete breakdown in the function of the fluid body and, as one osteopath has said, the fluid body is fractured, especially in infants and children. Resolution of imprinting in the fluid body must be treated first because its genesis preceded the development of the soma. Biodynamic therapy is simply following the sequence of normal development.

Context of Skin Contact

Touch has an effect on different centers of the brain, but especially the insular cortex (Olausson, et al., 2002). This is part of the OFC of the brain and, as I said in the first volume, the OFC is generally regarded as having self-regulatory control of the entire corticolimbic system and autonomic nervous system. This means that the client who is receiving physical contact, such as biodynamic craniosacral therapy, is unconsciously reading the context of the touch, as much as the sensation from the touch, which registers in a different center of the brain. The context filter was built in the original attachment experience and even earlier, in prenatal existence, according to researchers. Optimally the context is love, affection, pleasure, and intimacy. This is actually the optimal design of the sympathetic nervous system rather than fight-or-flight. If we do not experience love consistently in the prenatal and perinatal time of life, then touch can be imprinted as something negative and frequently hyperactivating or dissociating. Biodynamic practitioners must generate respect and reverence for the client's inner dilemma and aberrant life filters that result in anger or non-normal dissociation when touched. This occurs through an allegiance to the stillpoint and Primary Respiration in the practitioner first.

Powerful negative imprints such as shame, disgust, rage, terror, and hopelessness need to be identified as body sensations both in the client and the practitioner and then contained via the stillpoint and Primary Respiration. Negative imprinting is the building block for the effects of non-normal dissociation. This is because touch can trigger such strong emotions and these strong emotions are a huge double-bind for the client. In other words, the very thing (a skillful, therapeutic, loving touch) necessary to heal early wounding is perceived as, or triggers, the opposite effect in the brain and soma. Instead of feeling held and nurtured, the client may experience anger or dissociate. Typically, when a client expresses the emotion verbally, it is done so as a left-brain abstraction of the experience, rather than an expression of the actual sensation that is the substrate of the emotion. Practitioners must learn to help clients develop a vocabulary of fluid sensation, fluid shape, and fluid image in order to describe the lived experience of the fluid body, to uncouple from the emotional discomfort. By developing this ability, which uses the language of instinct located in the fluid body and tidal body, the client is able to develop a witness consciousness and therefore bring more of her OFC on-line. Then the practitioner teaches the client to flexibly move her attention from inside her body to outside and back at the tempo of Primary Respiration with an occasional stillpoint.

Safety

Any relationship, therapeutic or otherwise, must have safety and trust embodied in it as a conscious operating function of the heart. Safety is a lack of defensiveness in a relationship. Early imprinting frequently destroys safety. One does not feel able to cope or be resourced from early attachment stress. Trust is the cumulative effect of safety over time. Without safety and trust, preverbal imprinting is difficult but not impossible to overcome. In this way safety is linked to self-regulation. When there is safety and trust, positive emotions, feelings, and sensations amplified in a biodynamic relationship become healing, especially for those vital connections to self-regulatory centers that need to be rewired in the brain and heart. Heart ignition restores safety as the practitioner breathes heart to heart and blood to blood at the tempo of Primary Respiration. It starts and ends with a stillpoint in the heart (Ridley, 2006).

As Judith Lewis Herman (Herman, 1992) has said, the central task of the first stage of healing is the establishment of safety. The second stage is remembrance and mourning via the accurate mirroring of the practitioner back to the client. The client needs to know that she is being heard. Even an infant wants to tell the story of her conception and birth. Many gestures that an infant makes and body movements—repeatedly crawling back through the mother's legs, the type of toys she gravitates to, the people that she shies away from, and so on—are symbolic of the story she is telling. And she wants the caregiver to hear it, acknowledge it, and reflect it back, so she knows she has been heard. The story is held in the soma and the fluids of the body throughout the lifespan and can be heard at any time by a biodynamic practitioner whose ears are attuned to the voice of Primary Respiration. More important, the infant is showering her caregiver with love and wants to know it is being received by its reflection back to her. Finally, the third stage in Herman's trauma healing process is reconnection with ordinary life. The client gets on with her life normally and with grace, having worked through profound pain and suffering. Healing is a natural consequence of a safe container of body mind and spirit that is carried forward into each of life's situations.

Safety is, without a doubt, the most critical component of a therapeutic relationship, if there is going to be a more functional outcome for the client. Psychological safety, according to Sandra Bloom (Bloom, 1997), "refers to the ability to be safe with one's self, to rely on one's own ability to self-protect against any destructive impulses coming from within oneself or deriving from other people and to keep oneself out of harm's way" (p. 115). For a client to feel safe, she must first feel safe in her body and have a sense of being able to control her body. This builds autonomy or auto-regulation, which is dramatically missing in many who have had a misattuned attachment experience. At a deeper level, autonomy refers to the ability for the client to be able to self-regulate and restore her natural (slower) biological rhythms by the auto-regulatory function of the OFC, to reduce hyperarousal and non-normal dissociative effects when alone. Finally, autonomy is the phenomenological experience of the embryo. I can really only know my lived experience as the instinct of sentience with my fluid body, not someone else's fluid body. As an infant my contact with the world takes place in the confines of my soma and fluid body, which was enormously compressed in the birth experience just as it was in the embryo. Relationship is easy but autonomy is hard, as the reader will see in the next chapter.

Once a client can feel safety in her body via interdependent self-regulation through resonance with the practitioner's, then she can sense safety in her heart and mind. This is a more autonomous self-regulation because it is heart centered rather than neurologically centered. The practitioner as mother-person acts as the first line of environmental safety as a calm "sea around us." This establishes both somatic safety and interdependent self-regulation. This refers to how a client self-regulates when in the presence of another person(s). The affective neuroscience literature points out that these two faculties of interdependent self-regulation occurring in the first year and autonomous self-regulation occurring in the second year are developed in an infant's growing brain via her ability to have the OFC of the brain hooked up, which then gives the ability to consciously self-regulate her emotions. The hookup is based on the experiences with the caregiver(s). These two modes of self-regulation are designed to be in a balanced ratio of function throughout life. It is an important therapeutic consideration to know that one or both of these two modes of self-regulation are lacking in a client. The practitioner must establish his own field of normal autonomy via the stillpoint and Primary Respiration to be effective in the rehabilitation of the fluid body. Depending on the type of insecure attachment, the infant loses varying degrees of both autonomous and interdependent self-regulation. Therefore, reciprocal functioning may be impaired. This has strong consequences throughout the lifespan, including psychopathology, non-normal dissociation, and disease and chronic illnesses via inflammatory processes in the neuro-endocrine-immune system.

It is the responsibility of the practitioner to co-create the deepest sense of safety possible in the therapeutic relationship, through attunement to the interchange of stillness and Primary Respiration in himself first. Body safety that includes fluid sensibility and environmental safety lead to spiritual safety, which, along with empathy, leads to moral development. When a client can self-regulate appropriately, by herself and when in the company of another person(s), it is possible to have a deeper and more expanded spiritual connection to all of life through a functioning midline. Our ability to connect with greater meaning, to lead an ethical life, and to have advanced moral development is dependent on the establishment of the midline of body and environmental safety. It is possible to experience one's own divinity directly, but it is difficult to do so from a misattuned caregiving experience. That is a long circuitous route to wholeness and healing.

CHAPTER 22

Biodynamics of Self-Regulation, Part 2: Empathy, Shame, and Autonomous Self-Regulation

How do body-mind systems retain continuity while changing in response to developmental and environmental pressures (Demos and Kaplan, 1986, p. 156)? This is the guiding principle for the investigation of the development of the empathy-shame system and, consequently, the self- regulation of emotions during infancy and especially toddlerhood. Maintaining continuity of the self is a function of the orbitofrontal cortex (OFC) and its servant, the autonomic nervous system (ANS). This happens by the development of self-regulation of emotions as stated throughout this and the first volume. This is a growing feature of the OFC-ANS, especially during the period of toddlerhood (also called the practicing period) 10–18 months after birth. At the same time the complementary emotions of empathy and shame (both positive and negative empathy and positive and negative shame) begin to develop.

A critical point to recall throughout this chapter is that one's emotions are maintained and mediated in the soma by the ANS, as we also saw in the section on trauma. This is a foundation principle regarding brain development in the first two years of life after birth. Therefore all further developmental stages after infancy will be built upon an emotional foundation linked to the ANS and the OFC being wired together for the most part from the infant's experiences with her mother. I want the reader to know that the brain is a major player in development but by no means holds the exclusive patent on how behaviors develop.

John Krystal (Krystal, 1978) suggested that the subsequent emotional development after infancy evolves out of a state of contentment and a state of distress being held together. This polarity differentiates into two distinct developmental lines. These developmental lines are based upon whether an infant has a secure or insecure attachment. One developmental line is for an adult to end up with an infantile nonverbal emotional system and the other is for the adult to end up with an adult verbalized but undersomatized emotional system. *Undersomatized* means a withdrawal from intense arousal typical of the period of time 10–18 months after birth, resulting in an inability to access safe somatic sensation later in life. It is the OFC, particularly in the second year of life, that must learn to balance these two developmental lines. This is done by regular and repeated experiences of elation-arousal in the toddler's ANS that rapidly crash into an internalized state of withdrawal and reduction of affect-sensation.

How one learns to self-regulate emotions from the caregiving experience is the key to infancy in the first two years after birth. The infant must be able to regulate emotional expression and the expression will likely be different for each of the different emotions.

> Some affects represent alterations, transformations, specifications of earlier affect states, whereas others are first born at later stages in the developmental process when the psychological conditions for their emergence are met. These psychological conditions involve new learnings, new acquisitions of mental life, that have consequences for affective experiences. (Pine, 1980, p. 232)

This means that the development of emotions is sequential. The more primitive emotions of fear and terror arise immediately after birth via the amygdala followed by empathy, shame, humiliation, guilt, and so on.

This chapter is about empathy and shame—a sympathetic activation in the autonomic nervous system and the phenomenon of transference. Shame is a developmental line that precedes the development of guilt. It marks a transition from an external regulation of the ANS by the caregiver in the first nine months after birth to an internal regulation of the ANS 10–18 months after birth. First, shame is a withdrawal from the caregiver when she is not able to match or meet the child's joy (sympathetic nervous system activation). The toddler wants to be *met* or matched in the elation of exploring a larger and rapidly expanding universe. Second, shame involves a strong activation of the parasympathetic nervous system after a rapid deflation of the sympathetic nervous system. The internal sense of deflation is called "shame shock" and is subjectively experienced by the toddler as physical pain. Third, shame triggers the need for self-regulation in the toddler's OFC. When the shame-shock experience is contained, as in a secure attachment, the OFC gets wired together with the rest of the limbic system and then begins to realize one of its potentials—self-regulation of emotions autonomously. Fourth, in a secure attachment healthy or positive shame will involve an interactive repair by the caregiver that imprints the internal sense of the self as being inherently "repairable." Otherwise the toddler will need to use transference of the unconscious internal dilemma of "self as not repairable" on to other people in life. This involves a behavioral regression back to the first year after birth to rely on other people's ANS to self-regulate. As such a person grows older the imprint causes low self-esteem or grandiose, inflated narcissistic behaviors (that are still a manifestation of low self-esteem) that are necessary to control the environment by getting other people emotionally upset or involved with their life. Fifth, the cycle of misattunement-repair initializes the function of empathy in the toddler. Empathy represents the onset of moral development and is a component of compassion. Compassion is a function of the heart and empathy is a function of the OFC. The heart and the OFC are linked in this way. To understand healthy shame is to understand the foundation of compassion.

Infant emotions have three basic functions: first, to amplify and exaggerate behavior; second, to communicate information about internal states; and third, to obtain helpful responses from the mother (Sroufe, 1979). This is an important principle in the overall theory of attachment. Specifically, caregiver sensitivity and responsiveness to the child's emotional communications—attunement—are critical to the way the infant organizes and self-regulates her emotional experience. "The baby will become attached to the caregiver who can help to modulate and minimize the experience of the negative and who maximizes and expands opportunities for positive affect" (Demos and Kaplan, 1986, p. 169). Such attunement between the mother and child is a precursor of self-confidence and autonomy—the opposite of shame. This is a sense in the child that she is able to control and self-regulate those emotions normally. It is the responsibility of the caregiver to repair misattunements and help the infant transform her negative emotion and stress into a positive emotion. Thus, the child is able to develop her OFC through an internal representation of herself that is both positive and repairable. This also means that the child has an internal sensibility of her whole body that is reliable.

Shame and the Sympathetic Nervous System (SNS)

Shame is primarily a social emotion. Its hallmarks are blushing and embarrassment, observed in infants as early as twelve months. Such self-consciousness of emotion happens to coincide with the ability of the infant to stand up and begin exploring her environment by walking rather than crawling. The mobile infant is now able to explore her world and expand her range of attention. This is very exciting and consequently the SNS becomes quite active metabolically and physiologically. Metabolically the SNS must facilitate the distribution of oxygen to the extremities for the now-mobile infant. Every blood capillary in the body has a sympathetic nerve plexus. So the rate and flow of blood (and thus oxygen) are controlled via the SNS. At the level of physiology, the ANS operates via four basic stress pathways: one is between the hypothalamus and adrenal medulla; another, known as the HPA axis, is between the hypothalamus, pituitary gland, and adrenal cortex; third, there is the hypothalamic-pituitary-gonadal axis; and finally, the hypothalamus-pituitary-thyroid axis. The four physiological functions of the hypothalamus are fighting, fleeing, reproduction, and feeding. Bear in mind that the hypothalamus is immediately in back of the OFC. It is essential that the OFC be wired together with the hypothalamus so the OFC can regulate the hypothalamus and stress states. Thus, shame is very closely connected to the physiology of stress.

Stress, as is well known, is a physiological state associated with the autonomic nervous system. It is expressed through reactions such as sweating, greater body awareness, intense perception, uncoordinated muscle activity, spinal extension, shaking and trembling, cognitive impairment, and gaze aversion. This is shame at its most primitive. What occurs in the ANS during shame is a shocklike onset of parasympathetic blushing, causing the sympathetic nervous system and its excitement to suddenly and dramatically lower its tone and activate the parasympathetic component of the ANS. The ANS, and especially the parasympathetic branch, is therefore the physiological base of shame. Shame signals the early developing self-regulation system, especially the orbitofrontal cortex, the apex of the emotional limbic system, to terminate interest in whatever has come to her attention. Dr. Alan Schore proposes a model of shame in which the young toddler is in a hyperstimulated, elated state of sympathetic arousal at the time she is making a reconnection with her mom. "Despite an excited anticipation of a shared affect state, the self unexpectedly experiences an affective misattunement, which thereby triggers a sudden stress, shock-induced deflation" (Schore, 2003a, p.155). In other words, when the mother does not match the toddler's excitement, suddenly the sympathetics deflate the child and this activates the parasympathetic withdrawal system. This is a shock to the ANS and forms the physiological experience of shame. Whether the shame is positive or becomes adaptive (negative) and part of an infantile wounding will be determined by the cumulative effect of such mismatches over the time of the practicing period and the lack of interactive repair when such a mismatch occurs. When the toddler is consistently not met by the caregiver, the physiological will become the psychological.

During the practicing period, mobile infants show different emotions than previously. There is a significant increase in positive emotion and a decrease in negative emotion starting at about ten months after birth. Under the best conditions, such as a secure attachment, thresholds of stimulation decrease and the ability for a toddler to tolerate higher levels of stimulation increases. This is a major developmental task starting during the first year. An infant must evolve its ability to increase its tolerance of high arousal states in the sympathetic nervous system and consequent sudden dropping of arousal. This situation occurs during the attachment process with a well-attuned caregiver who is able to match and amplify the infant's high state of stimulation, excitement, and joy within a tolerable range, one that does not consistently overactivate the more primitive part of the vagus nerve of the parasympathetic nervous system. The ability to experience such strong levels of elation and interest-excitement depends upon the preceding experiences of merging with the all-important mother figure immediately after birth.

The sympathetic and parasympathetic components of the autonomic nervous system have different timetables of development. This results in a unique physiological organization at different stages after birth. The parasympathetic function of inhibiting heart and lung rate and withdrawal in general is expressed by two distinct parts of the PNS called the polyvagal system (Porges, Doussard-Roosevelt, and Maiti, 1994). Stephen Porges and colleagues out that the dorsal motor nucleus (DMNX) of the vagus located in the brain stem is responsible for metabolic shutdown and immobilization. This system puts a "brake" on the heart and slows down respiratory function following high sympathetic arousal. On the other hand, a more flexible part of the vagus takes six years to mature. This more "social" part of the PNS is located in the nucleus ambiguous (NAX). The vagus nerve is the tenth cranial nerve and Porges suggests that it represents the lion's share of what he calls the "social nervous system." The NAX innervates structures above the neck and the DMNX innervates structures below the neck.

The social nervous system is organized around the development of the pharynx and cranial base. It takes six years minimum after birth for ossification of the cranial bones to occur because of the gradual growth of the brain and especially the brain stem. The pharynx is responsible for organizing the air coming through it into unique sounds. The early sounds are called proto-conversation in the infant. Most sounds are expressions of emotion. Since the infant cannot talk, she must get the caregiver to feel and see what she is feeling, and this happens through the organization of air into sound coming through the pharynx.

The emotional, behavioral, and cognitive (attention span) aspects unique to the practicing period of a toddler's mobility are timed in a way that the empathy-shame system emerges at the same time of such dominant sympathetic hyperarousal and behavioral excitation. The empathy-shame system is thus a way that the brain evolves a type of *control mechanism* over these hyperstimulated states. Separation for the mother during the practicing period does not activate shame. Rather, it is the reunion between the toddler and the mother that serves to regulate levels of arousal whether high or low and whether the arousal can be self-organized into a more functional and attentive state (Brent and Resch, 1987). Ideally, the mother attempts to maintain her child's excitement and activation in a middle range that is not so intense as to cause distress and avoidance. The optimal reunion experience between a mother and her toddler lasts between thirty seconds and three minutes. These are the important moments of the child's daily experience associated with the development of self-regulation in the OFC.

However, during the reunion experience, which is face to face, intense interactive stress can occur. The highly aroused toddler looking for an attuned mother to match her state of excitement and joy may unexpectedly encounter a face that expresses a significant misattunement such as anger or depression. It is not possible for mom to be 100 percent available to her child. It need only be "good enough." This mismatch of emotion and excitement creates a break and a sudden shock-induced collapse of positive emotion. The toddler is thrown into a state that she cannot yet self-regulate. Shame represents this rapid transition from a previous positive state to a negative state of stress. Thus the toddler creates an association to an unfulfilled expectation (Wurmser, 1981). The shock of shame comes from the breach of the infant's expectation. The toddler must switch from being elated to being deflated, from being curious, positive, excited, and *having focused attention* to having unfocused attention and distress. Interest and attention to the external environment is suddenly terminated as a defensive and adaptive need. Thus shame represents a passive as opposed to an active resourcing strategy.

This state of the shame system is driven by the DMNX and especially associated with immobilization and withdrawal behaviors. This induces a separation stress response triggered by the presence of the mother. Activation theorists have shown that very low levels of arousal, just like high levels, are associated with uncomfortable negative emotional states and behavioral inefficiency (Cofer and Appley, 1964). Understimulation stress modulated by the vagus and overstimulation stress modulated by the sympathetics are perceived by the toddler as pain. Shame heightens these stress reactions. Understimulation stress modulated by the vagus is reflected in the psychological experience of helplessness, passivity, and painful sensitivity to the critical reactions of others (Morrison, 1985). Schore suggests that the normal experience of shame is associated with a decrease in PNS activity and elevated DMNX functioning. Humiliation, however, is a type of hyper-shame from an insecure attachment that involves both an elevated DMNX plus an activated sympathetic nervous system.

The autonomic nervous system has two coupled, reciprocally integrated circuits that control states of activation. Nuclei located in the brain stem have circuits that go from the brain stem through the limbic system to the orbitofrontal cortex. They are called dorsal and ventral tegmental circuits. The dorsal circuit is for the parasympathetic component of the autonomic system and the ventral circuit is for the sympathetic component. The sympathetic branch is catabolic, which means it is responsible for energy mobilizing excitation and activation. This includes heart rate acceleration. The parasympathetic branch, on the other hand, is anabolic. This means that it is involved in energy-conserving activity that inhibits function, especially heart rate deceleration (Porges, Doussard-Roosevelt, and Maiti, 1994). "The physiological expression of emotion is dependent, in part, upon both sympathetic and parasympathetic parts of the autonomic nervous system" (Truex and Carpenter, 1964, p. 431). Thus, the DMNX and its parasympathetic function are reflected in low-key emotions. The shame system is mediated by these two emotional autonomic systems. The language or social communication between a mother and her child is generated via the autonomic nervous system of both parties.

The period of toddlerhood represents a developmental phase of imbalance and unregulated sympathetic overexcitation. The dorsal tegmental circuit of the parasympathetic system must be built and connected all the way through to the OFC without too much unregulated shame-shock. The ventral sympathetic circuit is also growing forward to the OFC and during toddlerhood the hypothalamus is quite active. The balanced and emotional matching and regulatory capacity of the caregiver is what allows the neurons of the tegmental circuit of the infant to reach its apex in the OFC so that attention can be sustained, in a coupled reciprocal sympathetic and parasympathetic way. The distress of a mismatch with a caregiver decreases the vital self-regulatory capacity of attention in the OFC. The ability to sustain attention on an object of perception is related to the witness function of the OFC. Such attention slowly shifts dysregulated states toward normal. When properly wired up, the OFC is able to auto-regulate the "too high" of the distressed sympathetics and the "too low" of distressed parasympathetics through the containment of a mature caregiver. This is a critical component of the practicing period or toddlerhood 10–18 months after birth.

When the infant-mother bond is stressed, during the practicing period, the internal sense of self of the toddler no longer feels whole, but divided into parts or subpersonalities. Negative shame undermines the relationship process and unfortunately promotes a regressive effort to reestablish the earlier symbiotic type of relationship after birth (Broucek, 1982). The first ten months after birth feature symbiosis, or a merged state with the mother rather than a differentiated state that begins in toddlerhood. This is an important therapeutic understanding: a toddler, a client, or even a therapist when undergoing relationship stress, will behaviorally revert back to early infancy and the undifferentiated, merged state. This is unconscious preverbal behavior. Basically, during toddlerhood, the infant becomes more internal and switches from a shared autonomic emotional state to an intra-psychic state. The personal intrinsic regulation of emotions begins to "come on-line." Essentially, shame is a state of frustration because of the inability of the other person, in this case the mother, to react positively to one's communication (Basch, 1976).

Shame has two basic components. One component reduces hyperactivated sympathetic states, lowers expectations, and decreases self-esteem and interest; it interferes with cognition and increases the internal experience of shame as well as the parasympathetic resourcing of a depressed emotional tone. The second component reduces the conscious experience of shame, negative self-esteem, and low-toned depressive states, and initiates recovery of the sympathetic positive tined moods. This includes feelings of expansion of the self, increased self-esteem, and active resourcing. This describes the reciprocal coupled functioning of the autonomic nervous system when it is functioning optimally in the auto-regulation of emotions. It does this continuously in the face of changing environmental situations and relationships.

The caregiver modifies the toddler's shame system in the co-creation of a psychobiological bond of interactive self-regulation. This is facilitated by the caregiver in the interactive repair following an episode of misattunement. As stated, this switches off the toddler's DMNX that fuels a depressive withdrawn state in the child. The sympathetics can then reignite. The world can now be approached again with excitement. Children do this constantly as though they have completely forgotten the misattunement. The give and take of the infant-caregiver relationship facilitates a transition from the more primitive DMNX to the later maturing and flexible NAX in the developing brain. The DMNX shuts down metabolic activity causing immobilization, death feigning, and withdrawal behaviors in relationship to the amygdala. The NAX allows for communication via facial expressions that include mutual gazing, vocalizations (proto-conversation), and gestures based on social interactions. These transactions take place repeatedly throughout the practicing period of toddlerhood. It is a characteristic of this period that misattuned states and distressing emotions occur even in a secure attachment, which makes the development of shame normal.

The toddler internalizes the emotional and cognitive (capacity to pay attention) components of relationships and this defines the construction of internal working models of reality that will filter reality and influence all subsequent relationships (Pipp and Harmon, 1987). Internal working models are beliefs about the way the world works and directly related to implicit memories laid down in the right hemisphere in the preverbal time of infancy, as mentioned in the previous chapter. In other words, since the infant has no language, the corticolimbic system and the right hemisphere of the child create these models about the way the world works and how one's needs will be met in the future. They are imprinted by the quality and quantity of the caregiver's capacity to meet the infant's needs. These beliefs are coupled to behaviors about how the child and future adult need to manipulate, strategize, or otherwise control the environment (and other people) to get such needs met. These internal working models define the character of the self-regulation of emotion and provide the rules of engagement for regulating distressing emotions in the context of intimate relationships. Negative shame is imprinted into preverbal implicit memory and therefore is the source of deep transference patterns (Tulving, 1972).

Transference

Now I would like to discuss the fourth component of emotional development, started in the last chapter. There is a remarkable tendency to recapitulate our early experiences throughout life, thus reinforcing the original insult. The origin, which in the adult is now buried deep in the unconscious right hemisphere and numerous body symptoms, is heavily defended by what Donald Kalsched (Kalsched, 1996) calls the "negative self-care system," built during infancy and early childhood. The main defensive strategies or states of the negative self-care system, therefore, are dissociation, projection, and transference. Projection is the most natural fundamental strategy used by an infant in the first nine months after birth to get her needs met, as mentioned in the previous chapter. Transference emerges from negative shame used by the toddler in the adult who experienced an insecure attachment and not able to have her excitement consistently matched by the mother then or now. Transference is a projection that got hit by lightning, as my friend Judith Suarez often says. Transference is a projection that is overloaded with emotion. The person gripped by a transference is convinced that the other person is "making" her feel what she is feeling and that there is no choice about what she is feeling. This continues to occur as an imprint throughout life, especially in working and intimate relationships.

Therapeutically, both the client and the practitioner need to develop the ability to identify these imprints as they exist in their adult bodies—as sensation and "gut feelings"—while establishing a stillpoint and staying in the tempo of Primary Respiration.

Transference issues consistently arise in relationships. They are based on a misattunement between the practitioner and the client or a perceived break or rupture in the container of the relationship that mimics the toddler-caregiver relationship. Just as the practitioner has responsibility for maintaining awareness of his own countertransference issues, he must also maintain an awareness and ability to manage, repair, and return the developing transference coming from a client. All the triggers from the preverbal toddler imprinted in the adult brain and body will most certainly give rise to the complex development and activation of a transference onto the practitioner. It's automatic in any relationship to constellate the issues needing to be healed. Projection and transference are the working materials and mechanics of relationship.

The client must also be able to develop an intra-psychic structure of meaning in both her body and mind, which can re-own and reframe the transference placed on the practitioner. Quite frequently in biodynamic practice, the transference involves sensing the practitioner as the carrier of an emotion or the one who causes such emotion in the client, just as what happened early in childhood. In order to re-own transferences, it is helpful for the client to identify the person in her life, either historically or currently, who originally facilitated this emotion.

Biodynamic practitioners educate their clients nonverbally through Primary Respiration and stillness that these transference issues are deeply rooted in the organic compressional forces of the embryo and the inevitable the consequences of having a body and being born. Consequently, a transference issue is ultimately healed through synchronization with Primary Respiration and uncoupling it from the related imprinting of anger, fear, and negative shame, coupled to organic embryonic processes. This retrains the OFC to self-regulate to contain the emotion rather than using transference to rid oneself of unwanted emotions. When emotional processes become abstractions, they emerge as behaviors rooted in the preverbal history of the client and slowness and stillness become the enemy rather than the ally. It is through the stillpoint and attending to the exquisite ability of Primary Respiration to direct itself for healing that deeper change process occurs. The main focus for a biodynamic practitioner needs to be the ability to live in the fluid-instinctual world of both himself and the client. Accessing fluid shape, fluid sense, and fluid image are the basis for rewiring the fluid body to the soma and the soma to the OFC of the brain.

The body and its sensory, visceral processes can overwhelm or keep the right hemisphere of the brain overactive. The right hemisphere generates both strong emotion and builds defenses against those same emotions. Since the right hemisphere is largely unconscious, the body tends to "keep the score" as Besel van der Kolk (van der Kolk, 1996) has said. The top-down, conscious self-regulation of feelings and emotions coming from the OFC is missing or muted. It becomes transferred in a negative way onto the practitioner or those closest to the client in life. As I said earlier, it is quite easy to enter phases of misattunement in the therapeutic relationship when the practitioner is not grounded in his own stillpoint and Primary Respiration. The practitioner acts as the corpus collosum of the client's brain, that area between the right and left hemisphere. As a corpus collosum, the practitioner is like a large bundle of interconnecting neurons between the client's two hemispheres. When the practitioner is grounded in his own stillpoint and Primary Respiration, he is more able to facilitate such right-left hemisphere integration because his own brain state is self-regulated. When the practitioner is not attuned in this way to himself, he unconsciously breeches the client's self-regulatory capacity by merging with the client emotionally. This exacerbates an existing dysfunction or symptom just as the insecure mother-infant relationship did. It was unsuccessful then and it remains unsuccessful now.

The physiological self-regulatory function of the infant's ANS is initially performed by the mother in the first nine months. This is a phase of symbiosis. There is an intimate union of two dissimilar people that is absolutely necessary and advantageous to the baby. Then during toddlerhood the ANS is consequentially internalized by the child. The child brings the projected part of the ANS back into her brain. The opportunity for internalization of ANS function at that time then determines the structural development of the autonomous self-regulatory capacity of emotions in the OFC throughout the lifespan. Self-regulation provides consistency for modulating internal feeling and emotional states and therefore especially the self-regulation of mood. In securely attached infants relational distress does not last long, especially beyond the condition or stimulus that brought it on. There is a rapid recovery to positively toned sympathetic emotions. In contrast, insecure attachments cause distress for longer periods of time and typically way beyond the precipitating stimulus or provoking event (Gaensbauer, 1982). This is the hallmark of trauma in later life—a reaction does not match the stimulus.

The question becomes, then, how does one heal the transference that seems to be an organic metabolic and physiological process in the client-therapist relationship. The answer lies in the ability of the practitioner to sense her own body. The various practices and meditations given throughout this book and Volume One are primarily oriented around developing this simple skill of being grounded in one's own soma, fluid body, and tidal body. The ability of the practitioner to access Primary Respiration as a felt sense of wholeness in her own body allows the perception of the client's fluid body to intermingle with that of the practitioner's. This intermingling, when brought to conscious awareness, actually allows the practitioner to take on the shape of the client's trauma and stress and process it through the metabolic biodynamic forces in the fluid body. In essence, the practitioner is bypassing the autonomic nervous system by focusing on the active shaping processes and forces of the fluid body in relation to the movement of wholeness called Primary Respiration that is the central ordering and organizational dynamic of our entire biology. Transference happens, as the bumper sticker might say. And it must be contained through conscious awareness by the practitioner of the practitioner's own fluid body and tidal body. This, I believe, is the answer offered through the practice of biodynamic craniosacral therapy.

Rapprochement

At the end of toddlerhood, around eighteen months, is another major developmental transition from the practicing period to the rapprochement period. The vocabulary of a child at this point is approximately twenty-two words. Very shortly, emotionally descriptive language will emerge as the left hemisphere comes on-line. The emergence of new structure and function during this transition time is based upon successful passage through the preceding states of symbiosis in the first year and practicing in the second year. During this third developmental period, there is an important crisis. Separation anxiety is intensified because the mother is discovered to be a new object unto herself. The infant perceives the mother as different from herself. The child uses tantrums and narcissistic rages to regain control of that loss. Again, the response of the caregiver to such behavior is critical. Heinz Kohut (Kohut, 1971) "underscored the principle that a true sense of self is a product of the accommodation or neutralization of the individuals grandiosity and idealization" (Schore, 2003a, p. 170).

Schore states an important principle here. He says that the positive shame system that regulates hyperstimulation and other sympathetic states is critical to the ability to modulate these highly aroused narcissistic emotions characteristic of the period. Furthermore, the deflation of the child's sense of omnipotence and grandiosity via the evolved sympathetic state is supposed to resolve in the rapprochement phase. Narcissistic rages must be dealt with by the parents in a balanced way. This allows the child to have a heightened self-consciousness, protects her individuation and self-regulation development, and softens the boundaries and personal nature of the autonomous self. *Measured and repeated exposures to limitation* must be experienced in order to dilute the primary infantile narcissistic emotions and neutralize the primitive aggressive drives during this transition phase of rapprochement. It is during the practicing period that the repeated collapses from sympathetic excitement to parasympathetic withdrawal initiate the internal awareness of limitation and separation. No wonder childhood can be so painful.

Autonomous Self-Regulation

The capacity for autonomous self-regulation emerges during the middle of the second year (Fox and Davidson, 1984). It is at this time that the child develops the capacity to inhibit distress and other negative feelings and emotions. Thus, self-regulation is a type of "control/delay/inhibition process" (Pine, 1980). This principle of autonomous self-regulation emerging in the second year after birth is demonstrated by the ability to transform strong tantrums and rages into more focused and modulated anger. This is when the functional ability of the child to control sympathetic states of arousal occurs and thus a maturing of the OFC takes place. Self-regulation of anger in this particular phase of development is crucial. Sympathetic states of activation once containing joy and excitement now contain anger and rage. The rage interferes with the child's capacity to be alone. The ability to be alone is an important function of the OFC regarding the capacity to witness and pay attention to internal states without defaulting to freeze states or non-normal withdrawal of emotion.

People prone to negative shame have difficulty in internalizing or being autonomous. Unregulated hyperarousal interferes with learning and memory processes. This makes it very difficult to resolve the next transition crisis in childhood that occurs emotionally between the practicing period and the rapprochement period, toward the end of the second year. The word *rapprochment* comes from the French word *rapprocher*, which means "to cause to approach again." So the end of one developmental phase causes the growing toddler to re-approach the caregiver with even stronger emotions. Again, the success or lack of success at this transition will imprint the brain with even stronger memories that may last a lifetime as behaviors and attitudes.

Ultimately the caregiver's responses that deactivate and then reactivate sympathetic arousal are critical to the self-regulatory development in the OFC. It is expected that late in the second year the child will have greater autonomy and more ability to modulate strong emotions even in the absence of the caregiver. Autonomy then is the second half of self-regulation and its necessary connections in the OFC. The first half of self-regulation is relational and is learned in the first year after birth. Self-regulatory failure coming from this period of time (practicing and the transition to rapprochement) causes narcissism and stronger disorders related to self-esteem, co-dependency, inflated ego, and grandiosity. It appears as a type of perpetual adolescence or a Peter Pan syndrome in adults. Such wounding causes people to withdraw emotionally from their significant others in order to protect themselves "against the unconsciously anticipated painful experience of shame-humiliation" (Schore, 2003a, p. 177). Narcissistic wounding, then, results in repeated swings of one's self-esteem from high to low and unending attempts to repair the inner self without success. This is sometimes called the "mother complex." The job ultimately is to rid one's self of adaptive or negative shame when moving through life and intimate relationships by finding a midline to connect it all together, and is the subject of the last section of this book.

One of the functions of the OFC is to be able to measure itself. This is one of the key components of the OFC self-regulatory system. This means at one level that the brain is perceiving present time information coming from someone in the environment and comparing it to past events. The amplitude of the sensation and associated feelings together with the context of the situation must be compared with preexisting implicit memory (expectations, filters, models, and so forth). Shame is related to self-image and thus to self-esteem. Self-esteem is the emotional picture of one's self developed in the right hemisphere during the first two years of life and is continuously being compared and evaluated in the OFC throughout the lifespan. It is linked to the development of a body image at the same time through skin-to-skin contact with the caregiver. The skin is the boundary of the skin ego, which transmutes into the psychological ego later in life. The right hemisphere stores events that have meaning for the concept of self, including a three-dimensional image of the inside of the body, and are significant for the maintenance of self-esteem (Tulving, 1972). The OFC attempts to balance self-esteem (one's autobiography carried forward through successive stages of life) internally and to sustain autonomous emotional control especially in relationship stress. It is truly a delicate balancing act. Thus high self-esteem is considered very positive and low self-esteem very negative.

Phases of Self-Regulation

Self-regulation has several phases. Right after birth, it is externally managed by the caregiver as the infant biologically projects her need for regulation into the mother. During the succeeding phase of toddlerhood the previous stage of interactive self-regulation is internalized and emotional control gradually becomes auto-regulated by the toddler. This is the beginners' phase of autonomous self-regulation. The intermediate and advanced training continues through childhood into adulthood. The shame lessons from toddlerhood slowly develop the capacity to constantly monitor the self in relationship to others. These lessons occur from the failure of an expected response by the caregiver and later occur when intrapersonal self expectations, unconscious beliefs, values, and desires are not fulfilled. There is a painful, heightened self-consciousness associated with shame stress. Thus a major function of the OFC is to self-repair the injuries perceived as coming from someone else as slights or insults. This is a critical component of autonomous self-regulation.

Empathy and Compassion

Internal signs of self-regulation are preverbal and begin to manifest late in the second year of life. Infants and toddlers are capable of demonstrating moral behavior and having compassion for people in distress. Thus the self-regulatory function of the OFC is a stress-sensitive resourcing system for one's self and others. It involves comparing and contrasting previous states and memories with the current one and toning down strong emotions as well as negative emotions. Schore proposes that the "auto-regulatory system monitors, adjusts, and corrects emotional responses, thereby providing flexibility and unity in socioemotional function" (Schore, 2003a, p. 181). The modification of emotional responsiveness necessarily includes compassion and empathy. In this way the acquisition of shame is concurrent with that of empathy. Thus toddlerhood is about the development of an empathy-shame system from a brain-heart point of view.

The question, then, becomes how to identify and integrate the psychobiological states underneath unconscious right-brain behavior. To do this requires empathy, compassion, and love. Empathy, which is the way we sense and feel the dilemma of another person, is a function of right-brain attunement that begins to arise in the second year of life. It is connected to the heart hormonally and via the autonomic nervous system. Compassion starts as a resonance with another person. It is a felt state of warmth in the area around the heart. Gradually a perception of the other person's distress arises. Empathy emerges from compassion as an interpretation of the situation and clarity that what is experienced personally is indeed coming from another person (Iacoboni, et al., 2005; Carr, et al., 2003). The heart does compassion and the brain does empathy. Reaching out and offering solace is the fruition of the compassion-empathy reflex. This is loving kindness, the most innate function of being human. Taking in, absorbing, and mirroring the state of another person, and then reaching out to offer solace, arises naturally as part of being human and in relationship with other people. If there is an insecure attachment, the capacity for the empathy cycle is muted or developmentally delayed. With an impaired capacity to be empathetic to another person, the other person's projections become amplified and anger or withdrawal is generated mutually. Compassion flies out the window and the quality of love is strained.

To regenerate empathy there is a need to amplify positive emotions such as joy, which is also regulated sympathetically, while in relationship. This helps to uncouple the imprinting from thwarted developmental needs and wake up the compassion reflex, so to speak. Love is the state where we can give tenderness, care, concern, and kindness to another person in an effort to help the loved one be happy. It is also related to moral development. In other words, human beings must overcome their self-centered narcissism from early wounding in order to care for people and ultimately care for the planet in its totality. A lack of empathy, compassion, and love, when thwarted from the beginning at an individual level due to negative shame, impedes moral development in the long run.

To be compassionate, biodynamic practitioners need to be able to feel another person's inner ocean via the practitioner's own stillpoint and Primary Respiration. The practitioner's heart and arms become a satellite dish receiving the client's signals of wholeness via Primary Respiration. This requires the practitioner to be consciously self-aware, not only of his own stillpoint and Primary Respiration, but also of how he is metabolizing the client's emotions in his own heart and brain through the felt sense of heat and warmth. This process is called attunement and resonance to the interchange of slowness and stillness.

In physics, a property of resonance is harmonic sympathetic vibration, which is the tendency of one resonance system to enlarge and amplify through matching the resonance frequency pattern of another resonance system. The practitioner's empathetic ability to receive, resonate with, and amplify the patient's transient states of positive affect facilitates the interactive generation of higher and more enduring levels of positive states than the patient can autoregulate. (Schore, 2003a, p. 79)

Practically a biodynamic practitioner can consciously pendulate between the stillpoint in himself and its interchange with Primary Respiration. This allows the client to connect with her OFC since the client is unconsciously resonating with the practitioner's self-attunement. The biodynamic practitioner develops other ways to resonate with a client in the same way a mother and infant develop resonance. That is through skin-to-skin contact, which profoundly influences infant growth and development. The biodynamic practitioner who is well self-differentiated must recognize that touch is an extremely powerful tool since it lights up the right hemisphere of both his and the client's brain like a Christmas tree in Times Square. Touch and all its therapeutic varieties and modalities are extremely powerful tools in the hands of a skilled practitioner. The practitioner is literally plugging into the entire prenatal and perinatal history of the client with the practitioner's right brain, hands, and body. It is critical for the practitioner to access stillness and Primary Respiration in himself first and thus maintain autonomy during the session.

Buddhism

Any discussion of empathy and compassion must include the philosophical perspective from Buddhism. The Buddha taught that compassion is, first, the desire to eliminate the cause of pain and suffering in all human beings. Second, compassion is to take in and absorb others' suffering as much as possible or is practical. One's inner conflicting mental and emotional states, however, are considered the strongest sources of pain and suffering. To have compassion is to digest, so to speak, the pain and suffering, not only in oneself but in all others. Compassion, therefore, is supreme and lies at the root of all spiritual and moral endeavors.

Research points out that moral development proceeds in three stages (Wilber, 2000). The first stage is being self-centered, as in childhood and adolescence. The second stage is caring for the people around us—family and friends. Finally, we learn to care for the entire community we live in, which actually includes the whole planet. This is the altruistic attitude that takes a lifetime to develop. It starts in the emergent relationship between a mother and her embryo, then her fetus, and then her baby. Biodynamic practitioners can activate the compassion reflex by slowing the pace of interaction with clients via the stillpoint and Primary Respiration. This slow tempo in one's body and mind uncovers the compassion reflex. The key to compassion is slowing down so the heart and brain can recognize the pain and suffering in another person (Nyima and Shlim, 2004). Compassion and empathy then naturally arise in relationship. It is an innate system. It is the preexisting condition of our incarnation. The infant is naturally slow with her internal endogenous rhythm of growth.

Walking down the street, it is possible to encounter someone else's distress. We can see people in an ocean of Primary Respiration all around them. It is simple enough to consciously breathe in the thought of the distress in each person. This is done by taking a deep breath and imagining that the respiratory diaphragm is located in the upper left portion of the rib cage—right where the heart is located. This action alone will slow the brain down long enough for the compassion reflex to deepen in the heart. It only takes one conscious breath with a person on the street. I believe the compassion-empathy system is a complex interaction between the heart and brain of an individual that is yet to be fully understood or capable of being explained by the scientific community. I also believe that an explanation is forthcoming in my lifetime.

While working with someone biodynamically as a client, the practitioner can also breathe in the client's dilemma as a dark color into his heart and then exhale a light color and the thought of loving kindness to the client. Being a mother, a father, a therapist, and a human being requires a big heart connected to a conscious mind. It is interesting to note that the brain and heart begin as hollow organs and parallel each other's development. One needs the other almost symbiotically. The heart is the first or original organ to appear in the embryo. The original heart of the embryo differentiated at the top of the head as a fluid-filled space that, when it formed, became dynamically still for two days. Then the heart flexed forward and filled the space between the collarbones and tailbone since that space was also empty at the beginning, waiting for the heart to fill it. Those imprints of stillness, originality, and *being* in the whole middle of the human body are still there and we all have the innate potential to find our original heart. "Be still and know"—Psalm 47.[7]

Acknowledgments:

This chapter and the preceding one have been an attempt to bring forward the writing of Allan Schore to the community of biodynamic craniosacral therapists. The root texts I studied are Chapter 3, "Clinical Implications of a Psychoneuro-biological Model of Projective Identification," and Chapter 5, "Early Superego Development: The Emergence of Shame and Narcissistic Affect Regulation in the Practicing Period," which appear in *Affect Regulation and the Repair of the Self* (Schore 2003a). I am very grateful for his perseverance in spreading this vital knowledge of relationship building.

CHAPTER 23

The Change Process

In order to change beliefs, their life filters, and perceptions from attachment dysfunction, clients need well-bounded physical contact by the biodynamic practitioner. Attunement and resonance between the client and practitioner are the foundations of the change process. The practitioner works slowly, buoyantly, silently, and spaciously with the interchange between stillness and Primary Respiration in herself first, then the client, and then together pendulating attention back and forth between herself and the client. This creates a cumulative effect on the rewiring of the lower limbic (amygdala) and brain stem to the upper limbic orbitofrontal cortex (OFC) missing from misattuned infant-caregiver experiences. Thus the OFC can assume its proper function of self-regulation from the "top down" over the lower limbic structures. Biodynamic change process has different phases and sequences. This means that the residual effects of a misattuned attachment and prenatal stress are decompressed through the fluid body and its various subsystems such as the blood and lymph, at different rates and with different gradients of activity systemically. Then the autonomic nervous system will be able to respond to trauma in the soma without hyperarousal and states of freeze and collapse. When the fluid body and soma are ready to decompensate, it is called "automatic shifting" in biodynamic craniosacral therapy.

When change process occurs in biodynamic practice, the fluid body and soma automatically shift into a normal relationship with the midline. This shifting is oriented to a midline or fulcrum in the middle of the fluid body or the middle of the physiological system in the soma that is holding the trauma. Somatic trauma is held in relationship to that part of the limbic system that has the power to keep it organized at a low level of physiological function, such as the hypothalamus (immediately posterior to the OFC) and brain stem. Trauma is held in systemically in the fluid body and requires Primary Respiration to shift it into an appropriate relationship with its midline of the longitudinal fluctuation. The movement of the whole must occur first in the sequence of biodynamic practice in order for the fluid body to have a reference point for its original state in the embryo. Then the soma has a reference point for its origin and so forth.

The body is formed embryologically by two cavities (yolk sac and amnion), interconnected by a third (chorion). The early-forming visceral system (yolk sac) is followed by a fast-developing nervous system (amnion). They are connected by a circulatory system (chorion) and orienting midline. The circulatory system of the heart and vasculature needs muscles and bones as scaffolding to form an elastic matrix between the consciousness of outside and the consciousness of inside circulating in the blood of the embryo. A lasting healing response, at all levels, occurs within the client's Primary Respiration and not to any preconceived idea about Primary Respiration on the part of the practitioner. The practitioner must be patient and wait for the cumulative effect of the change process under the direction of Primary Respiration to be integrated from the fluid body to the soma. The biodynamic practitioner does this by holding the trauma as she senses it in her own body and mind and, at the same time, maintains an awareness of her own midline of stillness interchanging itself with Primary Respiration. Orientation to a midline of stillness as it translocates from outside the soma to inside and back out to the horizon is an essential therapeutic skill.

Witness Consciousness

This speaks to another important principle and that is the need to develop a self-reflective or witness consciousness. The witness can maintain attention on stillness and Primary Respiration for long periods of time. This is a critical component of the OFC that gets wired together in the preverbal time of life during the time of attachment and also through Buddhist meditation practice. The witness is associated with the conscious ability to sustain one's attention for prolonged periods of time, which results in the ability to internally weigh different options regarding a stimulus and thus control, inhibit, and slow down one's emotions and resultant states of mind. In other words, a functioning OFC gives a person choice over which emotional states are important and which are not, and to formulate a response that appropriately matches a stimulus from the outside world or another person. Hopelessness is the result of feeling there are no choices or controls over any of the circumstances in life. The witness has choices. The emerging field of neurotheology (Begley, 2001) has demonstrated that the capacity for sustained attention is also located in the OFC. MRI studies performed on long-term meditators using Buddhist mindfulness meditation show the OFC to be quite active during meditative states. Contemplative practices such as mindfulness meditation build witness consciousness, which is equated with a sense of equanimity, introspection, and non-attachment, especially to strong afflictive emotions. Mindfulness meditation reduces chronic pain, anxiety, and depression (Kabat-Zinn, et al., 1987).

It is now recognized in the research literature that practitioners need to develop the ability to synchronize with their own sensory experience first and any emotions that arise during therapeutic session work of any kind (Schore, 2003a). This requires the development of an interactive emotional-sensory regulation capacity that was intended to be wired into the brain before, during, and for the first two years after birth. The therapeutic task is to uncover and contain this imprinting, which is already present as a function of the right hemisphere in both brains of the client and the practitioner. In other words, the effects of a misattuned caregiving experience are already active and present constantly in the waking state. It is just below conscious awareness and only takes a slight nudge to bring it to consciousness. It is possible for someone to experience numerous episodes of fight-or-flight and the subsequent dissociation all day long and not even be consciously aware of it. All adult behavior has a psychometabolic origin coming from the prenatal and perinatal environment of the mother-person and the unique personality of the little one, who is growing and attempting to self-regulate with no language available to him.

Essentially, body sensation generates feeling tones and resultant emotions that, with proper training and education, can be consciously perceived. Bio-dynamic practice therefore is a perceptual study. Behaviors are the end result of working models (filters) of reality that an embryo, fetus, and infant develop through the process of imprinting, in a sentient relationship to her environment. The mother-person or caregiver is experienced both as an extension of the developing self and as a type of filter or a companion (an undifferentiated companion who is merged symbiotically) who is either friendly or not from a phenomenological point of view. In other words, if the womb and body of the mother are toxic during pregnancy with nicotine and alcohol, for example, then the embryo and later fetus owns the toxicity as part of her own body and developing self. The embryo is not aware that it is coming from the mother. The toxicity is imprinted on to the fluid body (which is a huge living fluid web) as a shape that condenses and a stillness that centers the toxicity. The embryo and fetus do not know that it is the mother's body. The mother's body is a phenomenon of the *periphery* of the embryo and fetus itself. This is the lived experience of the embryo.

Self-regulation is related psychologically to a personal drive for autonomy and freedom. This, of course, is one of the most challenging polarities that we ever encounter throughout life because it is learned while in relationship in early life. The unfolding of freedom through the lifespan happens in widely varying degrees depending on how a person experiences the mother-person.

Therapeutic Focus

There are many skills and competencies in biodynamic practice that facilitate the unfolding of freedom unique to each individual. Biodynamic practice operates under the embryological principles of growth and development. All growth and development in the human embryo and the adult body are ultimately oriented to a midline (located in the middle of the spine) and to several slow tempos found in the fluid body. The adult body is 70–75 percent fluid, the embryo 98 percent fluid. The long-term success or ability to achieve effective biodynamic therapeutic outcomes must account for these metabolic principles of embryonic origin. There must be a midline of stillness to relate to therapeutically and spiritually. A biodynamic therapeutic relationship needs to focus on the fluid body and tidal body so that emotions, as they arise, can be self-regulated by the client and reconnected to a functioning midline. Within a slow tempo a client is able to uncouple from his imprinting and understand the imprint as normal embryonic function. In this way, the practitioner gives back to the client the power or midline of internal self-regulation that was transferred onto her just as the client tried to do with his mother.

The issue frequently becomes: Is the practitioner willing to self-reveal her own internal sensory processes? What is the purpose and intention for doing so? In this case, there is a clear need for the client to know that the practitioner is a human being and has feelings of her own. Thus a mature brain is modeled and verbally reflected back to the client. Self-disclosure includes a caveat that the client does not have to take responsibility for the practitioner's feelings and emotions. There is mutual ownership and responsibility for the feelings and emotions of both the practitioner and the client. This can be challenging at first, as the therapeutic relationship navigates the ups and downs of the projection process. But a practitioner who is genuinely working on her own issues and is committed to her own self-differentiation and self-regulation can provide an enormous reflection of active maturity to the right hemisphere of the client. The client can then metabolize this maturity and learn to be in a collaborative relationship. This builds a foundation of safety and trust, as described in an earlier chapter, and allows much deeper material to emerge from the preverbal time of life and to be integrated with Primary Respiration.

Mutual respect and collaboration develops greater tolerance for deep issues to emerge in the fluid body and soma, be held and contained, and lead to more effective therapeutic outcomes. This takes time and patience. It most certainly requires generosity as well from the practitioner. All parts of the client can safely emerge in the relationship, be held in their totality of the tidal body and fluid body, and then be reflected back to the client. It is the responsibility of the practitioner to manage and maintain the container through stillness and Primary Respiration. This is of vital importance.

From the point of view of pre- and perinatal psychology, it is much more important to focus on right-brain processes than left-brain processes. Right-brain processes involve body sensation, gut feelings, spatial awareness, and the whole experience of the embryo, the fetus, the infant, and the child all rolled into one total adult client. Let us not forget to include the adolescent. Left-brain cognitions may be used as compensations and avoidance behaviors to the deeper material stacked up in the right hemisphere. The left hemisphere is exquisitely suited to experiment with symbolic language and even to lie. By this I mean the left hemisphere does not have a demand to be accurate. It can fudge the data, so to speak. On the other hand, the left-hemisphere skills that are vitally important in therapy involve keeping the client oriented in present time and helping the client sequence the body processes, memories, and experiences he is having. Language itself can be very grounding, especially in the middle of emotional affect. We live in a culture that has a relentless demand to be left-hemisphere dominant. Yet, the literature points to the fact that it is the right hemisphere that is dominant because it holds the whole history of the bodily sensorium and at the same time maintains an awareness of its totality from moment to moment. The right brain is even thought to control the amount of information it thinks the left brain can handle!

The right hemisphere is claimed to be largely unconscious, but anecdotally and in the research it is known that the right hemisphere has language and an ability to express its unique consciousness—for instance, through humor and art, not just strong affect. So, the practitioner must be able to see and understand the "gestures" of the right hemisphere in the therapeutic relationship. "The resonating practitioner must flexibly shift, in a timely manner, into a state of 'reparative withdrawal,' a self-regulating maneuver that allows continued access to a state in which a symbolizing process can take place, thereby enabling him/her to create a parallel affective and imagistic scenario that resonates with the patient's" (Freidman and Lavender, 1997). This "symbolizing process" is rooted in the sensorium of the body and the viscera; the entire last section of this book is dedicated to symbolizing and healing.

This means, in clinical practice, that the practitioner needs to be attending or attuned to her own right brain emotional functioning via her somatic sensation, because the client communicates unconsciously to the practitioner from his right hemisphere to hers. The right hemisphere stores a representation of the totality of our bodily self. The practitioner resonates via her right-hemisphere and creates an inner bodily representation of the client, as a sensory experience or an imagistic experience. Sands stated, "If I allow myself to be taken over by (the patient's) experience, successfully contain it (and wait until later to interpret it), she becomes calmer and more organized, and her need to communicate through me decreases in intensity" (Sands, 1997, p. 700).

I am advocating for a contemplative approach to biodynamic practice that utilizes this capacity to co-metabolize the client's emotional ups and downs. Very simply, the practice of "exchanging one's self for another" involves the practitioner consciously generating in her mind's eye an image of a sad event in her own life until she can sense a sensation of warmth around her heart. There is a whole chapter on this in my first volume. Then the practitioner imagines that she is breathing in a dark color that is full of all the difficult issues and dramas from the client into her heart at the tempo of Primary Respiration. The practitioner then breathes out a light color filled with well-being to the client from her heart at the same tempo. This generates both empathy and compassion consciously without having to wait unconsciously for it to emerge in the therapeutic session. It jump-starts the engine of love by bringing the witness consciousness down into the heart from the OFC. It is like a spiritual blood transfusion between practitioner and client. Paul Pearsall calls this "interpersonal cardiovascular systems" (Pearsall, 2007, p. 18).

It is imperative that the practitioner be able to focus first on the sensory aspects of her experience, and then the perception of the whole breathing with Primary Respiration. She must be able to hold the feeling long enough with a stillpoint in order for negative, preverbal belief systems (filters) to be transformed into positive belief systems regarding love, affection, tenderness, and well-being.

Conclusion

As stated throughout this section of the book, the style of the infant-mother attachment shapes the brain. The shaping process imprints emotions and beliefs that are carried through life as unconscious behaviors and working models of reality. The models are learned filters of experience that interpret reality coming from within the body and from the world outside the body. Filters include internalized images and story lines, since this is how the mind of a newborn works, rather than left-brain cognitions. As protective strategies against early wounding, filters inaccurately interpret reality and trigger mild, moderate, and severe reactions and emotions from rage and terror to negative shame and guilt. These imprinted emotions are usually very potent and can cause substantial mental affliction. Such strong affliction results in the need to freeze, collapse, project, and use transference to unload the unbearable internal pressure and conflict. All of this complex interpretation and response is largely below conscious awareness. The place to augment the therapeutic forces of Primary Respiration and the stillness is through the heart ignition process. Augmentation at this level fortifies the client's heart through the resonance with the still witness in the heart of the practitioner. The practitioner in this scenario is an equal partner in the two-way street of the therapeutic process.

Ultimately the practitioner and the client, through containment, holding, and witnessing, are able to generate meaning from preverbal experience, tolerate greater levels of uncertainty, rebuild the self-regulatory capacity of the OFC, and wake up the instinctual healing capacity of the fluid body. In other words, the practitioner forms a container and holds the client, patiently waiting, while she accesses her still witness in her gut, heart, and third ventricle. She then can cause the client to resonate with her stillpoint and slow tempo. This is enormously restorative for the client. Correct attunement is curative.

The practitioner-client relationship is designed to co-metabolize, ingest, and transform the emotional states of each individual. This builds greater tolerance for confusion and the ability to explore life more fully, including the ability to empathetically match emotions, states, imprinting, and perception in an appropriate context. Clients with PTSD symptoms frequently mistake or are misattuned with their emotions in relationship to the context or environment they are in at the present time. In other words, the response a person has to small life events often does not match the stimulus. When perception does not match the reality of a given situation, the disconnection becomes an enormous problem for any level of development, from the physical to the spiritual.

The development of a coherent self-concept originates in the OFC, the so-called "senior executive of the emotional brain" (Joseph, 1996). One's personal autobiography, etched as a memory in the nervous system and metabolism of the embryo, is dependent on a multitude of causes and conditions outside of one's control. A goal of the biodynamic therapeutic process is to rebuild and reintegrate the two modes of self-regulation, which may not have been invited into existence as an embryo or an infant. One mode of self-regulation is autonomous. The other is interdependent self-regulation. These two modes of self-regulation are necessary to deal with the relentless emotional content of life and the various stresses and dramas associated with postmodern living.

These two inherent capacities are necessary for self-differentiation and moral development. They exist as a polarity or as a possibility of a balanced ratio of activity between one and the other. First, I must overcome my insecure preverbal attachment (or, as it is sometimes called, "infantile narcissism"), then I must care for other people, and finally I must have care for the world community I live in. The capacity for self-regulation exists simultaneously in the psyche and in the unconscious, which I consider to be the human body. To self-regulate I must be able to consciously turn off strong emotions within myself, whether alone or in the presence of another. My fluid body must be able to automatically shift and fluctuate on its midline without overdensification. My heart must be able to sustain prolonged periods of settling and stilling.

The ability to have a self-reflective witness consciousness decreases the amount of negative projection of the unknown parts of the self onto other people and things. It decreases the power and the electricity of transferences that arise with a select group of people around the transferor. It decreases repetition compulsion and the pressure to reenact unconscious needs that were not met or regulated by a caregiver or mother-person. When I am unable to self-regulate, I am bound, so to speak, to get someone else to feel the unconsciousness of my state and help me to self-regulate, even if I don't get permission from the other person. I do this by gesture and behavior. Therefore, these two kinds of self-regulation and their biological substrates in the right hemisphere and OFC of the brain are crucial to the health and well-being of every human being. This includes the ability to maintain a coherent, tolerant, and flexible sense of self inside and outside the soma and a compassionate interconnectedness to the world, via the fluid body and the heart throughout the lifespan.

SECTION IV

. . .

Embryology

Client-Therapist Visualizations

The principle of center and periphery has a very direct homologue to the client-therapist relationship. In this chapter, my intention is to present a sequence of events that occur through the physical movement and shaping of the human embryo. Then it must be understood how that process is oriented to points of stillness in the fluids outside the central body of the embryo and the actual structure of the tubes that the blood flows through and the pericardium itself.

A homologue is defined as the origin of a function that remains throughout life, but differs depending on the context. In other words, when two people get together in a therapeutic relationship, the underlying metabolism of that relationship is directly related to the way in which the metabolic fields of the human embryo, especially the central and peripheral bodies of the embryo, relate to one another in the weeks following conception. I call this the self-self relationship. Following that are self-other relationships that the embryo forms with aspects of the maternal environment via the uterus. There are many such homologues to be found in the human embryo that can be extended into the therapeutic relationship, as described below.

- **Trophoblast-embryoblast (periphery to central body).** Imagine as you sit with a client that you are a cluster of cells and the client is a cluster of cells. Both of you are connected only by a sea of fluid inside a sphere that encloses both of you and extends several feet beyond both of your bodies. As a therapist, imagine that you are the cluster of cells that is going to become the gut first and the client is a cluster of cells that will function as the interface between the inner world of your gut and the outer world of the mother's womb. What is the nature of this connection by fluid only? Is it possible to sense the client as though both of you were resting in a fluid medium, both inside and outside of your body? At the same time, these two clusters of cells are moving as the sphere that contains both of you together is rolling down the fallopian tube. Is it possible to feel both you and the client moving as a single unit?

- **Endoderm-ectoderm.** Imagine now in the second week of embryonic development that the definitive cells forming the gut have differentiated first. Let the client be the gut. The therapist is the future nervous system, the ectoderm. The therapist as ectoderm has a sac of fluid attached to its dorsal surface. The client has endoderm as a sac of fluid attached to the ventral surface of his body. Imagine as the therapist that you have an enormous sac of clear fluid attached from the back of your head all the way down to the heels of your feet. This sac extends 6–12 feet in back of you. Meanwhile the client has an equally large sac extending from forehead down to toenails on the front of his body. This enormous sac of fluid engulfs you. Now the connection between the two of you is stronger and grows. There is still a sphere that surrounds both you and the client that is burrowing deeper and deeper into the uterine wall of the mother. Begin to sense how the space around you and the client has a texture and a tone to it that extends out to the walls of your office space and perhaps beyond. Tune into a very subtle tidal movement or subtle wind moving in these fluids.

- **Heart-blood.** The blood is the first organ to arise. It is outside of the central body of the embryo. Let the client be the blood as it circulates outside of your own body, but yet is contained on the inside surface of the chorionic cavity, the sphere that holds both of you. Let the client be the blood that circulates all around the inside surface of this sphere and all around the outside surface of your body and the client's body. This blood contains connective tissue and seeks to establish not only tubes for the blood to flow in but also a solid connecting stalk that links both of you to the womb and the Great Mother. The therapist is the heart. The heart begins to develop as two tubes that merge into one. Sense your body as one big heart from head to foot. This is the way it was toward the end of the second week and beginning of the third week of embryonic development. Your heart must get connected to the client's blood and begin a reciprocal flow moving at a very slow tempo. The sphere that contains both of you must now get grounded and rooted into the uterine wall in order to survive. Now switch places with the client. Let the client be a big heart and you be the blood. Notice any changes in tempo or feeling tone in the room.

- **Embryo-placenta.** Let the client be the placenta. The therapist is now the embryo. Both are connected by a strong connecting stalk and umbilical veins and arteries. The placenta allows nourishment in the form of molecules to come through its body and mix with the blood of the embryo. Imagine the molecules that make up the client's body are now slowly and in a tidelike manner migrating into your body. Likewise, a buildup of waste products from your body and blood are recirculating back into the client's body. This is normal metabolism. It is a much better way to imagine the psychic debris that therapists frequently complain that they have to ingest from their clients. The client is doing the same with the therapist. Reverse the roles. The client now becomes the embryo and the therapist is the placenta. Slowly, all of the cells of the body of the therapist are migrating slowly through an ocean of fluid into the inside of the client's body. Concentrate on love and compassion as surrounding every cell of your body and the client's body.

- **Heart-head.** In this contemplation, the therapist begins as the heart and the client is the nervous system and brain. The relationship of the heart to the brain is one of slowness to speed. The heart likes to be slow and consequently causes a lot of resistance in the brain growth that ultimately contributes to the formation of the brain's coverings including the muscles and bones. The therapist sits and imagines her whole body is a heart that is moving very slowly. The major veins and arteries of the heart extend out to the brain and nervous system of the client. Notice any resistance or tug in the space between yourself and the client. The principle action of the heart in this case is slowness. The principle action of the brain and nervous system is speed. Now reverse roles. The therapist now becomes the brain and nervous system. Likewise, the client becomes the heart. Imagine these large veins and arteries between your two bodies. Bring awareness and attention to the total surface volume of your skin as the therapist and notice if it is being pushed or pulled in any direction. What images or sensations arise on the inside of your body as you are connected to your heart, which is the client? The heart-brain relationship is a very strong relationship. Make sure that this flow has a very slow tempo and wait until the tempo disappears and all that's left is stillness and silence.

- **Embryo-womb.** In this contemplation, the therapist begins as the womb. The client is the embryo. What does the womb represent to you? Imagine this soft, warm, dark, supportive, and nurturing space. At the same time, this space is compressed, so imagine that the therapist as womb has a thick sphere of warm, dense material surrounding the client as well. Close your eyes briefly and imagine being in a dark space like a cave. What feelings come up? Is this scary or nurturing? Imagine an umbilical cord from your own umbilicus to the umbilicus of your client as the embryo. Imagine a movement of fluid from the core of your body moving out of your abdomen through the umbilical cord and into the client. Wait for the reversal of motion so the client and his essence moves from the core of his body out into the umbilical cord and into the therapist. Imagine that this liquid movement has the texture of liquid soap. As before, reverse the roles. Let the client become the womb that supports and nurtures the therapist. Let the therapist as the embryo bring attention to her abdomen and umbilicus. Imagine the flow of very rich nutrient coming from the client into the umbilicus of the therapist. Then let it reverse itself. Make sure that this flow has a very slow tempo and wait until the tempo disappears and all that's left is stillness and silence.

- **Metabolic field relationships.** An embryonic field is always in relationship to adjacent field(s). The client and therapist represent two metabolic fields in direct relationship to one another. This means that they have different tempos, directions, and densities of activity that are influencing each other. (1) The client is the fluid breathing oriented to the therapist as a fulcrum of stillness. (2) The client and therapist are reciprocally breathing. This means that when the therapist inhales, the client exhales, and vice versa. At some point, both the client and therapist will inhale together and exhale together. (3) At some point in the client-therapist relationship, either or both the therapist and client will experience all boundaries dissolving between each other. This may cause an awareness of expanding into open space. (4) Both the client and the therapist are resisting each other, as though they are having a tug of war pulling on a rope between the two of them with equal pressure. The therapist waits for the perception of stillness through this tension resistance. (5) Frequently, the client-therapist relationship feels very compressed and claustrophobic, and then releases and expands. This is a type of emotional breathing between the two metabolic fields. The compression-decompression may be limited to a headache or a backache or involve a more systemic cluster of sensations for either or both the client and therapist. (6) Frequently, either or both the client and therapist become uncomfortable in the position of sitting, standing, or lying. Consequently, either or both the therapist and client begins to shift position—crossing the legs, doing a stretch, or getting up and going for a glass of water. Any gross motor activity of the body's musculoskeletal system represents the felt sense of two embryonic metabolic fields relating to one another normally. The important principle of understanding these embryonic fields that condense into the structure of the human body is that they are all oriented to a center point of stillness and are connected by a very slow tempo, much like a Long Tide moving in the ocean for a minute in one direction and then a minute in the other direction. Whenever the therapist is compelled to move, she should do so very slowly and also instruct the client to move slowly.

- **Embryo-mother as a metabolic field.** Imagine that the client is an embryo at the time that the therapist as mother discovers she is pregnant with a new life. What feelings and sensations arise during this discovery process? Usually the most important part of the body being developed during the discovery process is the blood and heart. The relationship between the embryo and the mother is principally centered in the blood. Some cells, unencapsulated maternal DNA, and a host of molecules come from the mother into the embryo's blood. On the other hand, the embryo is also exchanging its cells' DNA and molecules with the mother. The immune system of the mother is active and the mother unconsciously resists the embryo and the embryo unconsciously resists the mother. It is as if the mother and embryo must work hard to maintain their own autonomy while embracing each other at such an intimate level. Is it possible for the therapist to sense the power of this polarity? This is an enormous resistance between a unified state and the necessity for autonomy.

You can see from this partial description that the embryo is constantly self-regulating itself through a bifurcation of its structure and function into two distinct metabolisms. One is the metabolism of autonomy and one is the metabolism of relationship. One will die at birth and be temporarily replaced by the mother-person and all subsequent relationships through a projection process. This bifurcation exists all the way from cell aggregations, organ differentiation, and maternal uterine relationships to the psychology of projection and transference in adult relationships. The principle is that metabolism becomes physiology and then becomes psychology. Embryonic metabolism has homologous links to adult structure and functional relationships. This includes especially the client-therapist relationship.

In conclusion, I would like to reiterate the importance of using the embryonic metaphor for the therapeutic relationship. The embryo strives to form a relationship with itself by dividing into two bodies during development. These two bodies, the central and peripheral bodies, form a self-self relationship and circulatory system for managing structure and function. Thus at one point of the client-therapist relationship, it seems that both the client and therapist are in a merged, undifferentiated state. This phase of the therapeutic relationship requires conscious awareness and containment within the fluid body of the practitioner, as stated in earlier chapters. Gradually, the embryo builds a relationship with the uterine environment in what I call the self-other phase of the therapeutic relationship. During this phase of biodynamic practice, the practitioner is able to make a clear distinction between herself and the client. Nonetheless, it is still a circulatory system based on the placenta while the self-self relationship gradually becomes based on the central body of the embryo and the yolk sac. By maintaining a three-dimensional awareness of the surface of the practitioner's skin, the ability to orient to a shifting state of stillness, and the hands and arms of the practitioner as a type of umbilical cord and connecting stalk, the practitioner can enter the biodynamic circulatory system called the client-therapist relationship.

CHAPTER 25

Early Formation of the Basicranium in Man

By Raymond F. Gasser, PhD

Over the past century there have been extensive studies on the developing skull including its basal portion. These studies have dealt with both its ontogeny and phylogeny. Most of the information available prior to 1937 was included in DeBeer's classical tome entitled *The Development of the Vertebrate Skull,* which included a section on the ontogenesis of the human skull. Since then, there have been numerous publications on the embryology of various parts of the skull in a variety of vertebrates.

Blechschmidt (Blechschmidt, 1961, 1969, 1973, 1974) has published extensively on the biokinetic aspect of human development including the skull. In 1961 he described the dural girdles or thickened bands in the embryonic skull. The development of the frontal bone was presented by him in 1969. His biokinetic principles and theories are the results of many years of precise and extensive investigations on a wealth of human embryonic material. He documented his new findings in 1973 with the publication of an atlas of very accurate total reconstructions of each system in embryos at critical stages of development. These findings were discussed and explained in a recent monograph (Blechschmidt, 1974). Special attention was given to the development of the *position, shape,* and *inner structure* of organs and were found to be closely related. He concludes that cells and tissues differentiate according to their particular location in the embryo where a particular set of biophysical phenomena exists. Hopefully, as a result of our coming together attention will be focused on these principles and theories. Because of them and, in light of recent experimental studies, human skull development should be reexamined especially its basal portion. Experimental studies have shown that parts of the head mesenchyma and its various skeletal derivations are normally formed by neural crest cells. Papers on this topic include those of Chibon (Chibon, 1964) on the amphibian embryo and Johnston (Johnston, 1966) on the avian embryo. The relationship between the formation of the cranial base and closure of the palate was investigated by Long, et al. (Long, Larsson, and Lohmander, 1973). Enlow and McNamara (Enlow and McNamara, 1973) described the relationship between the development and configuration of the brain and the formation of the cranial base. Overman and Peterson (Overman and Peterson, 1975) found that the brains of drug-induced cleft palate mice were reduced in size and lagged in development.

General

The human basicranium develops from the mesenchymal cells located during the fourth week between the cranial part of the neural tube and the foregut. Presumably, these cells originate from both the primitive streak and *cranial neural crests*. During the fifth and sixth weeks the mesenchymal cells increase in number and begin to collect in certain areas to form condensations. The condensations are collectively referred to as the *desmocranium* or blastemal stage of skull development. Some of the condensations will differentiate directly into membrane bone. Others will develop into cartilage most of which subsequently ossifies.

Cartilage formation is evident in human embryos by the seventh week. The cartilaginous part of the developing skull, the *chondrocranium,* reaches its height of development during the third month and arises through the fusion of a considerable number of cartilages originating from independent centers of chondrification. The chondrocranium is mainly but not completely replaced by bone. Ossification begins during the latter part of the second month. Most individual bones of the skull arise from two or more centers of ossification. Many are partly membranous and partly cartilaginous in origin. This is especially true of the bones that form the skull base.

At the beginning of the second month, mesenchyma at the ventral aspect of the neural tube forms a loose network of cells sometimes referred to as the *primitive meninx.* By the middle of the month, the basal and lateral parts of the primitive meninx differentiate into an outer, dense layer called the *ectomeninx* or brain capsule and an inner, loosely arranged layer called the *endomeninx* located adjacent to the brain. The ectomeninx gives rise to the dura mater and the cartilages and bones of the skull.

The precartilage condensations at the base of the brain are named mainly in relation to the midline notochord that terminates behind the hypophysis. A *parachordal* formation becomes evident on each side of the notochord extending from the hypophysis to near the caudal end of the rhombencephalon. It transforms into cartilage and fuses with its counterpart on the opposite side to form the *basal plate.* When the occipital sclerotomes fuse with the caudal end of the plate, the hypoglossal canal and nerve become incorporated into the plate. The *prechordal* formation is in and near the midline in front of the notochord. Here there are two pairs of chondrification centers: (1) the two fused *trabecular cartilages* which probably have a large neural crest component and (2) the two *polar hypophyseal cartilages,* one located on each side of the hypophyseal stem remnant. These four centers unite and join to the rostral margin of the basal plate. In addition to the para-and prechordal condensations, there are others located more laterally. They are the *otic* and *nasal sense capsules,* the *ala orbitalis* (orbitosphenoid) around the optic nerve, and the *ala temporalis* (alisphenoid) around the maxillary nerve as it arises from the trigeminal ganglion.

The Basicranial Region in Human Embryos Three through Eight Weeks of Age

The morphology of the basicranial region will be presented in staged human embryos beginning with a presomite, 18-day specimen and ending with a late embryonic, 54-day specimen when the chondrocranium is well developed and ossification centers have begun. Approximate ages of the specimens were based on the publications of Iffy, et al. (Iffy, et al., 1967) and O'Rahilly (O'Rahilly, 1972). Stages 8, 10, 13, 16, 19, and 23 will be described (O'Rahilly, 1973; Streeter, 1945, 1948, 1951; Heuser and Corner, 1957). The greatest length (GL) of the youngest embryo is approximately 1.5 mm (23–25 days). The crown-rump length (C-RL) of the oldest specimen is 30.7 mm (56 days). All of the specimens with one exception are from the Carnegie Collection now housed at the University of California, Davis. One 18-mm (C-RL) specimen is from the Hooker-Humphrey-Brown Collection at the University of Alabama Medical Center, Birmingham. Total wax or graphic reconstructions of each embryo and most of its systems were made. Line drawings taken from reconstructions of the head region indicate the level and plane of each micrograph.[8]

Third Week. The embryo is an arching disc of tissue between the amniotic and yolk sac cavities (Figure 25.1). The three primary germ layers become well defined as the primitive streak that extends caudally from the primitive knot gives rise to the loose intermediate layer of mesoderm. Toward the latter part of the week the notochordal process lies in the midline beneath the ectoderm from the cranial end of the disc to the primitive knot, elongating as the knot moves caudally. The notochordal process joins the underlying endoderm throughout most of its extent. A tiny canal in the notochordal process provides a communicating channel between the amniotic and yolk sac cavities. A shallow, median groove in the ectoderm overlying the notochordal process represents the first appearance of the brain anlage. The floor of the groove, the neural plate, is bound on each side by a neural fold. Mesenchymal tissue in front of the notochordal process at the edge of the disc gives rise to the primordial heart which will move ventrally and caudally as the head fold develops (Figure 25.1, arrow). Ectoderm covers the later aspect of the disc as the lateral body folds form.

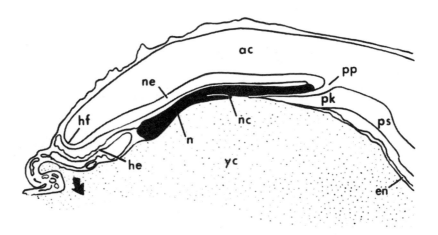

Figure 25.1. Midsagittal view of the cranial portion of a reconstructed pre-somite human embryo, stage 8, eighteen days. Arrow indicates direction of movement of head fold. ac, amniotic cavity; en, endoderm; he, heart primordium; hf, head fold; n, notochordal process; nc, notochordal canal; ne, neural plate ectoderm; pk, primitive knot; pp, primitive pit; ps, primitive streak; yc, yolk sac cavity.

Fourth Week. With further development of the head and lateral body folds, the cranial part of the endoderm forming the roof of the yolk sac cavity becomes molded into a blind tube, the foregut (Figure 25.2). The heart moves to a position ventral to the foregut. Dorsal to the foregut the neural folds approach each other in the midline and begin to fuse giving rise to the neural tube. A ventral bend in the brain anlage, the cephalic flexure, indicates the position of the mesencephalon with the prosencephalon in front and the rhombencephalon behind. Cells collect in the angle between the neural plate and the surface ectoderm giving rise to cranial neural crests. Trigeminal and the facioacoustic crests develop early.

Figure 25.2. Sagittal view of the cranial portion of a reconstructed 10-somite, 3.0-mm (GL) human embryo, stage 10, twenty-two days. Arrow indicates growth direction of brain. f, facio-acoustic neural crest; fg, foregot; he, heart; hf, head fold; m, mesencephalon; n, notochordal plate; op, oropharyngeal membrane; p, prosencephalon; pp, first pharyngeal pouch; r, rhombencephalon; st, stomodeum; t, trigeminal neural crest.

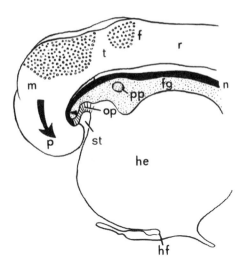

For a short period the notochordal process at most levels becomes a plate forming the median part of the dorsal foregut lining. It is also in close contact with the neural tube. After separation from these organs, it is referred to as the notochord. Its terminal portion lies near the prosmesencephalic junction in the oropharyngeal membrane (Figure 25.3). This membrane makes up the floor of the stomodeum separating the stomodeum from the foregut. The first aortic arch courses dorsally from the heart through the first pharyngeal arch to join the dorsal aorta above the foregut roof. An enlarged capillary channel in the mesenchymal tissue next to the ventral part of the neural tube represents the internal carotid artery. The primary head vein begins as a network of anastomosing capillary channels on the lateral surface of the brain anlage.

Figure 25.3. Sagittal view of the cranial half of a reconstructed 5.0-mm (C-RL) human embryo, stage 13, twenty-eight days. Arrows indicate brain movements. Triangles denote position of cephalic and cervical flexures. d, diencephalon; fg, foregut; h, hypophyseal pouch; he, heart; m, mesencephalon; n, notochord; o, primitive oral cavity; os, optic stalk; pc, parachordal condensation; r, rhombencephalon; te, telencephalon.

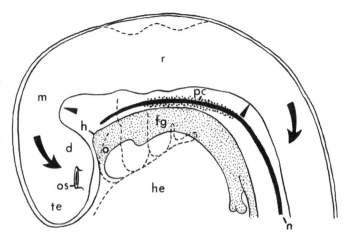

Fifth Week. As the embryo bends ventrally into a C-shape, the pharyngeal arches and grooves become distinct (Figure 25.4). The C-shaped neural tube closes completely and exhibits sharp ventral bends in the region of the mesencephalon (cephalic flexure) and at the junction region of the rhombencephalon with the spinal cord (cervical flexure) (Figure 25.5, arrows). The optic nerve begins as the stalk of the optic vesicle (outpouching of the prosencephalon). With this, the telencephalic and diencephalic brain subdivisions can be determined. A loose network of mesenchymal cells that are collectively referred to as the primitive meninx surrounds the brain.

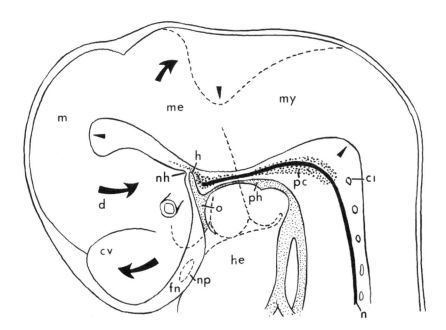

Figure 25.4. Sagittal view of the cranial half of a reconstructed 10.5-mm (C-RL) human embryo, stage 16, thirty-seven days. Arrows indicate brain movements. Triangles denote position of cephalic, pontine, and cervical flexures. C1, level of first cervical nerve; cv, cerebral vesicle; d, diencephalon; fn, frontonasal area; h, hypophyseal pouch; he, heart; m, mesencephalon; me, metencephalon; my, myelencephalon; n, notochord; nh, neurohypophyseal bud; np, nasal pit; o, primitive oral cavity; pc, parachordal condensation; ph, primitive pharynx.

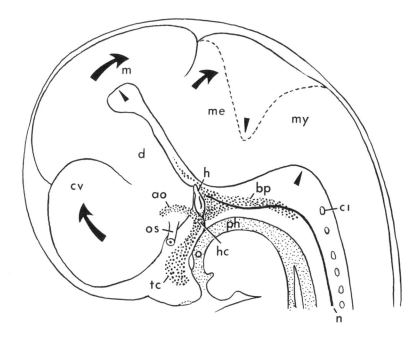

Figure 25.5. Sagittal view of the head region of a reconstructed 18.0-mm (C-RL) human embryo, stage 19, forty-six days. Arrows indicate brain movements. Triangles denote position of cephalic, pontine, and cervical flexures. ao, ala orbitalis; bp, basal plate; C1, level of first cervical nerve; cv, cerebral vesicle; d, diencephalon; h, hypophysis; hc, hypophyseal cartilage; m, mesencephalon; me, metencephalon; my, myelencephalon; n, notochord; o, primitive oral cavity; os, optic stalk; ph, primitive pharynx; tc, trabecular cartilage.

The notochord also becomes C-shaped along with the embryo and neural tube (Figure 25.5). It is composed of densely packed cells surrounded by a faint sheath as it detaches from the roof of the foregut. Mesenchymal cells begin to collect lateral to it in the vicinity of the rhombencephalon. This cell collection represents the parachordal condensation (Figure 25.5). The ventral and medial walls of the occipital somites break down as a result of cell proliferation to form a collection of cells that represents the occipital sclerotomes. This condensation develops lateral to the caudal part of the rhombencephalon in the vicinity of the hypoglossal nerve. Its ventral portion is closely related to the notochord and the caudal part of the parachordal condensation. With the complete disappearance of the oropharyngeal membrane, the ectodermal lining of the stomodeum is continuous with the endodermal lining of the foregut. The junction area is approximately at the cranial tip of the notochord. A broad shallow diverticulum that forms just rostral to the notochordal tip in the stomodeal ectoderm is the beginning of the hypophyseal (Rathke's) pouch. It is closely related to the diencephalon near the region of the cephalic flexure (Figure 25.5). The attachment of the notochordal tip to the epithelial lining of the pouch is transient. An internal carotid artery passes each side of the pouch.

Sixth Week. The cephalic and cervical brain flexures become more acute and a dorsal bend occurs in the rhombencephalon called the pontine flexure (Figure 25.6). The latter flexure delineates the metencephalic and myelencephalic subdivisions of the brain. The metencephalon moves dorsally and caudally (upper arrow). A cerebral vesicle appears on each side as a dorso-lateral outpouching of the telencephalon (lower arrow). The diencephalon bends dorsally and caudally as the cephalic flexure becomes more acute (middle arrow). At the base of the brain, the primitive meninx separates into an inner loosely arranged layer (endomeninx) and an outer condensed layer (ectomeninx) in which the desmocranium is forming. All twelve cranial nerves can be identified.

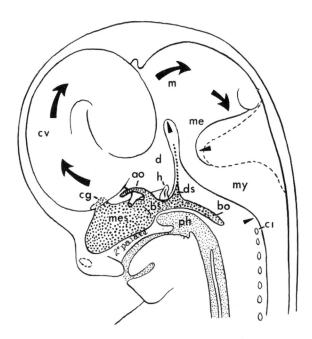

Figure 25.6. Sagittal view of the head region of reconstructed 30.7-mm (C-RL) human embryo, stage 23, fifty-four days. Arrows indicate brain movements. Triangles denote position of cephalic, pontine, and cervical flexures. ao, ala orbitalis; bo, basioccipital; bs, basisphenoid; C1, level of first cervical nerve; cg, crista galli; cv, cerebral vesicle; d, diencephalon; ds, dorsum sellae; h, hypophysis; m, mesencephalon; me, metencephalon; mes, mesethmoid; my, myelencephalon; ph, pharynx.

The hypophyseal pouch elongates but remains in communication with the former stomodeum that enlarges and becomes the primitive oral cavity. The point of communication is located behind the optic chiasma area. The epithelial wall of the pouch thickens and is closely associated with the neurohypophyseal bud of the diencephalon. Passing lateral to the lower part of the hypophysis is the internal carotid artery, which joins other arteries at the base of the brain to form the circle of Willis. The thickened ectoderm below the cerebral vesicle invaginates as the nasal pit (Figure 25.6). Mesenchymal cells collect between the nasal pits contributing to the formation of the frontonasal area.

The ventral bend in the cranial segment of the notochord is reduced as the pontine brain flexure develops (Figure 25.6). The parachordal condensation enlarges in the roof of the primitive pharynx and extends to the cranial tip of the notochord next to the hypophyseal pouch. The sclerotomic condensation from the occipital somites blends with the caudal end of the parachordal condensation. Rootlets of the hypoglossal nerve course through the sclerotomic part. Mesenchymal cells collect at the periphery of the expanding epithelial wall of the otocyst and nasal pit, thereby forming the otic and nasal capsules, respectively.

Seventh Week. The pontine brain flexure becomes more acute as the head begins to raise from the ventral chest wall and the expanding cerebral vesicle starts covering the diencephalon (Figure 25.6, arrows). The hypophyseal pouch no longer communicates with the primitive oral cavity, but for a short period its wall remains connected by a narrow stem remnant (Figure 25.6).

As the cerebral vesicles expand the midface region enlarges. The paired primitive nasal cavity develops from the deepened nasal pits and is separated from the primitive oral cavity by the primitive palate. With rupture of the oronasal membrane the two cavities communicate through the primitive choana. The inner aspect of the maxillary process bulges into the enlarging primitive oral cavity forming the lateral palatine process. The lateral palatine process is closely related to the lateral surface of the tongue that also protrudes into the cavity.

The chondrocranium begins to replace the desmocranium as the precartilage condensations transform into cartilage. The parachordal condensations together with the occipital sclerotomic condensations become the basal plate cartilage (Figure 25.6). The cartilaginous plate lies between the rhombencephalon and the primitive pharynx from the hypophysis to the first cervical nerve. Hypoglossal nerve rootlets course through a large canal in the caudal part of the basal plate. The notochord takes a slight S-shaped course through the basal plate with its middle segment located on the ventral surface. Cranial to this, it passes obliquely through the basal plate to terminate near the hypophysis. The caudal segment also passes obliquely through the basal plate to the dorsal surface near the occipito-cervical junction. The otic capsule is becoming cartilage and begins to fuse with the lateral aspect of the plate.

The basal plate is continuous rostrally with the prechordal condensations that are also transforming into cartilage but at a slower rate. Hypophyseal (polar) cartilages flank the stem remnant and join together in the midline between the stem remnant and the optic chiasma. The fused portion of the prechordal condensation gives rise to the trabecular cartilage that extends rostrally in the midline to become continuous with the nasal capsule condensation and primitive palate mesenchyma.

The ala orbitalis begins as a sickle-shaped condensation arching over the optic stalk (Figure 25.6). It quickly transforms into cartilage and joins the lateral aspect of the hypophyseal cartilage. The ala temporalis develops as an isolated condensation medial to the maxillary and mandibular nerves and lateral to the rostral portion of the basal plate.

Eighth Week. As the head continues to raise, the cervical brain flexure becomes less acute (Figure 25.6). The cephalic and pontine flexures do not change substantially but the entire front portion of the brain raises (arrows). The mesencephalon moves dorsally relative to its earlier position. The metencephalon and myelencephalon move from an almost horizontal position to an almost vertical one. The cerebral vesicle undergoes considerable expansion growing in a semi-circular direction (dorsally and caudally) and covering over much of the diencephalon.

Enlargement of the midface region continues to concur with the movements of the expanding brain (Figure 25.6). The lateral palatine processes move from a vertical position lateral to the tongue to a horizontal position above the tongue. The processes fuse with each other and the lower edge of the nasal septum, thereby forming the secondary palate.

Most of the desmocranium is replaced by the chondrocranium. The more rostral portion continues to lag behind differentiation of the more caudal portion. Midline components of the basicranium can be identified but not as separate cartilages. The basal plate forms the basioccipital cartilage. It is continuous rostrally with the basisphenoidal cartilage, which develops from the hypophyseal cartilages and contains a shallow fossa that houses the hypophysis. A prominent transverse ridge at the back of the fossa represents the dorsum sellae. The hypophyseal stem remnant usually completely disappears but occasionally lingers for a while in the center of the cartilage. More rostrally, the trabecular cartilage becomes a vertical cartilaginous plate within the nasal septum called the mesethmoid. This cartilage separates the epithelium of each side of the nasal cavity and connects the nasal capsule cartilage with the basisphenoid without a demarcating line. Its upper edge exhibits a prominent crista galli that separates the olfactory bulbs.

Two parts of the ala orbitalis can be identified, a basal part that joins the basisphenoid and a lateral sickle-shaped part that arches around the optic nerve. Projecting laterally from the basisphenoid is the ala temporalis which forms a small part of the very incomplete middle cranial fossa. The foramen rotundum can be identified.

Summary

The morphology of the basicranial region is presented in the representative stages of human embryonic development beginning with a presomite, three-week specimen and ending with a late embryonic, eight-week specimen, when the chondrocranium is well established. Attempts are made to correlate this morphology with the arrangement of related important structures, *viz.* the brain, meninges, hypophysis, notochord, the primitive pharyngeal, nasal, and oral cavities, certain cranial nerves, and blood vessels.[9]

CHAPTER 26

The Development of the Facial Muscles in Man

By Raymond F. Gasser, PhD

—ABSTRACT—Morphogenesis and histogenesis of the facial muscles are described in human embryos and fetuses 4.2–360.0 mm (crown-rump length, abbreviated C-RL). The microscopic study was performed on 50 specimens that had been variously serially-sectioned and stained. Graphic or wax reconstructions were made from transverse serial sections at eleven representative ages. Three late fetuses and a term infant were studied grossly.

Second branchial arch mesenchyme in early embryos (4.2–6.5 mm, 32 days postfertilization) becomes increasingly dense, but is not subdivided into distinct premuscle masses. By 8–20 mm (38–46 days postfertilization), sheetlike collections (laminae) of premyoblasts and early myoblasts extend from the superficial part of the arch into the temporal, occipital, cervical, and mandibular regions. Premuscle condensations deep in the arch become the stapedius, posterior digastric, and stylohyoid muscles. The infraorbital lamina and the occipital platysma appear by 20–23 mm (49–51 days postfertilization). The superficial muscles differentiate rapidly between 26 and 37 mm (end of the embryonic period to 56 days, and beginning of fetal period). Most are composed of myoblasts at 41 mm. By 80 mm, all the muscles contain myotubes and are in their definitive positions. At 80–140 mm the myotubes become young muscle fibers. From 140 mm to 360 mm (term) the muscles increase in size and gain definitive attachments. Superficial muscles differentiate later than the deep and those in the cervicomandibular and occipital regions differentiate earlier than those in the frontal and midfacial regions. The muscle masses form pari passu with the muscular branches of the facial nerve which develop deep to them.

This [article] presents a detailed description of the morphogenesis and histogenesis of the muscles innervated by the seventh cranial or facial nerve in man. Such a study may be helpful in understanding and explaining variations and anomalous arrangements of the facial musculature and the general patterns of development in the head and neck regions. Besides functioning to express the emotions of man, these muscles are also important in phonation, mastication, deglutition, audition, and vision. This may help explain their extensive development and their unusual degree of individualization in the human subject. In comparison to the important role this musculature plays in the postnatal life of man, its embryology has received little attention. Since the time of Rabl (Rabl, 1887) and Gegenbaur (Gegenbaur, 1890) the embryonic development of the facial muscles has been associated with the second branchial or hyoid arch. Futamura's (Futamura, 1906) paper is the most extensive report on the morphogenesis of these muscles and is widely quoted in the literature. He described the ontogeny of the muscles in the light of their phylogeny, which makes an already difficult subject more complex. In addition, the existence of primitive sphincter arrangements which he described at an early age around the eye, nose, mouth, and ear is questionable. Because Popowsky (Popowsky, 1895) and Huber (Huber, 1931) used mainly fetal dissections as the source of their information, they could not adequately cover the early morphogenesis of the facial muscles and even many of the muscles in the fetal specimens were overlooked. Zuckermann-Zicha (Zuckerman-Zicha, 1925) included statements on facial muscle histogenesis in their papers but more complete information during the early periods of prenatal life becomes significant in the light of Hooker's (Hooker, 1952, 1958) and Humphrey's (Humphrey, 1964) studies on the appearance of human fetal reflexes in the head and neck areas.

Materials and Methods

The head and neck of fifty serially sectioned human embryos and fetuses 4.2 to 146.0 mm crown-rump length (C-RL) were examined microscopically and segregated according to their state of development into four groups. Three aborted late fetuses (142, 210, and 270 mm C-RL) and a stillborn term infant (360 mm C-RL) were dissected. The three oldest dissected specimens comprised a fifth group. All future references to millimeter measurements in this [article] will pertain to C-RL. All references to ages of the specimens studied will be menstrual age calculated from the C-RL.

The distribution of the sectioned specimens is as follows: group I, 4 specimens 4.2 to 6.5 mm (29–33 days); group II, 20 specimens 8 to 20 mm (36–49 days); group III, 18 specimens 20 to 45 mm (49 days onward); group IV, 8 specimens 20 to 45 mm; group IV, 8 specimens 50 to 146 mm (fetal period). The material had been sectioned in various planes and at various thicknesses, but most were cut transversely at 10 μ. Most of the youngest specimens (4.2–13.5 mm) had been stained with hematoxylin and eosin; specimens 13.5 to 37.0 mm had been stained with a variety of techniques, usually either protargol or a quadruple stain of hematoxylin, orange g, aniline blue, and eosin. The 14 sectioned specimens over 37 mm had been stained with the quadruple stain.

The right sides of 11 transversely sectioned specimens at representative age levels were reconstructed, five graphically and six with wax. As many as 30 measurements were made on the right half of the projected image (17X to 70X) in the graphically reconstructed specimens. A graph was constructed which consisted of horizontal parallel lines. The distance between the lines depended upon the thickness of the sections, their magnification, and the number of sections measured. The measurements of the sections with the largest rostrodorsal diameter were the first plotted on the graph followed by sections cranial and caudal to them. The picture constructed in this manner is a lateral view of the right half of the head and neck. The sections were subsequently examined microscopically in order to determine the location, arrangement, and extent of the muscle precursors. Premuscle masses were plotted on graphs section by section in the form of dots (mesenchyme) and lines (myoblasts and myotubes). The lines had the same orientation as the premuscle cells in the sections.

The wax reconstructions resulted in essentially the same type of map with the added feature of having definite external contours. Their construction was similar to the method of Born (Born, 1883). Selected sections were projected (7X to 20X) onto sheets of dental tray spacer wax which had a uniform thickness (1.7 mm). The outlines of the projected images were cut into the wax sheets. Each sheet represented the same number of sections. The approximately 100 impressions were stacked in order and secured in position. The right side of the resulting model and a scale were photographed from a central lateral position and prints made at one-to-one magnification. The wax sheets in the model were represented in the print tracings as horizontal, parallel lines 1.7 mm apart. The sections were examined microscopically and the facial premuscle masses were plotted on the tracings in the same manner as above.

The dissected specimens were obtained relatively fresh and in good condition, embalmed by way of the umbilical vein with 10 percent buffered formalin, submerged in this fixative for two days, and then washed in tap water for 24 hours. Then they were wrapped in cotton previously soaked in Kaiserling III solution, placed in plastic bags, and stored as long as six months at 40°F. One week before their dissection, the heads and necks were lightly and carefully skinned and submerged in Bouin's fluid. At the time of their dissection, the fetuses were washed for one minute in water. The dissections were performed with a dissecting microscope at magnifications up to 40X using teasing needles, needle forceps, and a small pair of scissors.

The types of primordial muscle cells present in various regions of the facial muscle field were observed in ten variously stained, representative specimens 4.8 to 146.0 mm. After 26 mm, four regions were primarily observed, namely, occipital, orbicularis oris, orbicularis oculi, and buccinator. The definitions of the various terms used for stages of histogenesis differ considerably from one author to another. In order to avoid this confusion, the terms suggested by Boyd (Boyd, 1960) for the histogenesis of nonsomitic muscles have been used, namely *premyoblast, myoblast, myotube,* and *muscle fiber.* In order to facilitate a better understanding of facial muscle histogenesis some of Boyd's stages have been subdivided. The definition of each stage and substage is as follows:

1. *Premyoblast*—a primordial muscle cell which cannot be distinguished from associated fibroblasts and is without orientation.
   a. Early—an irregular stellate-shaped cell with little cytoplasm and a large, round, darkly staining nucleus.
   b. Late—an irregular stellate or spindle-shaped cell with scant cytoplasm and an oval nucleus that stains lightly with finely clumped chromatin.

2. *Myoblast*—the cell may be uni- or multinucleated, has become elongated but shows no visible transverse striations and little or no cytoplasmic structure. Many groups of nuclei are oriented in the same direction.
   a. Early—a uninucleated, short, spindle-shaped cell with the cytoplasm beginning to increase in amount and containing one oval or elongated, ellipsoidal nucleus with one or two nucleoli and finely clumped chromatin. No cytoplasmic structures are visible.
   b. Middle—a uni- or multinucleated, long, spindle-shaped cell with elongated, ellipsoidal nuclei containing finely clumped chromatin. No cytoplasmic structures are evident. Cell shape and nucleus are similar to a short, smooth muscle cell.
   c. Late—a multinucleated, very long, spindle-shaped cell with elongated nuclei containing finely clumped chromatin. Fine fibrils are sometimes evident in the cytoplasm. Groups of cells, in longitudinal section, have the appearance of long, parallel ribbons.

3. *Myotube*—a very elongated cell containing fibrils that show some transverse striations in the periphery and has an axial core of pale, homogeneous cytoplasm with ellipsoidal, central nuclei.

4. *Muscle fiber*—a multinucleated cell with fully established, transverse striations and nuclei situated at the periphery.
   a. Early—a muscle fiber with peripheral nuclei that are large in comparison to the total cross-section of the cell.
   b. Late—the definitive muscle fiber.

Developmental Observations

The sequence of development of the facial muscles is presented in five stages. Within each stage there are important developmental changes, yet there is a natural overlap between stages.

As individual muscles develop, they separate into a superficial and a deep group. When the separation becomes clear (Stage II), the development of the superficial muscles is presented before that of the deep muscles. The muscles innervated by the facial nerve are listed in Figure 26.1 where they are grouped according to their location (superficial or deep) and their common, premuscle condensation (lamina, mesenchymal collection, or complex). The definitive location of the muscles is illustrated in Figures 26.2 and 26.3 in the 80-mm fetus.

SUPERFICIAL MUSCLES
Temporal lamina
    Auricularis superior m Occipital lamina
    Occipital belly of occipitofrontalis m (occipitalis m)
    Auricularis posterior m
    Transversus nuchae m
Cervical lamina
    Cervical part of the platysma
Occipital platysma
    Occipital part of the platysma
Mandibular lamina
    Mandibular part of the platysma
    Depressor labii inferioris m
    Mentalis m
    Risorius m
    Depressor anguli oris m
    Inferior part of the orbicularis oris m
    Buccinator m
    Levator anguli oris m
Infraorbital lamina
    Zygomaticus major m
    Zygomaticus minor m

Levator labii superioris m
    Levator labii superioris alaeque nasi m
    Superior part of the orbicularis oris m
    Compressor naris m
    Dilator naris m
    Depressor septi m
    Orbicularis oculi m
    Frontal belly occipitofrontalis m (frontalis m)
    Corrugator supercilii m
    Procerus m
Mesenchymal cells adjacent to the first branchial groove
    Auricularis anterior m
DEEP MUSCLES
Posterior digastric complex
    Stapedius m
    Posterior belly of digastric m (posterior digastric m)
    Stylohyoid m
Digastric tendon
    Note: A definite premuscle mass from the second branchial arch was not evident for the muscles with a question mark. However, each of these muscles probably develops from the precursor indicated.

Figure 26.1. The superficial and deep facial muscles

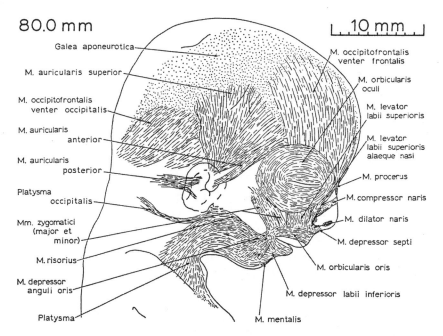

Figure 26.2. The superficial facial muscles of an 80.0-mm fetus, 14.5 weeks. Quadruple stain. Taken from a wax reconstruction. Fibroblasts (galea aponeurotica) are shown as stipple; myotubes are shown as lines.

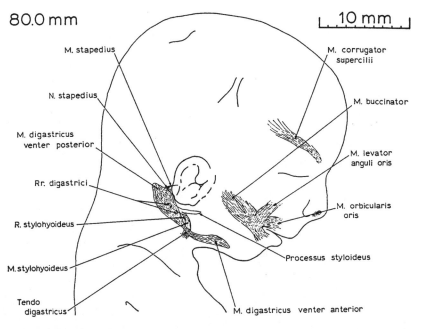

Figure 26.3. The deep facial muscles and the deeper superficial facial muscles in the same 80.0-mm fetus. The outline of the stapedius muscle and styloid process deep to the posterior digastric muscle is shown as stipple.

Stage I: Second Branchial Arch Mesenchyme (4.2 to 6.5 mm)

The mesenchyme of the second branchial arch in 4.2–6.5 mm embryos is most densely cellular in the middle and ventral regions of the arch. Midway in the arch it extends medially to join with the mesenchyme of the arch on the opposite side. When traced dorsally from the middle area it becomes less and less cellular (Figure 26.4). At the termination of the facial nerve, the mesenchyme surrounds the nerve and, at the level of the second arch epibranchial placode, it is located deep and caudal to the nerve. Dorsal to the arch, the mesenchyme is very much scattered with the cells becoming less numerous. The cells become slightly more numerous in the area lateral to the otic vesicle. No discrete condensations are present in the arch. The cells that will develop into muscle are in an early premyoblast state. Deep to the branchial grooves the mesenchyme is continuous with that of the adjacent arches. This is also true for the sparse mesenchyme dorsal to the arch.

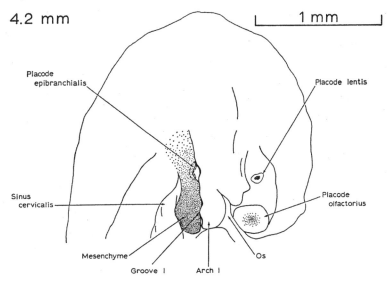

Figure 26.4. The second branchial arch of a 4.2-mm embryo, six weeks. Holmes' silver stain. Taken from a graphic reconstruction. The mesenchymal cells in the second arch are shown as stipple.

Stage II: Facial Premuscle Masses (8 to 20 mm)

The first mesenchymal condensation in the second arch is observed in an 8.0-mm embryo (34 days) and represents the primordium of the second branchial (Reichert's) cartilage. It is located medial to the facial nerve, just dorsal to the origin of the chorda tympani nerve. At 9.5–10.5 mm the primordium enlarges and is slightly rostral to the facial nerve. It extends ventrally and medially to an area which is rostral to the caudalmost part of the pharynx and is circular to oval in transverse sections.

Superficial. A superficial condensation appears in the caudolateral part of the arch by 10.5 mm (40 days). Its border is not well defined but is roughly fusiform to oval on transverse section. Ventrally it blends with the dense mesenchyme in the arch. By 10.6–14.0 mm the condensation is developing extensions into the region caudal to the second arch (Figure 26.5). This caudal extension is most prominent at its dorsal and ventral extremes. The dorsal part spreads into the future occipital and posterior auricular regions and is designated the *occipital lamina*. It is more apparent in 18.0-mm embryos (49 days) but is less dense than the mesenchyme within the arch (Figures 26.7 and 26.8). The posterior auricular branch of the facial nerve is developing deep to the lamina. The ventral part of the caudal extension that is present at 14.0 mm (Figure 26.5, 45 days) grows into the rostrolateral aspect of the upper cervical region and is designated the *cervical lamina*. A collection of mesenchymal cells also extends rostrally into the mandibular arch region and is designated the *mandibular lamina*. It is not well defined at 14.0 mm, but becomes more apparent at 15.0 and 16.0 mm, and at 18.0 mm it is continuous with the *cervical lamina* (Figures 26.7 and 26.11). In 14.0-mm embryos, the mesenchyme in the dorsal part of the arch is slightly more cellular than the loose mesenchyme dorsal to the arch. At 18.0 mm, this more cellular mesenchyme appears as another extension from the second arch and spreads in a dorsal direction as a *temporal lamina* (Figures 26.7 and 26.9).

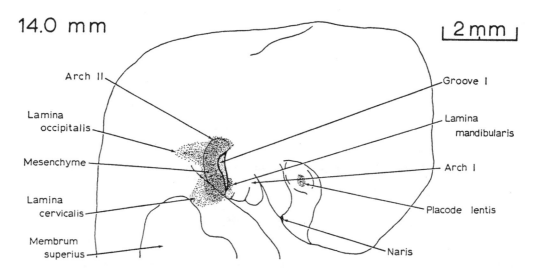

Figure 26.5. The superficial part of the second branchial arch of a 14.0-mm embryo, eight weeks. Bodian's protargol stain. Taken from a graphic reconstruction. The mesenchymal cells in the superficial part of the arch with their extensions are shown as stipple.

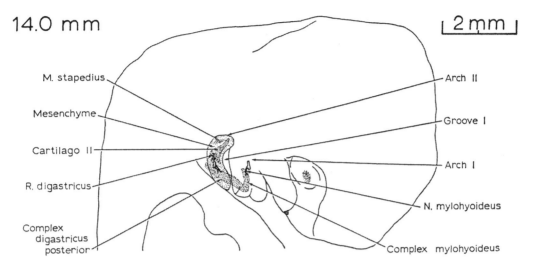

Figure 26.6. The deep part of the second branchial arch of the same 14.0-mm embryo. All mesenchymal condensations in the deep part of the second arch and one of the condensations in the first arch are shown as stipple.

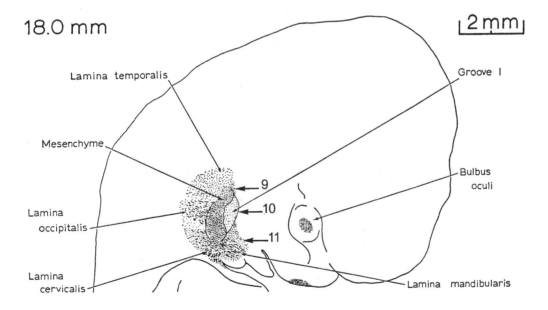

Figure 26.7. The superficial facial muscle masses of an 18.0-mm embryo, 8.5 weeks. Bodian's protargol stain. Taken from a graphic reconstruction. Mesenchymal cells and premyoblasts are shown as stipple; myoblasts are shown as interrupted dashes with the direction of the lines indicating the myoblasts' orientation. See Figures 26.9, 26.10, and 26.11 for explanation of numbered arrows.

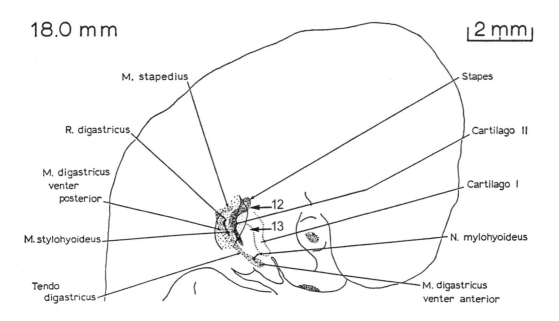

Figure 26.8. The deep facial muscle masses of the same 18.0-mm embryo. See Figures 26.12 and 26.13 for explanation of numbered arrows.

Figure 26.9. A section through the temporal lamina (T) of the same 18.0 mm as in Figure 26.7. 8.5 weeks. Bodian's protargol stain. 10 μ. Scale = 300 μ. Arrow 9 in Figure 26.7 indicates level and plane of section.

Figure 26.10. A section through the occipital lamina (O) of the same 18.0-mm embryo shown in Figure 26.7. Scale = 300 μ. Arrow 13 in Figure 26.7 indicates level and plane of section. CT, chorda tympani nerve; D, posterior digastric muscle; F, facial nerve; G, first branchial groove; P, posterior auricular nerve.

Figure 26.11. A section through the cervical (C) and mandibular (M) laminae of the same embryo as in figure 26.7. Scale = 300 μ. Arrow 11 in Figure 26.7 indicates level and plane of section. CI, first branchial (Meckel's) cartilage; F, terminal branches of facial nerve.

Figure 26.12. A section through the stapedius muscle (S) of the same 18.0-mm embryo shown in Figure 26.8. Scale = 100 μ. Arrow 12 in Figure 26.8 indicates level and plane of section. C2, second branchial (Reichert's) cartilage; F, facial nerve.

Figure 26.13. A section through the posterior digastric muscle (D) of the same 18.0-mm embryo. Scale = 100 μ. Arrow 13 in Figure 26.8 indicates level and plane of section. C2, second branchial (Reichert's) cartilage; F, facial nerve; SH, stylohyoid muscle.

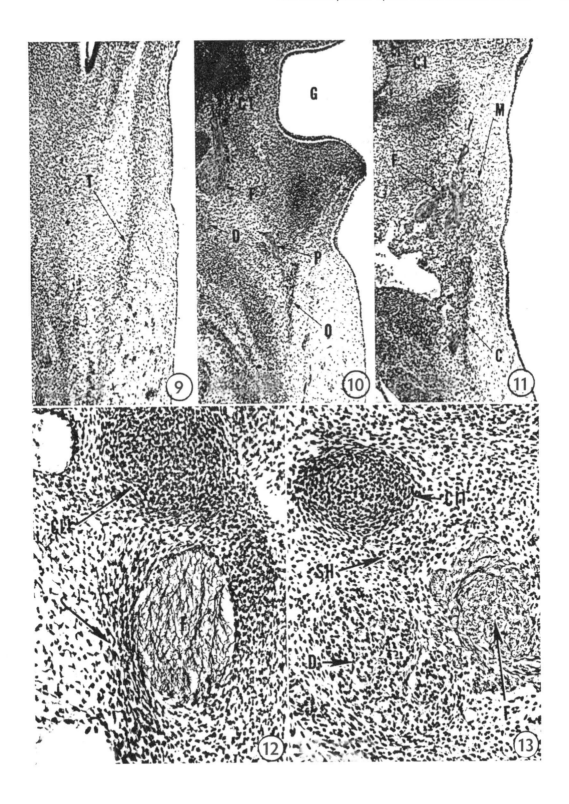

Deep. The most discrete second arch premuscle condensation in 10.5–14.0 mm embryos is located caudal and medial to the facial nerve in the deep part of the arch and is designated the *posterior digastric complex* (Figure 26.6). At 14 mm it is continuous laterally with the deep aspect of the *cervical lamina.* The complex increases in size as it courses ventrally and then becomes slightly constricted as it proceeds into the mandibular arch where it is continuous with another densely cellular concentration, the *mylohyoid complex.* The *posterior digastric complex* receives a series of small, diffuse branches from the caudal aspect of the facial nerve. These branches can be traced ventrally within the complex to the region of the first branchial groove. They could not be traced beyond the constricted part of the condensation in any of the embryos examined. The most dorsal part of the *mylohyoid complex* receives a small, single branch from the mandibular division of the trigeminal nerve. This continuous group of condensations represents the first appearance of the digastric, stylohyoid, and mylohyoid muscles. By 18 mm the dorsal part is dividing into the posterior belly of the digastric (posterior digastric) and stylohyoid muscles (Figures 26.8 and 26.13). The ventral part is dividing into the anterior belly of the digastric (anterior digastric) and mylohyoid muscles. The intermediate region becomes more constricted and is developing into the digastric tendon. The stylohyoid muscle develops form the rostral part of the *posterior digastric complex* immediately caudal to the second arch cartilage.

The dorsal extent of the *posterior digastric complex* is continuous on the medial side of the facial nerve with the dorsal part of the second branchial cartilage. In this region will develop the stapedius muscle and the stapes of the middle ear. At 18 mm the stapes is forming in an area adjacent to the dorsal end of the second arch cartilage (Figure 26.8). The stapes at this time is a ring-like condensation with the stapedial artery coursing through it. A small collection of late premyoblasts is located caudal to the dorsal tip of the second arch cartilage in 14-mm embryos (Figure 26.6, 29 days) and is the first appearance of the stapedius muscle. These premyoblasts are adjacent to the medial side of the facial nerve and course rostrally to the vicinity of the second arch cartilage. At 18–20 mm the stapedius muscle is better defined (Figures 26.8 and 26.12) and is composed mostly of early myoblasts which join the cells connecting the stapes and the second arch cartilage.

Histogenesis. Most of the premuscle cells in 14–16-mm embryos are late premyoblasts. None of the cells are mature myoblasts. By 18 mm many of the cells are early myoblasts and the most mature premuscle cells in the second arch area are located in the *occipital lamina* and in the dorsal part of the *posterior digastric complex.* The cells in both of these regions are closely related to branches of the facial nerve. By 18–20 mm the myoblasts increase in number and are more mature; some have become middle myoblasts. Since the myoblasts are numerous, the laminae and deeper muscle masses are easier to outline, trace, and identify.

Stage III: Facial Muscle Differentiation (20 to 45 mm)

Superficial muscles. The superficial laminae present in earlier embryos are well developed in 20–23-mm (49–53 days) specimens and two additional structures, the *infraorbital lamina* and the *occipital platysma,* appear (Figure 26.14). The directions of development of each of the laminae present at 22.2 mm (50 days) are illustrated in Figure 26.15 by groups of arrows. At 24–26 mm (53 days) the laminae extend farther from the second arch region where the auricle is forming (Figure 26.16) and by 27–45 mm (beginning fetal period) they subdivide into individual muscles at variable distances from the auricle (Figure 26.17).

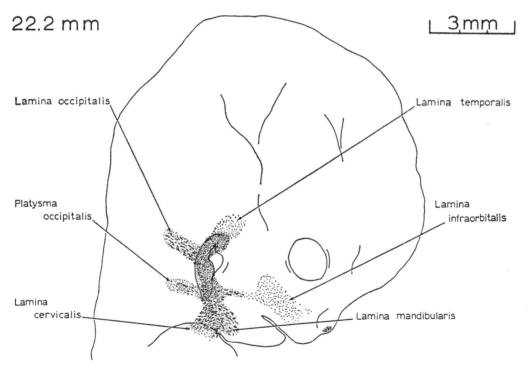

Figure 26.14. The superficial facial muscle masses of a 22.2-mm embryo, nine weeks. Bodian's protargol stain. Taken from a wax reconstruction. Mesenchymal cells and premyoblasts are shown as stipple; myoblasts are shown as interrupted dashes.

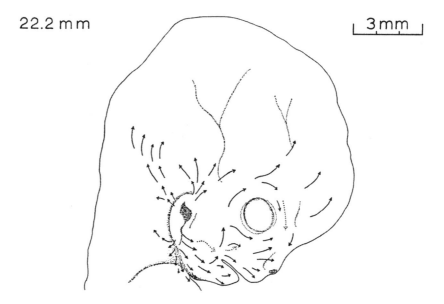

Figure 26.15. Groups of arrows superimposed on the same 22.2-mm embryo indicate the future location and apparent direction of growth of the superficial laminae. The stipple and arrows in the supraorbital, infraorbital, and buccal regions indicate the regions where the corrugator supercilii, levator anguli oris, and buccinator muscles, respectively, appear to form by delamination from the deep surface of the more superficial layer of muscle.

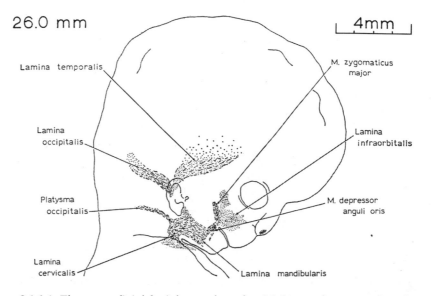

Figure 26.16. The superficial facial muscles of a 26.0-mm fetus, ten weeks. Erythrosine and toluidin blue stain. Taken from a wax reconstruction. Mesenchymal cells and premyoblasts are shown as stipple; myoblasts are shown as interrupted lines.

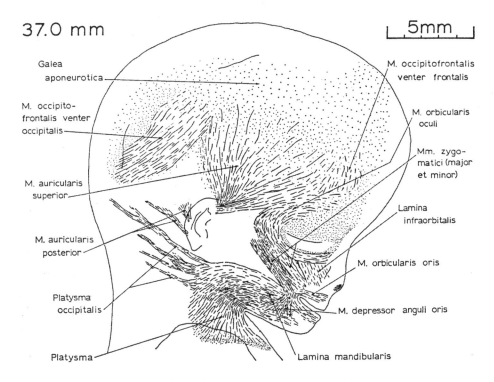

Figure 26.17. The superficial facial muscles of a 37.0-mm fetus, eleven weeks. Bodian's protargol and erythrosine stain. Taken from a wax reconstruction. Fibroblasts and premyoblasts are shown as stipple; myoblasts are shown as interrupted lines. The closeness of the lines is proportional to the relative concentration of premuscle cells.

The *temporal lamina* is composed of loosely arranged late premyoblasts at 20–23 mm. It is better developed by 26 mm (53 days) where it courses rostrally and cranially and is composed of many premyoblasts and some early myoblasts. In 27–40-mm fetuses (31 mm is considered the end of the embryonic period) the lamina is a thin layer of myoblasts which has spread into the temporal region forming the auricularis superior muscle (Figure 26.17). As the lamina courses cranially it is gradually replaced by premyoblasts or active fibroblasts. The auricularis anterior muscle is present at 40–45 mm as a small collection of cells immediately rostral to the auricle. It does not develop from the *temporal lamina* but from mesenchyme adjacent to the first branchial groove.

The *occipital lamina* contains occasional early myoblasts at 20–23 mm and courses dorsally toward the occipital region. The number of myoblasts increases by 26 mm. The major part of the lamina forms the occipital belly of the occipitofrontalis (occipitalis) muscle but both bellies of the auricularis posterior muscle also apparently develop from it between 27 and 40 mm (Figure 26.17). In one specimen the two muscles were continuous. Many of the cells of the occipitalis muscle in 40–45-mm fetuses are myotubes and are the best differentiated of any of the premuscle cells in the superficial muscles at this time.

In 20–23-mm specimens (49–53 days) a small band of late premyoblasts and early myoblasts, the *occipital platysma,* courses dorsally from the caudal part of the developing auricled and represents the precursor of the occipital part of the platysma. By 26 mm it is a narrow band that blends with the dorsal border of the *cervical lamina.* It is composed of several narrow bundles of myoblasts in 37–45 mm fetuses that course into the occipital region. They are superficial to the sternomastoid muscle and in some fetuses are continuous with the ventral border of the trapezius muscle.

Ventral to the first branchial groove at 20–23 mm the *cervical* and *mandibular laminae* are united in a continuous thick layer of middle myoblasts and many premyoblasts. The layer of cells extends into the ventral part of the upper cervical region *(cervical lamina)* and also into the mandibular arch *(mandibular lamina).* Most of the myoblasts in the mandibular part are directed rostrally and ventrally; those in the cervical part are directed caudally. The myoblasts in the junction region are essentially horizontal in their orientation. Most of the superficial myoblasts in 24–26-mm specimens are concentrated in united *cervical* and *mandibular laminae.* The entire *cervical lamina* develops into the cervical part of the platysma and much of the *mandibular lamina* forms its mandibular extension. The premyoblasts are gradually replaced by myoblasts. The premuscle cells are continuous with dense collections of mesenchymal cells in the auricular region. The *mandibular lamina* extends almost to the angle of the mouth. By 27–40 mm the platysma is thinner and slightly broader as it extends to the shoulder region. At its caudal border the myoblasts are gradually replaced with premyoblasts or mesenchymal cells which can be traced to the level of the developing clavicle. At 40–45 mm the platysma extends to the midline in the mental and submental regions, but not in the cervical region.

A triangular group of myoblasts is located at the rostral termination of the *mandibular lamina* at 26 mm which extends to the angle of the mouth. It is on a plane superficial to the *mandibular lamina* and represents the first appearance of the depressor anguli oris muscle. The direction of the myoblasts differs from those in the *mandibular lamina* by 90 degrees. The myoblasts are more closely packed as they approach the angle of the mouth. The muscle is well defined between 27 and 45 mm and is superficial to the platysma.

The orbicularis oris muscle has begun to develop by 37 mm (fetal period) where it is a loose collection of middle myoblasts which is thicker in the upper than in the lower lip. The myoblasts are sparse in the midline. By 40–45 mm the muscle is made up of late myoblasts and completely encircles the mouth.

In 20–23-mm specimens the *mandibular lamina* is continuous with a loose collection of mesenchymal cells in the infraorbital region, the *infraorbital lamina*. The region of continuity is narrow and is limited to the area immediately rostral to the ventral part of the first branchial groove. Since the *infraorbital lamina* is highly vascular, it is difficult to determine if its component cells are forming facial muscles or blood vessels. Considerable changes take place by 24–26 mm (53 days). In the most lateral aspect of the infraorbital region, a discrete band of myoblasts has formed. It is round to oval in transverse section and represents the first appearance of the zygomaticus major muscle. The muscle courses from the region of the developing zygoma to the angle of the mouth where it is continuous with the depressor anguli oris muscle. Medial to the zygomaticus major muscle the *infraorbital lamina* is composed of premyoblasts and myoblasts which are superficial to the infraorbital plexus of nerves. The lamina extends laterally and dorsally into the area immediately above the zygomaticus major muscle in a very prominent band that is continuous along its medial border with the zygomaticus and orbicularis oculi muscles. The zygomaticus minor muscle is continuous medially with a sheet of myoblasts that courses into the upper lip and lateral aspect of the nose. No definite levator labial or nasal muscles are identifiable.

At 37 mm, the orbicularis oculi muscle is developing around the eye, but does not yet completely encircle it. The muscle is thickest laterally and thins as it spreads dorsally. The infraorbital portion is partly superficial to the zygomaticus muscles and *infraorbital lamina*. It courses medially and disappears at the side of the nose. Mesenchymal cells, probably premyoblasts, are arranged in a layer in the superior palpebrum and in the medial part of the orbital region. Only the most medial portion of the orbital part of the orbicularis oculi muscle is deficient in 40–45-mm fetuses. Myoblasts are present in most of the orbital part, but the palpebral part remains in a premyoblastic state.

The frontal belly of the occipitofrontalis (frontalis) muscle begins to develop in 27–45-mm fetuses, but is not well defined. Its premuscle cells are mainly premyoblasts which show little orientation. The majority of the cells cranial to the frontal, temporal, and occipital regions are premyoblasts or active fibroblasts which form a thin layer superficial to the developing calvarium. In 40–45-mm specimens, this layer extends to the vertex of the head, but thins in the midline in the frontoparietal and occipitoparietal regions. As development proceeds, the cells become oriented mainly in a rostrodorsal direction and form the galea aponeurotica. Myoblasts connecting the frontalis and occipitalis muscles were not observed in any of the specimens.

The buccinator muscle first appears at 26 mm, but is difficult to outline since it is primarily composed of premyoblasts and early myoblasts. Its dorsal boundary is especially difficult to define since it gradually blends with the mesenchymal cells lateral to the pharynx. The buccinator mass becomes superficial as it approaches the angle of the mouth where it joins the deep aspect of the more superficial muscle masses in the region. A nerve supply to the muscle was not observed until 37 mm. At this time, the muscle is more apparent and is divided in its dorsal half into a large caudal and a small cranial portion with the parotid duct coursing between them. The caudal portion extends farther dorsally, and between 37 and 45 mm, it blends with the superior constrictor of the pharynx. At this age, the muscle is completely pierced by the buccal branch of the mandibular nerve.

By 37 mm, the levator anguli oris muscle has formed deep to the caudal and lateral part of the infraorbital plexus. It begins cranially adjacent to the developing maxillary bone and courses caudally and laterally to join with the zygomaticus and buccinator muscles at the angle of the mouth. Caudal to the angle of the mouth, the muscle is sometimes continuous with the mandibular part of the platysma and the depressor anguli oris muscle.

Deep muscles. All of the deep facial muscles are recognizable in the previous stage but in the present stage they become more distinct and increase in size. Between 20 and 26 mm, the cranial end of the posterior digastric muscle is immediately caudal to the dorsal end of the stapedius muscle. As development proceeds, this distance becomes greater. The stapedius muscle remains close to the medial aspect of the facial nerve, sometimes receiving a short, but obvious, branch from the nerve. It is made up of early and middle myoblasts which terminate medial to the hyostapedial connection between the stapes and cranial end of the second arch cartilage.

The stylohyoid muscle is rostral to the caudal half of the posterior digastric muscle and dorsal to the second arch cartilage. As it proceeds caudally, it is sometimes lateral to the posterior digastric muscle and sometimes surrounds it before terminating in mesenchyme of the hyoid region. The digastric tendon is a dense collection of darkly staining cells that courses into the depths of both the posterior and anterior parts of the digastric muscle.

Stage IV: Definitive Location of the Facial Muscles (50 to 146 mm)

Superficial muscles. Additional superficial muscles can be identified between 50 and 58 mm and all of these muscles can be recognized and outlined at 80 mm in their definitive position (Figure 26.2).

At 58 mm, the auricularis anterior muscle is a short band of myoblasts coursing cranially from the rostral aspect of the auricle, and at 80 mm it is adjacent to the rostral border of the auricularis superior muscle. No separation could be seen between these two muscles at 142 mm. Dorsal to the auricularis posterior muscle a thin and small sheet of muscle is occasionally present in the lower occipital or upper cervical region. Its muscle cells are mostly directed transversely and compose the transverses nuchae muscle.

Between 58 and 80 mm, the *occipital platysma* is a single, discrete band which takes a variable path from the platysma into the occipital region. This muscle could not be identified in the grossly dissected 142-mm fetus. At 58 mm, the mandibular part of the platysma extends into the mental region where it is continuous with vertically directed muscle cells that extend into the lower lip and represent the depressor labii inferioris muscle. This arrangement is observed better at 80 mm where the mentalis muscle is defined for the first time. The risorius muscle develops as a thickening along the cranial border of the platysma. Its state of development is variable.

At 58 mm, the buccinator muscle extends farther dorsally, and by 80 mm it extends to the region of the lateral pterygoid plate (Figure 26.3). Between 101 and 146 mm, it unites dorsally with the superior pharyngeal constrictor muscle. A decussation of its muscle cells at the angle of the mouth is apparent at 80 mm. By 142 mm, a large fat pad has developed superficial to the buccinator but deep to the risorius and platysma muscles. The levator anguli oris muscle grows considerably in thickness and length deep to the infraorbital plexus of nerves.

In 58–80-mm fetuses, the orbicularis oris muscle is well developed, completely encircles the mouth, but is difficult to divide into superficial and deep parts. It has become thicker and is continuous with the perioral muscles. Its medial part in the upper lip lags in development.

The zygomaticus major and minor muscles are sometimes separate between 50 and 58 mm, but become more difficult to separate from each other by 80–142 mm. The levator labii superioris muscle is identifiable in the infraorbital region of 50–58-mm fetuses and is often separated by blood vessels into superficial and deep parts. The superficial part is continuous cranially with the orbicularis oculi muscle and the deep part attaches to the maxillary bone immediately caudal to the orbit. Both parts unite as they pass into the upper lip and are superficial to the infraorbital plexus of nerves. A sheet of myoblasts in the lateral nasal area is also separated into two parts by blood vessels. The myoblasts course caudally toward the upper lip and form, by 80 mm, the levator labii superioris alaeque nasi muscle. At this time, the compressor naris muscle is present on the lateral aspect of the nose. It courses from the bridge of the nose, passing deep to the levator labii superioris alaeque nasi muscle, and ending adjacent to the maxillary bone. The dilator naris muscle is evident at the lower, lateral part of the nose.

It is obliquely situated and blends with the deeper part of the orbicularis oris muscle. The depressor septi muscle is caudal to the nasal septum and courses in a vertical direction. At 142 mm, it courses from the naris into the upper lip where the fibers pass deep to the orbicularis oris muscle to attach to the maxillary bone.

The orbital part of the orbicularis oculi muscle is easily defined at 50–58 mm, but the palpebral part remains poorly developed. The myoblasts disappear at the periphery of the eyelids and are most numerous laterally and craniomedially. The craniomedial part joins with the frontalis muscle and both extend onto the bridge of the nose as the procerus muscle. The corrugator supercilii muscle appears deep to the supraorbital part of the orbicularis oculi muscle. It becomes larger by 80 mm and extends as a thick band into the lateral aspect of the supraorbital region (Figure 26.3). At this same time, the medial part of the orbicularis oculi muscle surrounds the lacrimal sac and canaliculi, and the palpebral part is present throughout the major portion of the eyelids.

Between 50 and 58 mm, the frontalis muscle is a thin sheet of myoblasts covering the major part of the frontal region, but is not continuous across the midline until 80 mm. The muscle is thin as it approaches the vertex of the head and the myoblasts are gradually replaced by active fibroblasts. At the vertex, the galea aponeurotica is represented as a layer of fibroblasts. The layer is not only continuous peripherally with the frontalis, but also with the occipitalis and auricularis superior muscles.

Deep muscles. The stapedius muscle is very large at 58 and 80 mm in comparison with the middle ear region and is oriented in an almost vertical plane (Figure 26.3). No significant changes occur in the posterior digastric and stylohyoid muscles. In 80 and 146-mm fetuses, the posterior digastric muscle is large, while the stylohyoid muscle is correspondingly small.

The cells of the facial muscles at 50–58 mm are late myoblasts and myotubes. By 80 mm, they are primarily myotubes, and by 146 mm, they are early muscle fibers. The bony or cartilaginous attachments of the muscles are not very apparent. Occasionally, connective tissue fibers are present which partially anchor the muscle cells to the periosteum of developing bone.

Stage V: Facial Muscles in Dissected Late Fetuses (210, 270, and 360 mm)

The muscles increase in size and extent as the head and neck regions become larger and, in most cases, the boundaries between individual muscles become more prominent. Since the muscles reach their definitive location as early as 58 mm, only gradual changes occur between 146 mm and term.

Superficial muscles. The transversus nuchae muscle is present in the 210 and 270 mm fetuses and is almost continuous with the auricularis posterior muscle. The latter muscle is composed of two bellies in all three specimens. The occipital platysma muscle could not be identified. In the term infant, the platysma extends caudally to the level of the nipple. A distinct, thickened risorius muscle is not always present. The boundary between the zygomaticus muscles is difficult to define, but there is usually a small gap between the zygomaticus minor and levator labii superioris muscles. All of the superficial muscles are delicate and most are deep to a layer of subcutaneous fat, but superficial to their nerve supply. Most of the bony attachments are established, but are not firmly anchored.

Deep muscles. The stylohyoid muscle is smaller and its fibers are less tightly bound together than those of the digastric muscle. All of the deep muscles are attached to bone or cartilage and their attachments are generally more firmly anchored than are the superficial muscles.

Discussion

1. Muscles of Expression

Futamura (Futamura, 1906) stated that by 31 to 34 days (9–13 mm) the superficial muscle blastemal becomes voluminous and spreads out dorsally, ventrally, and orally. These early, superficial extensions have been designated the occipital (dorsally), cervical (ventrally), and mandibular (orally) laminae. As the neck develops and increases in length, the cervical lamina expands to produce the platysma. This manner of development is similar to that described by Rabl (Rabl, 1887) and Futamura (Futamura, 1906). According to Bryce (Bryce, 1923), bundles of fiber sometimes are found in the definitive state extending from the dorsal border of the platysma to the cervical fascia over the sternomastoid and trapezius muscles, and even to the mastoid process. This inconsistent strip of muscle, the occipital platysma, appears very early in development (22.2 mm, 49 days), but diminishes in size as development progresses and could not be found in late fetuses. Huber (Huber, 1931) stated that it is a vestige of the nuchal portion of the platysma which reflects our primate ancestry.

At 6 weeks (18–24 mm), Futamura (Futamura, 1906) described two layers of premuscle tissue; a deep layer that he identified with the sphincter colli of lower vertebrates and a superficial layer which he looked upon as the platysma (colli) of lower forms. In the present study, no attempt is made to describe the ontogeny of the facial muscles on the basis of their phylogeny. The muscles are divided into groups according to their manner of development and definitive location. Futamura (Futamura, 1906) described the deep layer as giving origin to primitive sphincter arrangements around the eye, nose, mouth, and ear, and except in the case of the mouth, these early sphincters disappear and are replaced by new formations from the superficial layer. The present study did not reveal sphincters at 18–24 mm in any of these regions (Figures 26.7 and 26.14). Sphincters completely encircling the nose and auricle were never observed and the orbicularis oris and oculi muscles do not become complete sphincters until approximately 40–45 mm.

Popowsky (Popowsky, 1895) found no superficial muscles at 28 mm except the cervical portion of the platysma (cervical lamina). Huber (Huber, 1931) demonstrated the presence of an additional muscle (auricularis posterior) which is identified in the present work as the occipital lamina. The present technique revealed additional regions of muscle development, the temporal and infraorbital laminae and the occipital platysma, as early as 18–22 mm (Figures 26.7 and 26.14).

Futamura (Futamura, 1906) observed the anlage of the quadratus labii superioris muscle at 6 weeks (18–24 mm), which is similar to what is identified here as the infraorbital lamina. A small connection exists between the infraorbital lamina and the second arch region at 22 mm (Figure 26.14), which is less evident at 26 mm (Figure 26.16), when the lamina is more prominent. The origin of the premuscle cells in the lamina and exactly which muscles on the face develop from the lamina is questionable (Figure 26.1). The cells of the infraorbital lamina could be descendants of cells in the second branchial arch, their migration taking place at an earlier time when they could not be recognized as premuscle cells and did not form a discrete condensation. The infraorbital lamina gives origin to all of the muscles in the infraorbital region and probably contributes to the formation of the muscles of the nose, most of the orbicularis oculi and some of the orbicularis oris muscles.

By 8 to 9 weeks (32–36 mm), Futamura (Futamura, 1906) reported the facial muscles to be well differentiated for the most part. Huber (Huber, 1931) pointed out that the critical period of development is between the second and third months of prenatal life. There is a sudden surge in facial muscle differentiation between 26 and 37 mm, but deficiencies are present in the palpebral part (eyelid) of the orbicularis oculi and in all of the muscles close to the middle of the face. The present findings agree with Zuckermann-Zicha's (Zuckerman-Zicha, 1925) report that the palpebral part of the orbicularis oculi muscle differentiates between 55 and 80 mm.

The origin of the premuscle cells of the buccinator muscle is questionable. They probably migrated from the deep aspect of the mandibular lamina at an earlier age. The cells of the levator anguli oris muscle most likely have the same origin as those in the buccinator muscle.

2. Occipitofrontalis and Auricularis Superior Muscles

Although both bellies of the occipitofrontalis muscles are described definitively as components of a single muscle, they develop separately. At 37 mm (Figure 26.17), the occipital belly and the auricularis posterior muscle have replaced the occipital lamina. Bryce (Bryce, 1923) mentioned that these two muscles are sometimes united in the definitive condition. The frontal belly differentiates later in the frontal region and its origin is difficult to establish. The corrugator supercilii muscle probably originates from its deep surface. The auricularis superior muscle develops from the temporal lamina. The muscles of the scalp gradually thin as they approach the vertex of the head and become continuous with a layer of fibroblasts from which the galea aponeurotica develops. According to Bryce (Bryce, 1923), some authors regard the aponeurosis as representing the degenerated portion of a primitive fronto-occipital sheet. A continuous layer of myoblasts connecting the frontal and occipital areas was not observed in any of the specimens. It is difficult to consider the fibroblasts as dedifferentiated myoblasts; they probably differentiated directly from mesenchymal cells.

3. Deep Muscles

A concept of the posterior digastric complex from which the posterior digastric, stylohyoid, and stapedius muscles develop was presented by Rabl in 1887. Futamura (Futamura, 1906) reported seeing twigs from the facial nerve coursing to the complex at 35–36 days (13–15 mm). At this early age, some of the fibers course into the most ventral and slightly constricted part of the complex to the caudal aspect of the mandibular arch. No fibers continue into the mylohyoid complex since it already receives an innervation from a poorly developed inferior dental nerve. These findings indicate a dual origin for the digastric muscle, the posterior belly from the posterior digastric complex of the second arch and the anterior belly from the mylohyoid complex of the first arch. However, each complex is always continuous with one another deep to the first branchial groove. Gegenbaur (Gegenbaur, 1890) and Futamura (Futamura, 1906) believed that the digastric muscle develops from two independent parts. Some investigators consider the muscle to develop as a separation from the sternomastoid muscle. A union with this latter muscle was not observed in any of the specimens. Consideration of past and present data suggests that the posterior digastric muscle as well as the digastric tendon develop from the second arch, and the anterior digastric muscle develops along with the mylohyoid muscle in the ventral part of the first arch.

Ruge (Ruge, 1910) and Bryce (Bryce, 1923) pointed out the rare occurrence of a definitive muscular connection between the occipital fascia and the posterior digastric muscle. This connection probably represents a retention of an earlier connection (14 mm) between the posterior digastric complex and the cervical lamina.

The time and manner of development of the stapedius muscle agrees with Futamura's (Futamura, 1906) and Schimert's (Schimert, 1933) descriptions, but disagrees with Broman (Broman, 1898), who believed the muscle develops from the connection between the stapes and the second arch (Reichert's) cartilage. No explanation can be given for the variability in the size and orientation of this muscle during development.

4. Histogenesis and Pattern of Differentiation

In his studies on the labial muscles, Futamura (Futamura, 1906) saw no transverse striations at 22 weeks (170 mm), faint striations at 26 weeks (220 mm), and distinct striations at 30 weeks (250 mm). The present work reveals transverse striations in myotubes (e.g., orbicularis oris muscle) at 58 mm, which become very apparent at 80 mm. Early muscle fibers are present at 146 mm.

Contrary to the statements of Popowsky (Popowsky, 1895), the superficial musculature at the end of the third month (58 mm) is already differentiated. This is substantiated by Huber (Huber, 1931), who produced contractions of the muscles in a living 55-mm fetus through electrical stimulation. In their studies on the appearance of human fetal reflexes, Hooker (Hooker, 1952, 1958) and Humphrey (Humphrey, 1964, 1965) observed, at 37–47 mm, a squint-type reflex produced by contraction of the orbicularis oculi muscle. The orbital part of the muscle almost completely surrounds the eye at 41 mm and is composed of late myoblasts. At 47–49 mm, these investigators produced a scowl-type reflex by contraction of the corrugator supercilii muscle. This muscle is well differentiated by 58 mm when it is composed of late myoblasts and occasional myotubes. By 60–64 mm, Hooker (Hooker, 1952, 1958) and Humphrey (Humphrey, 1964, 1965) produced momentary lip closure and at 74–79 mm, lip closure was maintained. At 58 mm, the orbicularis oris muscle is well developed, completely encircles the mouth and is composed mostly of late myoblasts with some myotubes. They observed a sneer-type reflex produced by an elevation of the angle of the mouth and ala of the nose at 74 to 88 mm. All of the facial muscles, including the infraorbital ones, have differentiated by 80 mm and are made up of myotubes. Comparison of the degree of histogenetic development of the premuscle cells with the age at which reflexes can be elicited lends support to the view that late myoblasts, with unstriated fibrils in their cytoplasm, are not only able to contract, but that their contractions are influenced to some degree by nerve impulses.

A definite pattern of differentiation is evident in the formation of the facial muscles. The present investigation supports Futamura's (Futamura, 1906) findings that differentiation of the muscles begins earlier in the deep than in the superficial regions and earlier in the lower lateral than in the upper medial regions. In addition, studies show that the muscles in the occipital region (e.g., occipitalis) differentiate and become striated earlier than the lateral facial muscles (e.g., zygomaticus and depressor anguli oris) which in turn differentiate before the muscles close to the midline of the face.

Superficial muscle masses spread from the region of the second arch in all directions except one that is directly rostrally (Figure 26.15). The most likely reason for this is the presence of the external auditory meatus which is replacing the first branchial groove. The deep meatus probably causes cells from the second arch to migrate around it so that cell groups must extend first cranially or caudally before they can course rostrally.

In most of the specimens studied, the development of the peripheral branches of the facial nerve follow *pari passu* the development of the facial muscle masses (Gasser, 1967). A close relationship exists between the muscles and the nerve throughout development and each appears to influence the histogenesis and morphogenesis of the other. As the muscle masses form, the nerve supply to them differentiates. The premuscle cells in the vicinity of the nerve fibers are further differentiated than those more distant from the nerve fibers.[10]

CHAPTER 27

The Development of the
Facial Nerve in Man

By Raymond F. Gasser, PhD

This detailed description of the morphogenesis of the intracranial and extracranial parts of the facial nerve encompasses the formation of its roots, geniculate ganglion, branches, interanastomoses, and anastomoses with other nerves in the head and neck regions. Such a study may be helpful in understanding and explaining variations and anomalous arrangements of the nerves and general patterns of development in the head and neck regions. Since the description of Rabl (Rabl, 1887) and Gegenbaur (Gegenbaur, 1890), the embryonic development of this nerve has been associated with the second branchial or hyoid arch. The embryology of the seventh cranial nerve, especially its peripheral development, has received little attention in man in comparison to the important role it plays in postnatal life.

Materials and Methods

The right facial nerves of 31 serially sectioned, normal, human embryos and fetuses' 4.2- to 146.0-mm crown-rump (C-R) length were examined microscopically. Figure 27.1 lists the reconstructed specimens by their C-R length and menstrual age and gives specifications of histological preparation. They are grouped into four stages based on their state of development. The menstrual age in weeks was determined from their C-R length according to the tables of Mall (Mall, 1918). All references to millimeter measurements in this [article] pertain to C-R length unless otherwise indicated.

Reconstructed embryos and fetuses

C-R LENGTH IN MILLIMETERS	MENSTRUAL AGE IN WEEKS	PLANE OF SECTION*	THICKNESS OF SECTIONS IN M	TECHNIQUE**
Stage I				
4.2†	6.0	T	10	Holmes silver
4.8†	6.5	T	10	H & E
Stage II				
14.0†	8.0	T	10	Bodian's protargol
18.0†	8.5	T	10	Bodian's protargol
Stage III				
22.2‡	9.0	T	10	Bodian's protargol
26.0‡	10.0	T	10	erythrosin & TB
37.0‡	11.0	T	10	Bodian's protargol
41.0‡	11.0	T	20	quadruple
Stage IV				
58.0‡	13.0	T	10	quadruple
80.0‡	14.5	T	20	quadruple

Notes:

*T, transverse

** H & E, hematoxylin and eosin; TB, toluidin blue; quadruple, a stain of hematoxylin, aniline blue, orange G and eosin

† Graphically reconstructed

‡ Reconstructed in wax

Figure 27.1. Table of reconstructed embryos and fetuses, with sizes and ages

The head and neck regions of ten representative ages were reconstructed from transverse sections; four graphically and six by means of wax sheets. Seven of these are used for illustrations.

The serial sections of the graphically reconstructed embryos were projected onto white paper. The projected image of the sections was measured with a millimeter ruler. Approximately 25–30 measurements were made on the right half of each selected projection. A graph was constructed which consisted of parallel horizontal lines, one to two millimeters apart, depending upon the thickness of the sections, their magnification, and the number of sections measured. Each line was labeled with the appropriate section number. The sections with the largest rostrodorsal diameter were first plotted on the graph followed by sections cranial and caudal to them. Close attention was given to the location of the auricle, the eye, and the brain to obtain accuracy in placing the measurements above one another on the graph. Plotted measurements which represented the same structure were joined together with a solid line so that a drawing of the right lateral view of the head and neck was constructed. The serial sections were examined under a microscope and the location, the arrangement, and the extent of the facial nerve were plotted on the graph, section by section. The protargol silver methods of histological preparation permitted more accurate tracing of the nerves.

The wax reconstructions were made in a manner similar to that of Born (Born, 1883, 1888). The center of the right side of each wax model and a scale were photographed. Print tracings were made in which the wax sheets of the model were represented as parallel lines with a corresponding section number. The configuration of the facial nerve was determined microscopically and plotted on the tracings in a manner identical to that used for the graphic reconstructions.

Observations

The sequence of development of the facial nerve is presented in four stages. Within each stage there are important developmental changes, yet there is a natural overlap between stages.

Stage I: Facioacoustic Primordium and Placode of the Second Branchial (Hyoid) Arch (4.2–6.5 mm)

In a 4.2–mm embryo (29–32 days), the facial nerve arises in common with the eighth cranial or acoustic nerve (Figure 27.2) and is attached to the metencephalon just rostral to the otic vesicle. This facioacoustic primordium (acousticofacial crest) is fibrous at its attachment, but soon becomes cellular as it courses ventrally. It passes rostral to the otic vesicle and, at the lower part of the vesicle, the acoustic division arises. The major division of the primordium (facial part) continues ventrally, becomes more cellular and compact, and appears as a column of cells. As the facial division proceeds ventrally, it becomes superficial and slightly rostral, and terminates adjacent to the deep surface of the epibranchial placode (Figures 27.4 and 27.5) that lines the dorsal and caudal part of the first branchial groove. The cells making up the epibranchial placode are columnar in shape and are more closely packed than the cells in the adjacent single layered ectodermal epithelium. Loosely arranged cells are present on the deep surface of the placode which are continuous with the cellular column of the facial division of the primordium. Ventral to the placode the facial division cannot be identified but disappears into the surrounding mesenchyme. The columnlike arrangement of cells gives off no branches and the geniculate ganglion cannot be identified.

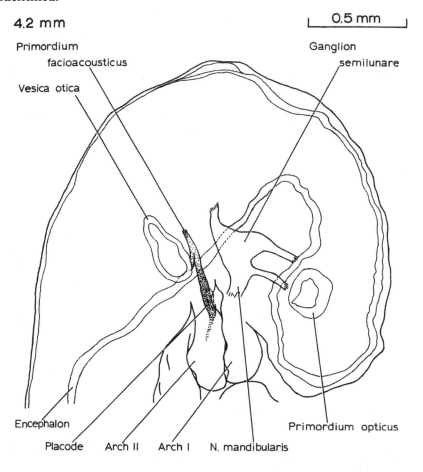

Figure 27.2. A 4.2-mm embryo with a menstrual age of six weeks. Age group XIII (Streeter, 1945). Holmes' silver method of impregnation. Neural crest cells of the facioacoustic primordium are shown as stipple. Outline of the epibranchial placode of the second arch is indicated by an interrupted line, within the stipple.

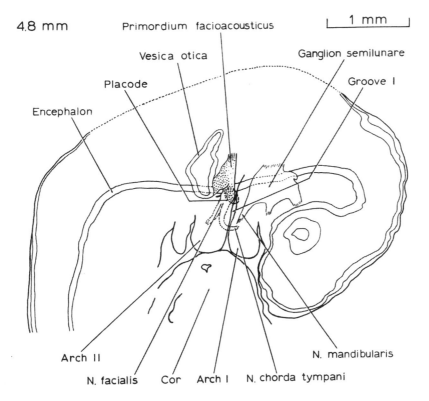

Figure 27.3. A 4.8-mm embryo with a menstrual age of 6.5 weeks. Age group
XIV (Streeter, 1945). Hematoxylin and eosin stains. Neuroblasts in the developing geniculate and acoustic ganglia are shown as stipple. Outline of the
epibranchial placode and the facial nerve in the second arch is indicated
by interrupted lines [below the stippled area]. Embryo is very mature for its
crown-rump (C-R) length.

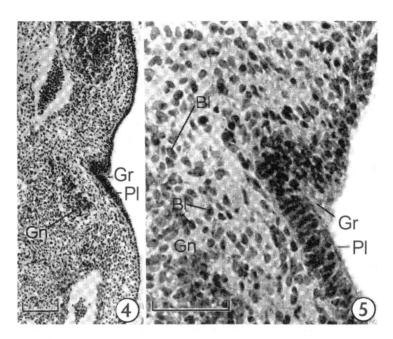

Figure 27.4. Low-power photomicrograph of a transverse section of the second arch epibranchial placode (Pl) in a 6.0-mm embryo with a menstrual age of 6.5 weeks. Stained with hematoxylin and eosin. Age group XIV (Streeter, 1945). Scale = 100 μ. GN, the developing geniculate ganglion; GR, the first branchial groove.

Figure 27.5. High-power photomicrograph of Figure 27.3. Scale = 100 Ì. Bl, cells that appear to be developing into neuroblasts of the geniculate ganglion.

In 4.8- to 6.5-mm embryos (Figure 27.3) the facial division of the facio-acoustic primordium is less cellular than the acoustic division and, as it courses ventrally, it is partially surrounded by the developing acoustic ganglion. Ventral to the acoustic ganglion the facial division becomes more cellular and lies in close proximity to the deep surface of the placode (Figure 27.3). Many of the nuclei within the cellular column at the level of the placode are round or oval in outline and are darkly staining (Figure 27.5, Bl). They are slightly larger than the nuclei of the surrounding mesenchymal cells and they appear to be developing into the neuroblasts of the geniculate ganglion. Ventral to the placode the facial division is difficult to follow due to the increased density of the mesenchyme in this region. The facial division separates into two almost equal parts. The caudal part, which constitutes the main trunk of the facial nerve, shortly disappears into the surrounding mesenchyme. The rostral part enters the mandibular arch by passing ventral to the first pharyngeal pouch and will become the chorda tympani nerve, the first branch of the facial nerve to develop.

Stage II: Proximal Nerve Growth, Branches, and Communications (8–20 mm)

The proximal part of the facioacoustic primordium begins to separate into two distinct nerves in 8.0- to 10.6-mm embryos (36–39 days). A complete separation appears at 14.0 mm (Figure 27.6) and a discrete nervus intermedius is present at 16.5 mm (45–46 days). In 18.0-mm embryos (46–49 days) the nervus intermedius is considerably smaller than the motor root of the facial nerve (Figure 27.7) and is arranged as one or two main bundles that pass from the geniculate ganglion to the brain stem between the motor facial root and the acoustic nerve.

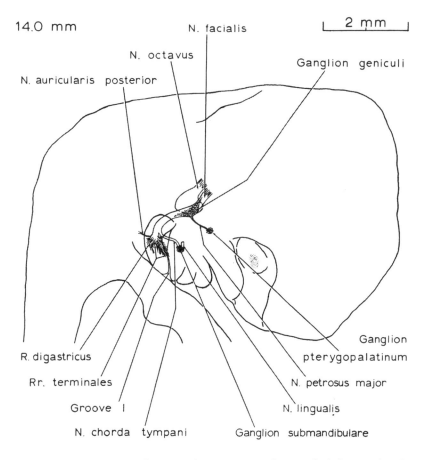

Figure 27.6. A 14.0-mm embryo with a menstrual age of eight weeks. Age group XVIII (Streeter, 1948). Bodian's protargol method of impregnation. Neuroblasts in the geniculate, pterygopalatine, and submandibular ganglia are shown as stipple.

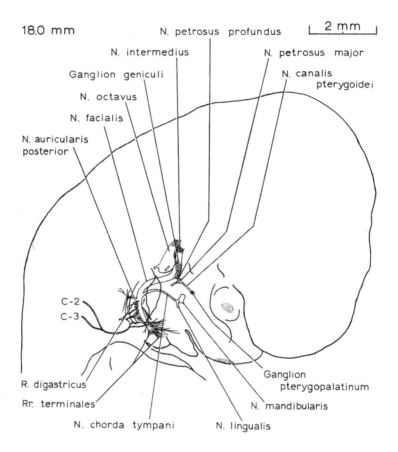

18.0 mm

N. petrosus profundus

2 mm

N. intermedius

N. petrosus major

Ganglion geniculi

N. canalis
pterygoidei

N. octavus

N. facialis

N. auricularis
posterior

C-2

C-3

R. digastricus

Ganglion
pterygopalatinum

Rr. terminales

N. mandibularis

N. chorda tympani

N. lingualis

Figure 27.7. An 18.0-mm embryo with a menstrual age of 8.5 weeks. Age group XIX (Streeter, 1951). Bodian's protargol method of impregnation. Neuroblasts in the geniculate and pterygopalatine ganglia are shown as stipple. C-2 and C-3, ventral primary rami from the second and third cervical ganglia, respectively.

In 8.0- to 10.6-mm embryos the geniculate ganglion lies rostral and lateral to the acoustic ganglion and at some levels it is adjacent to this ganglion. A small placode lines the first branchial groove opposite the most ventral part of the geniculate ganglion. The deep surface of the placode is separated from the ganglion by a small amount of loosely arranged cells. The placode has disappeared and the geniculate ganglion is well defined in 11.0- to 13.5-mm embryos (41 days).

The greater petrosal nerve is present in 8.0- to 10.6-mm embryos and is well developed by 14.0 mm (Figure 27.6). It leaves the most ventral part of the geniculate ganglion and courses rostrally and slightly ventrally to the lateral aspect of the developing internal carotid artery where it joins with the deep petrosal nerve, if the latter is present. It then continues rostrally as the nerve of the pterygoid canal and after a short distance disappears in a dense collection of cells, the future pterygopalatine ganglion.

In a 16.5-mm embryo, a branch arises from the ventral aspect of the geniculate ganglion near the origin of the greater petrosal nerve. This branch courses caudally and dorsally to join the undivided glossopharyngeal ganglion. Later in development (22.2 to 26.0 mm, 51–53 days) the tympanic plexus and the lesser petrosal nerve will form along the branch, changing the facial end of the branch into a communication (Figures 27.8 and 27.9).

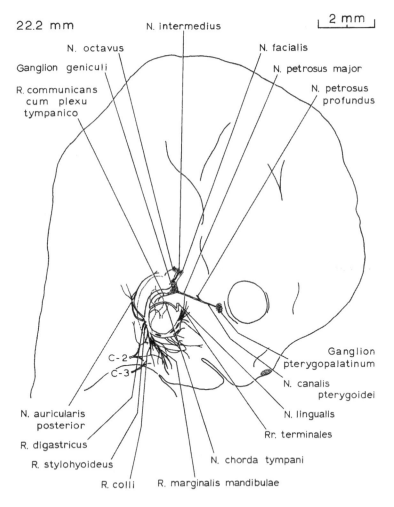

Figure 27.8. A 22.2-mm embryo with a menstrual age of nine weeks. Age group XXI (Streeter, 1951). Bodian's protargol method of impregnation. See legend of Figure 27.7 for further explanation.

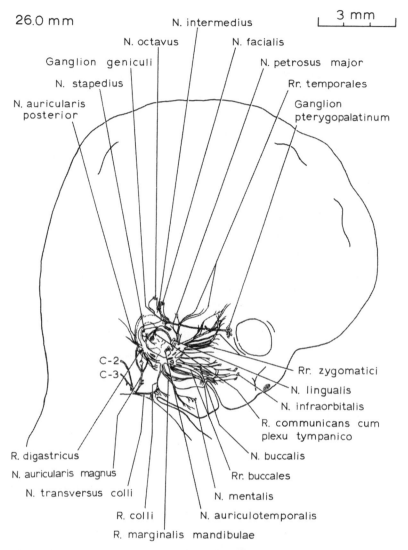

26.0 mm

N. intermedius

N. octavus

N. facialis

Ganglion geniculi

N. petrosus major

N. stapedius

Rr. temporales

N. auricularis posterior

Ganglion pterygopalatinum

3 mm

C-2
C-3

Rr. zygomatici

N. lingualis

N. infraorbitalis

R. communicans cum plexu tympanico

N. buccalis

R. digastricus

Rr. buccales

N. auricularis magnus

N. mentalis

N. transversus colli

N. auriculotemporalis

R. colli

R. marginalis mandibulae

Figure 27.9. A 26.0-mm fetus with a menstrual age of ten weeks. Age group XXII (Streeter, 1951). Erythrosin and toluidin blue stains. Some of the nerves with which the facial nerve communicates are only partially shown. See legend of Figure 27.7 for further explanation.

Distal to the geniculate ganglion, the facial nerve in 8- to 14-mm embryos loses its cellular character and inclines caudally and then ventrally in the medial part of the arch (Figure 27.6). In 8.0- to 10.6-mm embryos the chorda tympani nerve is a large and well-defined bundle that enters the mandibular arch where it terminates in the same region as does a branch of the mandibular nerve (the future lingual nerve). In a 14-mm embryo, the chorda tympani and lingual nerves terminate in a region where the submandibular ganglion is forming (Figure 27.6). These two nerves are united for the first time in an 18.0-mm embryo (Figure 27.7) where the submandibular ganglion is distal to the union.

In 8- to 14-mm embryos the posterior auricular nerve arises from the facial nerve in the same vicinity as does the chorda tympani nerve (Figure 27.6). It is a small ill-defined bundle which passes caudally and laterally for a short distance before it terminates. A prominent posterior auricular nerve arises distal to the chorda tympani in an 18.0-mm embryo and, after a short dorsal course, divides into cranial and caudal branches (Figure 27.7). The caudal branches communicate with nerves that originate from the second and third cervical ganglia.

Distal to the origin of the posterior auricular nerve in 8- to 14-mm embryos, the facial gives off a series of medially directed, ill-defined twigs that terminate in the posterior digastric premuscle mass (Figure 27.6). The facial nerve continues ventrally for a short distance and terminates by becoming a loose network of intermingling fibers that gradually become lost in the surrounding mesenchyme. Some of the fibers in the network reunite only to split again around other cells. Part of the fibers in a 16.5-mm embryo course rostrally for a short distance and terminate in the superficial and caudal part of the mandibular arch. In 18.0-mm embryos, the peripheral part of the facial nerve divides into several bundles (Figure 27.7). The most caudal bundles communicate with nerves from the second and third cervical ganglia in a plexus located in the caudal and ventral part of the second arch. Another bundle of the facial nerve, the future cervical branch, pursues a ventral course and terminates just deep to the myoblastic lamina from which the platysma muscle develops. The remaining peripheral bundles of the facial nerve pass either to the caudal and superficial part of the mandibular arch or farther rostrally to the angle of the mouth. In an 18.9-mm embryo, some of the peripheral branches course as far rostrally as the infraorbital region. Very few of the branches appear to turn dorsally in their rostral course. Those fibers destined for the zygomatic and the temporal regions arise from the facial nerve at higher levels. All of the peripheral branches lie close to the deep surface of the myoblastic laminae which will form the facial muscles.

Stage III: Distal Nerve Growth, Branches, and Communications (20.2–41.0 mm)

The facial nerve becomes proportionally smaller in relation to the total cranial region and its peripheral branches gradually approach the definitive condition. Proximally the facial nerve is round or oval on transverse section although peripherally, in some areas of the face, it is flat.

In a 26-mm specimen a short, thin branch is distributed to the stapedius muscle from the facial nerve as the latter begins its caudal descent through the petrous area (Figure 27.9). In specimens earlier than 26 mm the stapedius muscle is adjacent to the medial side of the facial nerve and only after the two become separated can the stapedius branch be seen. A small branch also arises from the rostral side of the facial nerve immediately distal to the stapedius branch and passes to the region of the external auditory meatus. In its course, the branch sends a few fibers to a plexus located lateral to the glossopharyngeal and vagus nerves and rostral to the internal jugular vein. This branch probably represents the communication between the facial nerve and the glossopharyngeal and vagus nerves.

As the facial nerve emerges from the region of the developing temporal bone, in 20.0- to 22.2-mm specimens, a large posterior auricular nerve is given off (Figure 27.8). In a fetus of 37 mm, this nerve courses into the occipital region, with one of its branches passing into the dorsal part of the auricle. When the posterior digastric and the stylohyoid muscles are separate muscle masses, the nerve fibers to them are arranged into a definite bundle. Each muscle may receive a separate branch from the facial nerve or a common nerve may innervate both muscles.

The interanastomoses of the peripheral branches first appear as separations in the main trunk of the facial nerve and become accentuated as development progresses. The separations are first observed at 22.2 mm and are increased in size and number by 26.0 mm (Figures 27.8 and 27.9). Some of the peripheral branches begin their course cranially toward the temporal and the zygomatic region as short, thin branches, the future temporal and zygomatic divisions. Approximately one-half of the peripheral branches pass caudally from the facial nerve toward the cervical region and the angle of the mouth to form the buccal, the mandibular, and the cervical divisions. All of the peripheral divisions of the facial nerve can be identified in the 26-mm specimen, but temporal branches do not yet extend into the frontal region. Branches from the temporal division of the facial nerve approach the frontal region in a 37-mm fetus but as yet no peripheral branches are distributed to the fused eyelids.

By 26 mm, communications are established with the infraorbital, the buccal, the auriculotemporal, and the mental branches of the trigeminal nerve. Branches of the second and the third cervical ganglia, which previously communicated with the facial nerve, become established as the great auricular and the transverse cervical nerves.

Stage IV: Definitive Arrangement (58–146 mm)

In fetuses of 58 and 80 mm, the peripheral part of the facial nerve branches considerably and some of its divisions course almost to the midline of the face (Figure 27.10). Since most of the peripheral branches of the facial nerve in the infraorbital and perioral regions communicate freely with those of the trigeminal nerve, the majority of the rami in these regions contain fibers from both of these cranial nerves.

In the 80-mm fetus, the nervus intermedius is between the acoustic and the motor root of the facial nerve and communicates with both of them. The external petrosal nerve is present as a tiny branch that arises from the facial nerve just distal to the geniculate ganglion and travels with an arterial branch of the middle meningeal artery. Two minute branches arise from the dorsomedial aspect of the facial nerve between the origins of the stapedius and chorda tympani nerves. After a short course, they join together and then communicate with the superior ganglia of the glossopharyngeal and vagus nerves. A small nerve arises from this communication to emerge from the skull between the developing mastoid bone and the tympanic plate (future tympanomastoid fissure) and to distribute to a subcutaneous area in the region of the external auditory canal. This nerve is the auricular branch of the vagus. Several small ganglia are scattered along its course through the developing petrous bone.

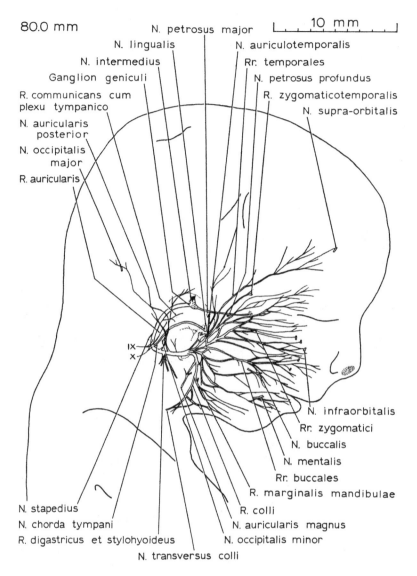

80.0 mm

N. petrosus major

10 mm

N. lingualis

N. auriculotemporalis

N. intermedius

Rr. temporales

Ganglion geniculi

N. petrosus profundus

R. communicans cum
plexu tympanico

R. zygomaticotemporalis

N. supra-orbitalis

N. auricularis
posterior

N. occipitalis
major

R. auricularis

IX
X

N. infraorbitalis

Rr. zygomatici

N. buccalis

N. mentalis

Rr. buccales

R. marginalis mandibulae

N. stapedius

R. colli

N. chorda tympani

N. auricularis magnus

R. digastricus et stylohyoideus

N. occipitalis minor

N. transversus colli

Figure 27.10. An 80.0-mm fetus with a menstrual age of 14.5 weeks. Quadruple stain. IX and X, branches from the ninth and tenth cranial nerves, respectively. The cervical part of the facial nerve could not be traced farther caudally because of a block cut that separated parts of the cervical region. See legend of Figure 27.9 for further explanation.

All but four of the numerous anastomoses of the facial nerve are present in the 80-mm fetus. The four exceptions are the communications with the zygomaticofacial, lacrimal, infratrochlear, and external nasal nerves. Branches from the temporal division of the facial nerve course in to the frontal region deep to the frontalis muscle. Tiny branches can be traced into the lateral aspect of the eyelids. A poorly established communication exists with the zygomaticotemporal nerve. The previous communications with branches from the second and the third cervical ganglia are now communications with the great auricular, the transverse cervical and the lesser occipital nerves. All of the definitive communications are established in the 146-mm fetus.

Comment

Although the derivation of the cells in the geniculate and other ganglia related to the facial nerve could not be determined in the present study, the close proximity of the developing geniculate ganglion to the second arch placode, plus the observation that the placode disappears as the ganglion becomes evident, are indications that the placode plays an important role in the development of the ganglion. Following the formation of the geniculate ganglion, an analysis of the facial nerve roots can be accomplished since the nervus intermedius arises from this ganglion. His (His, 1889) stated that up to the third month no nerve arises between the facial and the acoustic, and he concluded that the nervus intermedius, until that time, must run in the trunk of these two nerves. Streeter (Streeter, 1907) found the nervus intermedius (and geniculate ganglion) in a 7-mm embryo and stated that it could be distinguished as early as 3.0 to 4.3 mm. According to him, the nerve at 7 mm is fully as large as the motor root, but the proportion is gradually reversed in the older stages. The present study revealed a well-defined geniculate ganglion in 11.0- to 13.5-mm embryos and, in 16.5- to 18.0-mm embryos, a discrete nervus intermedius which is considerably smaller than the motor root. Pearson (Pearson, 1947) found the nervus intermedius fibers most often grouped into a number of smaller bundles that enter the brain stem separately, whereas in the present observations they were arranged as one or two main bundles.

The first branch of the facial nerve to develop is the chorda tympani followed closely by the greater petrosal nerve. Both Rabl (Rabl, 1887) and Futamura (Futamura, 1906) previously reported these two nerves to be the first branches of the facial nerve to form. Soon after developing (4.8 mm), the chorda tympani is almost the size of the main trunk of the facial nerve (Figure 27.3). This condition was also observed by Rabl (Rabl, 1887) and compares favorably with Streeter's (Streeter, 1907) description of a large nervus intermedius at this early age, since the latter nerve carries the sensory part of the chorda tympani. The chorda tympani and lingual nerves terminate in a region where the submandibular ganglion is forming in a 14-mm embryo (Figure 27.6). Dixon (Dixon, 1896) observed this in a 9.1-mm embryo. At 18 mm (Figure 27.7) the chorda tympani and the lingual nerves are joined and the ganglion is distal to the point of fusion. Futamura (Futamura, 1906) noted fusion of the two nerves at a similar age. The manner of formation of the lesser petrosal nerve described in this study agrees with that presented by Futamura and explains the definitive arrangement of the nerve as illustrated by Schäfer and Symington. (Schäfer and Symington, 1909)

Schimert (Schimert, 1933) found the stapedius muscle to be innervated at 35 mm (grösster Länge) [its greatest length]. This muscle very likely has an innervation when it begins to form at the medial side of the facial nerve, but only after it increases in size and separates from the nerve can a discrete branch going to the muscle be identified (26 mm).

That the posterior auricular nerve is one of the first, if not the first, extracranial branch to form was previously reported by Popowsky (Popowsky, 1895) and Futamura (Futamura, 1906). The premuscle lamina which develops in the occipital region superficial to the nerve also differentiates very early. Similarly, branches to the rapidly differentiating posterior digastric premuscle mass appear as the premuscle mass forms. These observations point out the close interrelation of muscle and nerve differentiation. As the premuscle laminae which form the facial muscles spread from the hyoid arch, the fibers of the facial nerve follow *pari passu*. This condition has been mentioned previously by Rabl (Rabl, 1887), Popowsky (Popowsky, 1895), Futamura (Futamura, 1906), and Bryce (Bryce, 1923). The peripheral branches of the facial nerve develop deep to the myoblastic laminae from which the muscles of facial expression are derived, with the exception of the buccinator muscle. The facial branches develop superficial to the buccinator muscle, including the branch that supplies it. With few exceptions the peripheral branches develop as the muscles differentiate.

The present study shows that the time at which the various branches appear is much earlier than the time at which Popowsky (Popowsky, 1895) first observed them. Popowsky gave a detailed description of the relations between the formation of the peripheral branches of the facial nerve and the facial muscles. He and Futamura stated that the complicated interanastomoses among the peripheral branches resulted from the shifting and the rearrangement of the muscles during development. The present work shows that interanastomoses form as separations in the main trunk of the facial nerve. These separations become accentuated as development progresses (Figures 27.8, 27.9, and 27.10).

At 35–36 days (13–15 mm) Futamura observed that the terminal part of the facial nerve divided into three small, short branches, which, he concluded, probably correspond to the temporal, the zygomatic, and the cervicomandibular branches of the definitive nerve. A facial nerve divided into three discrete terminal branches was not observed in the present study. A combined marginal mandibular and cervical branch is present at 22.2 mm (Figure 27.8), and at 26.0 mm (Figure 27.9), a portion of each definitive peripheral division is represented as groups of branches.

Little information is available on the development of the connections between the peripheral part of the facial nerve and other nerves in the head and neck regions. The definitive facial nerve has connections with several cervical nerves that take origin from the second and the third cervical ganglia. Numerous connections also exist between the peripheral branches of the facial and the branches of all three major divisions of the trigeminal nerve. These peripheral connections were not included in Dixon's detailed study on the early development of the trigeminal nerve. Popowsky stated that he was not able to find a connection between the nervus subcutaneous colli superior (cervical branch of the facial nerve) and the nervus subcutaneous colli medius (great auricular nerve) in human fetuses and even in some newborns. The present study shows that connections between the facial nerve and branches from the second and third cervical ganglia are the first to form (Figure 27.7, 18 mm) and that, later in development, they become the connections with the great auricular, the transverse cervical and the lesser occipital nerves. Popowsky could prove the existence of anastomoses between the peripheral branches of the facial and the trigeminal nerves at the end of the eighth or the beginning of the ninth month of prenatal life but the present work reveals that as early as 26 mm or 10 weeks (menstrual age) facial branches communicate with the infraorbital, the buccal, the auriculotemporal and the mental branches of the trigeminal nerve. Popowsky concluded that the majority of the anastomoses with the trigeminal do not occur until after birth. As the present study shows, most of the frequently occurring connections between the peripheral branches of these two nerves are present at 80 mm or 14.5 weeks menstrual age (Figure 27.10). The exceptions are the connections between the facial nerve and zygomaticofacial, lacrimal, infratrochlear and external nasal branches of the trigeminal nerve. These connections are present at 146 mm. Dixon stated that the malar nerve (zygomaticofacial) does not come so close to the surface during early development as does the temporal nerve (zygomaticotemporal). This anatomical relationship may explain the earlier development of the connection between the facial nerve and the zygomaticotemporal branch. At 80 mm, zygomaticofacial, lacrimal, infratrochlear and external nasal branches do not yet course completely through the developing skull to the superficial parts of the face.

Summary

This [article] presents the morphogenesis of the intracranial and extracranial parts of the facial nerve in human embryos. Included are the development of the roots, the geniculate ganglion, the branches, the interanastomoses and the anastomoses between the facial and other nerves in the head and neck regions.

1. The facial nerve develops from the facioacoustic primordium of the second branchial or hyoid arch (4.2 to 8.0 mm) in close proximity to the placode of the arch.

2. The facial division of the primordium separates from the acoustic division by 8.0 to 10.6 mm and develops a geniculate ganglion that becomes evident as the placode disappears.

3. The chorda tympani and the greater petrosal nerves are the first branches to form followed by the posterior auricular and posterior digastric nerves. The facial nerve terminates peripherally in early embryos as a loose network of intermingling fibers.

4. By 14 to 20 mm the nervus intermedius can be recognized, the chorda tympani joins with the lingual nerve, and connections are made between the facial nerve and the branches of the second and the third cervical ganglia. The terminal branches of the facial nerve course into occipital, cervical, mandibular, and infraorbital regions.

5. The muscular branches of the facial nerve follow *pari passu* the formation of the facial muscle masses and, in most cases, develop deep to them.

6. The peripheral divisions of the facial nerve are present at 26 mm and communications exist with infraorbital, buccal, auriculotemporal, and mental branches of the trigeminal nerve.

7. All of the common communications between the branches of the facial and of other nerves are formed by 80 mm with the exception of the zygomatico-facial, lacrimal, infratrochlear, and external nasal branches of the trigeminal nerve, which are present at 146 mm. Branches of the second and the third cervical ganglia, which communicate early with the facial nerve, become established later as the great auricular, the transverse cervical, and the lesser occipital nerves.[11]

CHAPTER 28

Metabolic Fields: Palpation and Sensory Experience

> The field concept defined development in dynamic instead of geographical terms. Every aspect of ontogeny had to be viewed in a double light, as the result of "interactions between the material whole with its field properties on the one hand, and the material parts on the other." Field factors themselves showed definite order: they were three-dimensional heterogeneous systems. The idea of a center, around which field intensity gradually graded off, led to the concept of field gradients. (Haraway, 2004, p. 178)

The subject of this chapter is the metabolic fields of the embryo, as named by Dr. Blechschmidt in all of his writings. It is my contention that the metabolic fields of the human embryo represent the most basic activity or work of the fluid body in biodynamic craniosacral therapy. The notion of metabolic fields refers to the process of congealing and densification of the fluid body into the various structures of the embryo and their final fates in the adult body under the influence of the outside presence of Primary Respiration first and then the genes (Ingber, 2006). The genes themselves are responsible for the final form that the body takes and a process called remodeling of the embryo is described in the twenty-three Carnegie stages of human embryonic development. Please refer to the epilogue for a chart describing the differences between the four stages of dynamic morphology, the eight metabolic fields of the fluid body, and the twenty-three Carnegie stages of somatic development.

Dr. Blechschmidt defined eight types of metabolic fields having to do with their *position* in the embryo, their *relationship* to one another via *ordered movement* in the fluids, and the resulting *shaping* of the cells and their aggregates into specific structures. This is a biokinetic process requiring the space to perform such differentiations (location) and the precise timing involved in each differentiation. A practitioner must be able to imagine that the embryo is empty of any structure on the inside and filled with fluid. This is the starting point of palpating and sensing the metabolic fields. The practitioner visualizes the perfect structure of the body in its initial frame or scaffolding as a transparent, living, ordered gel. It is the responsibility of the practitioner to maintain a three-dimensional sense and image of his own fluid body and its transparency, as well as that of the client.

There are progressive stages of sensing the metabolic fields of the embryo in your own body or the embryo in the client's body. At first, the embryo is just a cognitive construct and beautiful to behold in an embryology textbook. It is the systemic fluid movement of the embryo, its image, age, and shape that the practitioner is interested in. It is the stillpoint around which the movement occurs that the practitioner is interested in. Thus the rhythmic balanced interchange between the stillness and Primary Respiration begins the exploration of the embryo in the adult body. This interchange is linked to the first four metabolic fields in the embryo, the so-called early embryo, when it was all fluid.

Then the practitioner begins to explore the fluid body as it condenses with the systemic motions of compression-decompression and flexion-extension, as a whole movement in the practitioner's body and that of the client's. These are the last four metabolic fields—they have to do with how, for example, the blood relates to the heart, or the heart relates to the tubes that it's flowing through, as a particular direction and dimension of experience. Then, finally, the muscles, cartilage, and bones condense in the late embryo and early fetus. Metabolic fields are very alive and trigger both images and sensations when contacted with Primary Respiration. The key to feeling the personal embryo and that of the client is to sense the whole as a breathing three-dimensional sphere, go to stillpoint, and be drawn to the activity of the fields in the fluid body. It is the movement of the whole that is the first work done as a biodynamic craniosacral therapist. So, sensing the embryo in self and other has to do with qualities of sensing systemic movement at different rates and rhythms in the tidal body and fluid body and differential pressure placement of the practitioner's hands. The early metabolic fields require the buoyant and transparent hands to palpate. The late fields require buoyant hands that can be submerged briefly in the fluid structure of membranes and bones to palpate. It is possible for the hands to be applying more pressure without causing a false fulcrum in the client. The fluid body may stillpoint and the practitioner waits for that stillpoint to resolve itself before moving on. I think sometimes that practitioners expect that a book image of the embryo will suddenly appear as a template on the client's body. More likely, the quality of the movement and direction cue the practitioner to the age of the embryo and trigger an image and process in the practitioner's mind. The other level of experiencing the embryo is that its presence reveals the felt sense of loving kindness or the flow of unconditional love as warmth and heat. This requires that the practitioner have a relatively "happy mind," which means being open to revelation. I hope this is helpful. It does require imagination and some academic study to find your embryo.

Any discussion or perceptual process having to do with the metabolic fields of the embryo must be placed in the context of the basic principles of biodynamics. Primary Respiration cannot be broken down into separate categories, yet the fluid body and soma arise out of the embryo and are managed, so to speak, by the whole. In other words, Primary Respiration is the brain of the fluid body and soma. So the question is: What is the relationship between the whole and the unique differentiations in the metabolic fields that are occurring moment by moment in a precise, orderly manner? The second question would have to be: What does this relationship have to do with the healing process in the client-therapist relationship, in the context of biodynamic craniosacral therapy? In order to answer these questions I need to do a little review.

The specific biodynamic forces I am referring to are the presence of Primary Respiration as a living movement constantly generating, maintaining, and repairing the wholeness of the embryo in all of its developmental stages and fields of activity during its construction. The embryo is the visible form of the invisible movement of Primary Respiration. First, as a rule, at any stage of development, cell aggregations and the primordia *(anlagen)* of all the organs act according to the qualities that they acquire during that stage of development throughout the lifespan. Second, the unique shapes of all of the organs are dependent upon where the organ is located in the embryo because of differential rates of growth and different fluid densities at any given time and place in the embryo. As a result of this, normal directions of differentiation occur without exception because of the outside presence of Primary Respiration catalyzing different shapes, pressures, and densities in the fluid body. The conditions differ according to the location of each differentiation in question. This is called biokinetics, or the material process of condensing specific shapes in the metabolic fields of the embryo.

Every element of a cell, its delimiting membrane, especially the living water in the cytoplasm, the nucleus, and the extracellular matrix (ECM) participate in the developmental movements of the metabolic fields under the guidance of Primary Respiration. It is therefore important to understand that the developmental movement of Primary Respiration is causative or what would formerly have been called an inducer to the subsequent differentiations within the embryo. There is also an intermediate zone of fluid activity between the biodynamic (whole movement) and biokinetic (differentiation of inter related components) of the embryo. Think of the whole as being a field of different densities and gradients of fluid activity rather than parts that are sewn together like a quilt.

> A field is primarily an entity and not a mosaic. This property covered field pattern and self-conservation of the system. A field district is characterized by the fact that none of its elements can be identified with any particular component of the field, although the field as a whole is a definite property of the district as a whole. (Haraway, 2004, p. 178)

One fundamental direction of the fluid flow in the embryo is along the long axis of a limiting membrane. A second fundamental flow is perpendicular to the long axis of a limiting membrane such as the plate of the ectoderm when the primitive streak arises (longitudinal fluctuation). Because the embryo has such high water content and the whole embryo grows as a result of differential pressure gradients between its compartments, living water can flow right through a limiting membrane. Fourth, the fluids are moving in a spiral as an intrinsic property of the living water in the embryo. All cells, cell aggregates, and so forth down to the shape of the adult body are curved. It is to be understood that development then arises from influences outside the cell nucleus toward the inside simply in the sense that the genes themselves are not self-activating but must be "pressured" into activity from the outside. This lends itself to the biodynamic principle that Primary Respiration is said to be acting from the outside of the soma to the inside of the soma.

Biokinetics is the study of the fluid body as an interconnected system of metabolic fields, in the context of the embryo being a self-organizing whole (biodynamics). The metabolic fields cause the fluid body to differentiate into different compartments, whether they are fluid compartments (blood, lymph, and so on) or more densified structures such as muscles, bones, and cartilage. This activity is related not only to conception ignition, heart ignition, and birth ignition, but the ignition of the soma as a whole into its final form. The fluid body is a body of condensing and expanding fluids building the structure of the soma. It is a tensile field of intelligent protoplasm responding to the priorities of Primary Respiration on the outside and the genes on the inside. What is being described below are some of the key elements of the ignition process and therefore, when working with the fluid body level of understanding in biodynamic craniosacral therapy, the developmental motions and relationships between the fields are important considerations in the healing process as the embryo in the adult continues to generate its form, maintain its form, and repair its form moment to moment.

Healing would consist of well-bounded contact, synchronized with Primary Respiration, holding and containing the original function of the metabolic fields so that any imprinted memory of stress or trauma that occurred at that time could be uncoupled and resolved into the process of a stillpoint, its interchange with Primary Respiration, and reoriented to the midline.

I have arranged this discussion of the metabolic fields in the sequence that they arise in the embryo, although this is not precise because some of them arise simultaneously with each other. I have further subdivided the metabolic fields into two distinct categories. The early fields of suction, corrosion, dilation, and retention are the first, or early, category of fields. The second are densation, contusion, distusion, and detraction, which are associated with the later developing embryo. It is typical in the formation of the late embryo that this second category of fields can arise adjacent to one another or even within one another. This is especially in relationship to cartilage, tendon, muscle tissue, and bone. We'll look first at the four fields that belong to the first, or early, formations in the embryo. Then we'll move to the second category, the later developing fields.

Suction Fields

The suction field is the first metabolic field to arise in the embryo. It starts at conception and possibly earlier when the egg itself differentiates, many years preceding fertilization. The gesture of the suction field is the gesture of respiratory breathing. The image is that of a bellows being pulled apart and rhythmically pushed back to stoke the fire in the fireplace. This creates a differentiation between low pressure on one side of the fluid membrane of the zygote and high pressure on the other side. This is demonstrated by the motion observed in a newly conceived human embryo. The zygote begins to flex itself and stretches out in three dimensions and then back rhythmically. There is a pulsatory deformation in the zygote that mimics breathing and is recapitulated in all subsequent stages of embryonic development and fetal development. This occurs later in the embryo through the experience of one membrane rhythmically being pulled apart from another membrane. It begins when the surface layer of the embryo begins to expand, but the inner membrane layer does not. As a principle it must be stated that all adult function is preexercised in the embryo. Thus, respiratory function is the oldest and earliest human function to come on-line. The principle of preexercising of adult function will be accurate with all the metabolic fields, as will be shown. Healing requires an ability to contact this original function and normalize it with Primary Respiration in biodynamic craniosacral therapy.

Ultimately, the entire three-dimensional surface of the skin of the fluid body in all stages of human development exhibits a spatially ordered metabolic suction field. The skin of the fluid body is sometimes up against the skin of the soma but usually is located off the soma. In the embryo the amnion and chorion were the first skin of the fluid body and a short distance off the surface of the embryo, and in the adult that would proportionally be 12–14 inches off the surface of the soma. The suction field of the fluid body mediates gradients of high pressure and low pressure of the fluids in the core of the embryo and the amnion and chorion pressure dynamics on the outside surface of the surface membrane of the embryo and fetus in utero. The sweat glands in the skin of the soma are the formal part of the suction field in embryonic development and the blood in the capillaries under the surface of the skin. It is important to bear in mind the importance of the suction field being the first metabolic field that arises in the human embryo.

The heart primordium (future pericardium) also arises as a suction field. Even the endocrine glands are the result of suction fields in large part because the yolk sac acts as the original endocrine gland in the embryo and are imprinted with that swelling-receding breathing function of the yolk sac. The large organs in the visceral system, such as the lung (respiration), liver, pancreas, and kidneys are formed from a suction field. Not only does the suction field begin the preexercising of respiratory function at conception, but several weeks later builds the structure of the lungs in which that function will also take place. Thus another important embryonic principle of function preceding structure is seen here. The gesture of the suction field is the movement associated with reciprocal breathing or respiratory tidal movement whether it is an ocean tide or a zygote.

The later writings of Dr. Blechschmidt suggested that the suction field was a "loosening" field. When you consider that in the early embryo the reciprocal movement of the fluid conceptus would loosen adjacent structures, this makes sense. It is especially evident at the end of the first week when the conceptus must hatch itself from the shell of the zona pellucida. The zona pellucida develops cracks in it while it rolls down the fallopian tube but at the same time requires the internal energy of the suction movements to free itself and attach to the uterine wall. The gesture is similar to breathing techniques that seek to relax the nervous system and loosen soft-tissue restrictions (which Dr. Sutherland was fond of using). These adult stress reduction strategies are based on the original metabolism of the embryo.

> Proper use of fields in biology requires understanding of organization, increasing complexity, hierarchy, and transformations over time. (Haraway, 2004, p. 61)

Exploration: Breathing

With a partner who is supine on the table, synchronize your attention with your own skin and the movement of Primary Respiration moving in and out of your body. Gently place your hands on the skin of your partner's arms or legs. The suction field causes an undulating movement slightly underneath the skin in the capillary beds, like a bed of plankton moving on the surface of the ocean. One's hands must be very buoyant and spacious as Primary Respiration moves through them and causes the subdermal layers of the skin to undulate. Once you begin to sense the undulation under the skin, resynchronize your attention with Primary Respiration and get a three-dimensional sense of the entire surface of the partner's (or client's) skin. You may need to visualize the parts of the body that you can't see that are in touch with the treatment table.

The next step is to place your hands 12–14 inches off your partner's body and imagine you are holding a bowl of water as big as your partner and an imaginary bubble around your client that extends 12–15 inches off the body. This is called the skin of the fluid body. The sense here is to see if you can feel your partner's embryo at the end of the first week of development and the whole second week as the fluid cavities of the embryo were being built as a sphere outside the embryo's body. That particular suction field was especially strong all through the first and second weeks of development. At the same time that you are sensing the skin of your partner's fluid body breathing at a slow tempo, pendulate back to your own sense of Primary Respiration and find your own fluid body.

The next step is to discover the fulcrum of your fluid body, which will typically be shifting between the umbilicus, the heart, or the third ventricle. Then discover which fulcrum your partner's fluid body is oriented to. Finally, watch both spheres of the fluid bodies and see how they relate to one another. Do they want to merge? Do they want to stay separate in a twin dynamic? Do they want to differentiate into a later stage of development? How do they differentiate based on fluid image, fluid shape, and fluid sense?

Corrosion Fields

A corrosion field is established when two layers of embryonic tissue are compressed together to form a thin, double-layered membrane that begins to dissolve, like the development of the mouth. During development, these tissues are nourished only through the underlying inner tissue. They both release waste products into the adjacent fluids between them and outside of them. Consequently, there is a metabolic gradient between the inner tissue and the fluid in between. When this metabolic gradient is strong enough such that the waste products cannot escape, a rupture zone is created. Such rupture zones are found quite frequently in the embryo. There is a perforation between the two layers of tissue and the fluid gradient on either side of the tissue begins to balance and change. Examples of corrosion fields can be observed between the notochord and the underlying endoderm, as well as between the palatine processes in the mouth, the mouth itself, and the region of the anus called the cloacal membrane.

In other words, a corrosion field occurs when two membranes push against each other and dissolve their boundaries. This is also the way the chambers of the heart tube are formed. The basic gesture of the corrosion field is seen in the development of the heart when the paired cardiac tubes fuse into one tube in the middle. This fusion takes place inside the primordium (pericardium) while the ends of the two tubes become fixed at the boundaries of the primordium. It almost gives the early heart the appearance of having two arms and two legs. The corrosion field of the heart tubes is the gesture of dissolving boundaries as the two become one. In order for the cardiac tubes to merge together, the epithelial lining must disintegrate within the gradient of the fluid medium on the outside of the tubes and that on the inside of the tubes. A corrosion field has a pressure differential on either side of the two tissues. Later the heart develops from one tube to having two chambers and then four chambers. During this process the atrial-ventricular opening, the interatrial septa, and interventricular septa occur because of corrosion fields as well.

Exploration: Contact Boundary

How do two become one? With your partner standing across the room, face each other and find a stillpoint in your heart. Each of you take one step forward and describe any response that your autonomic nervous system might have or any felt sense of resistance around the area of the heart. Then take another step forward and repeat. Gradually, find the distance where each of you senses around the heart and gut the greatest resistance to coming closer to one another. Now imagine that the structure on the surface of your mutual bodies is dissolving. Now imagine the bones and muscles are dissolving, starting around the area of the chest and expanding in all directions in the body. Now imagine that only your two hearts are left in contact with one another. What is it like to have your two hearts touching together? Now imagine that arteries and veins start to connect the two hearts as blood starts to circulate between the two hearts. What is the sense of that dissolving and connection? Now have your partner lie down on a table and go through the same process as though your partner is your client. The aim is to have your two hearts merge together and be connected.

Another consideration for this exploration is that frequently it involves a projection process when one meets the boundary of self and other. It is important to notice any emotions or feelings, especially any subtle mental thoughts you have about the motivation and intention of the other person in front of you, especially a client or spouse. It's important in this exploration to see clearly that projected thought, feeling, perception, or emotion without any interpretation or judgment from each other. This is done by finding a stillpoint in your heart. Find the radiance and heat intrinsic to the heart itself that automatically seeks connection and dissolving of boundaries. It is not necessary that partners come into physical contact with one another, either in the standing part or the client-therapist table part, but rather go through two or three responses to the felt sense of a boundary arising and dissolving. Where does the contact boundary arise in the body and what manages that boundary? In other words, is it the autonomic nervous system? Is it your emotions? Thought processes? What is the boundary that need not be dissolved right now? Find the rhythm of making a boundary and dissolving a boundary.

Exploration: Conception Ignition

This practice will properly allow the client-therapist relationship to experience a corrosion field with Primary Respiration. Synchronize your attention with Primary Respiration as follows:

- **Practitioner's perception.** This starts with the two-dimensional perception of its outside presence or inside presence and the merging of those two into a single state of Primary Respiration. This means that the practitioner is perceiving Primary Respiration on a horizontal plane from her third ventricle, heart, or umbilicus out to the horizon and back through the front of her soma. This then turns into a three-dimensional perception of Primary Respiration and possibly the simultaneous perception of the inhalation phase and the exhalation phase occurring at the same time.

- **Practitioner's perception of the client.** The practitioner is able to clearly distinguish the expansion and contraction phases of Primary Respiration in the client as distinct from her own, using the area around the practitioner's chest and shoulders to sense the client's Primary Respiration. In addition, the practitioner may sense specific vector patterns of Primary Respiration in the client, especially on the vertical midline of the notochord, the long bones, the transverse axis of the cranium, and so forth.

- **Self-other.** Initially, the practitioner senses her Primary Respiration and that of the client's to be separate. This gradually changes into a sense of their being related and complementing one another. This then develops into a sense of both of the Primary Respirations mirroring one another, such that both are inhaling or exhaling together or one is inhaling and the other is exhaling. They may be sensed to be moving together in the same phase, or they may be sensed to be moving in opposite phases to one another. At this point the practitioner can begin to visualize more actively that her soma is actually the egg she was conceived from and breathing three-dimensionally with Primary Respiration.

- **Unified.** By maintaining a sense of her egg, a quantum event takes place and the sense of two Primary Respirations becomes one. This is the corrosion field of Primary Respiration. The practitioner and client breathe together as one egg or one heart. At this point, it is critical for the practitioner to stay differentiated from the client but not from their Primary Respiration. One osteopath calls this divided attention. This supports the client's autonomy and self-regulation. The practitioner can achieve this sense of differentiation by maintaining an awareness of stillness in her heart, bare attention on her thoracic respiration, or suspending attention to include the holding environment of the office and surrounding environment. This corrosion field encompasses the therapeutic process called conception ignition.

Dilation Fields

This field initially involves tissue being stretched in a way that develops muscle tissue because of two factors. One is the opportunity for tissues to expand and the second is the tensile stress that expansion causes. In other words, there is open space in the embryo that allows a rapid expansion. The original dilation field is a spatially and kinetically highly organized field of activity that starts between the ectoderm and the endoderm layers of the embryo. When inner tissue is stretched by a longitudinal pull without transverse compression, muscle tissue develops. This is also a type of shearing motion as the one layer of tissue is being pulled in one direction and the other layer of tissue is being pulled in the opposite direction; this type of motion is responsible for the tensile stress associated with a dilation field.

There are two types of dilation fields: early and late. I will refer mainly to the early dilation fields of the embryo, especially the development of its tube structures in the cardiovascular system. The late dilation fields include the muscles as an organ of locomotion that is always preceded by cartilage formation. The best example of an early dilation field is the heart, and, second, the gastrointestinal tract. The early heart becomes filled with and distended by precursor blood cells under high pressure because the tubes leading into the heart go from a small diameter into a larger diameter where they are attached to the primordium (pericardium), thus causing the fluid to move more rapidly as it is in the process of forming. The primordium is a kind of perimeter boundary circling the largest-diameter tubes that eventually become the heart. This causes a greater pressure on the inside of the fused cardiac tube discussed above in the corrosion field. Because there is less pressure in the space of the coelomic fluid on the outside, the heart is able to dilate (expand), which can be seen in embryos of only 3 millimeters! The image I often get is that of a rodeo rider being let out of the holding pen into the small riding arena of the primordium. The developmental sequence of rapid growth of the cardiac tube (rider on a bucking bronco) is as follows: It expands in diameter while lengthening, bends, turns upside down, twists to the left, and finally turns downside up. This is due partly to the fact that the atria initially start on the bottom of the heart while the ventricles are on top. The heart starts upside down because the primordium (arena) also starts upside down when it differentiates on top of the embryonic head. Imagine a globe on top of your head with a north pole and a south pole. When the embryo starts to flex and bring the primordium down into the center of the body cavity to surround the cardiac tubes, it ends up upside down. So, in development with the dilation field, the heart has to turn itself bottom side up. It has the space to do that, which is the good news. These are the basic gestures of the heart while it develops into a four-chambered organ. Because it is fixed at each end of the primordium on the walls of the thoracic cavity, it bends from an alpha shape into an omega shape inside the primordium. Thus the second gesture of a dilation field in the heart space is the gesture of the alpha and omega—the beginning and the end.

All dilation fields are characterized not only by the longitudinal dilation of the immature cells, but also, to a lesser extent, dilation perpendicular to the longitudinal axis. Thus there is a transverse bulging, which is also a feature of myotomes in later skeletal musculature. Overall, a dilation field means that muscles originate by having a passive growing function (extension) before they are able to actively contract (flexion) at the end of the embryonic period and fetal period. The most active part of the muscle building process is the distusion (lengthening) growth itself, which stimulates the biochemistry of actin and myosin regarding contraction and expansion of the tissue (Gasser, 2006). Muscles need the biokinetic and morphological circumstances of space and stretch to stimulate their function. Organs of shape and movement always differentiate by subdivision of the whole (subwholes) and never by the composition of isolated parts. The heart grows in an open space of the heart primordium and consequently has room to do so.

> … fields were distinguished from simple geographic regions of the embryo by three criteria: any given point within the field force had to possess a given quality, a given direction, and a given intensity. Fields were judged in terms of instability and successive equilibrium positions. Waddington reasoned that "a field is a system of order such that the position taken up by unstable entities in one portion of the system bears a definite relation to the position taken up by unstable entities in other portions." Behavior of cells was, within certain boundaries, a function of position within the whole. Many of the organizational forces of fields were "to some extent on a suprachemical level." (Haraway, 2004, p. 124)

A principle feature of the early dilation field is that it occurs around the expanding system of endoderm together with its neighboring vascular system. In such a field, the early muscle cells have a growth direction that is mainly circular, with the basic movement gesture of peristalsis because of the endoderm relationships. Thus the heart tissue as it forms has its original movement as a form of peristalsis from inferior to superior inside the heart primordium as a function of its relationship to the underlying endoderm. The upward growing movement of the heart tube is also induced genetically by the primitive streak. The primitive streak is a strong biodynamic, upward-growing, and structuring process from the future anus all the way up to the neck of the embryo. It ends where the future atrioventricular (AV) node of the heart will be and then recedes back to the top of the sacrum. The primitive streak itself arises biodynamically as a result of the longitudinal fluctuation of fluids as the embryo has turned itself through a growth gesture in a way that aligns the connecting stalk to the caudal end of the embryo. This creates fluid pressure and a canal zone of flow on the top of the ectoderm that invites the primitive streak to arise. So it could be said that the growth movement of the heart is influenced by all four things—the endoderm, the genes, the primitive streak, and the longitudinal fluctuation of the fluid body—but initiated by the fluid flow rather than the genes. The genes are induced by pressure from the fluids.

Another example of a dilation field is the entire gastrointestinal tract, as mentioned. Endoderm peristalsis is a movement from superior to inferior. Initially, the proximal segment of the gut tube (mouth and throat) is wide and the caudal segment in the pelvic floor is narrow in the embryonic colon because the mouth-head area is growing faster. It is only toward the end of the embryonic period when these dimensions reverse themselves because of the accelerated growth being reversed, and the pelvic floor grows quickly. At first the growth in the cranial end is rapid and the pelvic end slow. This gradually reverses itself and consequently the shape and diameter of the colon ultimately becomes larger than the mouth and throat.

Exploration: Heart Ignition 1

Now that we have palpated the suction field as a pattern of undulation on the surface of the skin and immediately underneath it, followed by the formation of a single heart tube, we will bring our attention to the ignition of the muscle tissue of the heart. Have your partner lie supine on the table and synchronize your attention with Primary Respiration in yourself. Comfortably place the pads of your fingers of one hand over the xiphoid process and the pads of your fingers of the other hand over the sternoclavicular notch. Bring your attention to the skin, as we did with the suction field. Now allow your attention to get into the bone, the cartilage, and the muscles underneath and around the rib cage and in the pericardium. Allow yourself to sense the total contents of the thoracic cavity to be moving as a peristaltic wave from the central tendon of the diaphragm through the pericardium and heart all the way up to the clavicles and neck. Remember that the heart tube goes through a series of bends, twists, and folds, so it will not be unusual for the peristalsis to have different convolutions in it.

Stay centered in your sense of Primary Respiration and periodically go right to a stillpoint in your own heart to orient in this perceptual exploration. Your own heart space may begin to move and produce increased sensation. As the peristalsis of the partner's (or client's) heart tube reveals itself in the tempo of the fluid body, wait for it to achieve a stillpoint. The stillpoint is the main feature of heart ignitions because the primordium was originally still. The first imprint on the entire cardiovascular system is stillness. Feel how the heart wants to expand into the stillness. Imagine that the entire thoracic cavity is a vast sphere of stillness in which all the movement of breathing and blood circulation takes place. Sense the disengagement of tissues in their ability to expand. This is an aspect of heart ignition.

Retention Fields

A retention field is a field of Dynamic Stillness where inner tissues (the lining or boundary of the protoplasm) are tensed and stilled through growth resistance at either end of the tissue. The growth in a particular direction is slower than that of adjacent tissues and thus a biomechanical resistance to stretching occurs. This causes a gradually increasing biomechanical counterpull against the tugging of the neighboring tissue. This pulsatory movement of push-pull, lengthening and narrowing and shearing between adjacent tissue fields is the kinetic activity of the retention field. It is dynamic in a way that causes the stretched tissue to periodically achieve a state of balanced stillness from the longitudinal pull and a transverse compression. The stillness acts as the inducer of growth.

At the level of the fluid body, intercellular fluids are squeezed out as though coming out of a porous sac when the sac is pulled longitudinally. The gesture is that of a sponge being squeezed by a hand. Liquid precollagen is initially observed between these types of cells, forming a scaffolding of the future structure as a jellylike matrix of shape. There is an intelligence manifesting in the fluid body that creates shape prior to the expression of genes. Then gradually the precollagen solidifies to form collagen fibers with the help of the genes. Thus all ligaments, tendons, and joint capsules are formed in retention fields and are considered fulcrums of stillness in biodynamic practice. The activity of the other adjacent metabolic fields is oriented to the stillness of the retention field.

Another image is related to how the notochordal midline forms. It is like two groups of people pulling on a rope that does not yield, because the rope that is attempting to be stretched is tension-proof and exerts a greater resistance against the forces that are pulling at either end of the rope. I remember growing up playing "tug-of-war" with friends and classmates with a long length of rope. Long before one group of us got tired and gave in, there was a significant amount of dynamic pushing, pulling, and pulsing at the ends but the rope itself remained dynamically still. This is the gesture of the retention field—Dynamic Stillness. Every single movement and motion that we did at either end of the rope was because of the stillness of the rope and not each other. This is the fundamental developmental feature of the notochord and all midlines in general. The other image is the Chinese finger-pulling toy. I remember putting it on opposing fingers and stretching it and my fingers were locked into place, unable to move. Thus all growth and development is oriented to the stillness of the retention field. Dr. Blechschmidt said that the stillness of the notochord is the cause of growth and differentiation in the whole embryo. The retention field becomes prominent in the second and third week of dynamic morphology.

The retention field has a secondary gesture of acting as a restrainer. During the embryonic time of development, stretched inner tissue generally remains short. The gesture of resistance is more than can be explained by the biochemistry of collagen. Tensile resistance of stretched connective tissue is critical during early development. Restraining embryonic growth is the mechanism of pacing and titration for the other complex metabolic fields in the embryo to stay in register with each other. The respiratory diaphragm develops as a restrainer. It must mediate the structural relationship of the heart to the liver by being compressed in the middle and stretched at the periphery. This goes on functionally as a growth process long before the diaphragm moves with breathing. The frame of the house goes up first.

Ultimately, the whole vascular system and heart act as a restraining mechanism against the rapid development of the brain. This is one reason why the embryo flexes beginning at the fourth week, because the heart pulls the brain down. The gesture is one of obedience that the brain has toward the nourishment of the heart. As the heart flexes into its position of middle in the embryo, it is the gesture of humility to move from the top of the midline and the top of the head down into the middle. It is the journey of humility.

The formation of the lacunae during implantation in the second week post-fertilization is another good example of a retention field. The lacunae take shape between the expanding trophoblast of the embryo and the uterine vascular system of the mother. The fuel for the expansion of the trophoblast (peripheral body of the embryo) is the cells of the uterus that are dying off. They feed the expansive growth of the future placenta. The tension between the uterus and the trophoblast causes fluid-filled lagoons to form in the trophoblast itself. These lagoons of nontidal fluid (fluid stillness) attract the vascular system of the mother to connect to them as an intermediate stage in the connection of the two vascular systems. In this way, as in the corrosion field above, the two become one as a result of growth resistance. But instead of a rupture between the two beings (embryo and mother) in the corrosion field, there is actually a uniting of the two blood vascular systems by way of the mother's vascular system being invited by the stillness of the embryo to share her blood. By uniting the blood vascular system, the embryo and the mother can now begin a complex exchange of hormones and neurochemicals, especially catecholamines. The presence of catecholamines causes the blood vessels and heart of the embryo to pulse and thus circulate blood. Even though there is a merging of the blood vascular system of the embryo and mother, this remains localized to the area of the lagoons, which will soon become the placenta. Meanwhile, the embryo builds its own vascular system and must manage a complex system of molecular and some cellular input from the early placenta, as well the circulation within its own vascular system. The embryo's own vascular system is growing in two directions from the inside of the chorion. It rather aggressively sprouts blood vessels in the second week to connect to the mother's uterine blood supply and it is also growing blood vessels to connect itself to the central body of the embryo, first for stability of a connecting stalk and then connecting peripheral blood vessels to a not-yet-developed heart.

Retention fields are also called restraining fields, as mentioned. Again, let's discuss the embryo's vascular system. The blood is the first organ to differentiate in the embryo and it surrounds the underside of the trophoblast (peripheral body of the embryo). The embryo's own blood forms the inner lining of the chorion in the second week postfertilization without a heart present. The blood must form channels and tubes and grow toward the heart in the direction of the central body of the embryo simultaneously building a filtration system for the molecules of nutrition coming from the mother's blood on the other side of the trophoblast.

The connective tissue lining of all blood vessels develops as a retention field. Inherent within the embryo's blood itself and later the whole vascular system is a restraining function or a gesture of the vascular system that says to all the tissues of the body, "slow down." To restrain means to slow down and orient to stillness for proper growth and differentiation to take place. It is possible to imagine in this scenario that the blood becomes the gesture of Primary Respiration wrapped in sleeves of connective tissue (arteries and veins). The embryo's blood on the periphery of the chorion carries the connective tissue building materials that will make the tubes that it flows through and enough to build a connecting stalk that ultimately becomes the umbilical cord.

The formation of the heart primordium (pericardium) also occurs in a retention field. As the early mesoderm primordium forms on top of the ectoderm, it is pulled in opposite directions by the amnion and chorion on the one hand and the inflexible pharyngeal membrane (future mouth) on the other. As a result of this restraining function of these membranes that surround the original heart space, the space fills with fluid and for a couple of days, the fluid remains dynamically still, while on the outside, opposing motions are taking place as this space or container for the heart swings down into the thoracic cavity. At that point, as the container meets the cardiac tube, the heart tube within the space begins to grow exponentially, as mentioned earlier. However, it must be remembered that the earliest imprint in the heart is that of a stillpoint. One author (Ridley, 2006) suggests that the stillpoint is now located directly in the AV node of the adult heart. Whether the stillpoint has a specific structure associated with it or is an imprint in the whole space itself is irrelevant, as long as the practitioner can access the stillpoint in the area of the heart in the thorax and manage the process of heart ignition, which is the disengagement and expansion of loving kindness and compassion.

A characteristic feature of late retention fields is that the growth resistance increases in the main direction of the inner tissue (tissue that is not in contact with the amnion or chorion), which is also narrower. This causes horizontal clefts and pouches in layers of embryonic tissue, especially in the fourth stage of dynamic morphology involved in the flexion and extension of the embryo. The most important horizontal clefts and pouches are called the pharyngeal arches, but in biodynamic craniosacral therapy are called embryonic seams. Retention fields cause important seams to form between the nose and the frontal bone where the interorbital ligament is located, the maxillae, the temporomandibular joint, the ramus of the mandible, and also around the development of the hyoid bone. Because of the retention field between the nose and the frontal bone, the eyes are pulled around from the sides of the head toward their position in the center of the face. Likewise, seams are formed for the nose, the inner ears, and jaw. Because of the retention field around the hyoid bone, lymphatic fluid becomes congested, which is necessary in order for lymph nodes to develop. Overall, the configuration of the face changes from a broad, horizontally aligned area to one that is narrow and vertically aligned, and thus characteristically human. During the horizontal structural time a series of clefts, pouches, and seams are displayed between the heart and the brain. Some are associated with the pharyngeal arches and arch arteries. This understanding is critical to the practice of biodynamic craniosacral therapy.

Exploration: Heart Ignition 2

With your partner in a supine position, place your hands under your partner's scapulae and sense the stillness of the blood vessels themselves and how the Primary Respiration in blood orients to the stillness of the blood vessels around the heart. Let the stillness connect to the stillness in the whole thorax. Now expand your awareness around the heart itself and sense the imprint of stillness in the container of the pericardium. It is the space and fluids of the pericardium that are imprinted with stillness. The heart arose from that stillness and those fluids. Now sense your way into the heart and imagine it is one chamber rather than four. Perhaps you sense the heart beating and within that is a stillpoint between each beat of the heart that can grow and fill the heart. It is important to pendulate constantly back to your own heart and sense the stillpoint located there.

The heart spiral is associated with the circulation of the embryonic blood in the peripheral body (inside surface of the chorionic cavity) and then the establishment of a heart tube in the central body of the embryo at the beginning of the third week of development. So, to begin, the practitioner imagines that blood is flowing toward her soma from all directions and covering the outside of her soma as it does in the embryo. The practice then moves to sensing the blood underneath the surface of the skin in the capillary beds. The whole musculoskeletal system is imagined as being a sponge filled with blood all spiraling toward the heart and head. The soma covered with embryonic blood on the outside, moving at the rate of Primary Respiration, invites a spiral on the inside of the fluid body to move up toward the top of the head. The spiral invites a canalization zone to form along the banks of the neural crest in the shape of a horseshoe.

The main focus of the heart spiral is to sense the strong current of fluid coming up from the pelvic floor throughout the entire core of the fluid body and organizing the tubular heart in the chest cavity as the middle legs of the horseshoe merge together into a single tube with a loop on top for the brain. This loop or top of the horseshoe includes the aortic sac, arch arteries, and cardinal veins and arteries into the top of the neural tube. It is as though there is one spiral from the floor of the pelvis to the top of the head, from the back of the soma including the spine to the anterior surface of the soma, and it bulges, rotates, elongates, shortens, twists, and side-bends all in front of the pharynx. This is where the heart tube and spiral were located in the embryo with the original fulcrum of the heart being located at C3. It is called the cardio-craniofacial module in embryology. In our adult body, it consumes the entire space of the trunk, neck, face, and head as a perception of a spiral.

Exploration: The Breathing Face and Pelvis

With your partner in a supine position, you will be placing the pads of your index and middle fingers lateral of the hyoid bone, then on the ramus of the mandible, then on the inferior border of the zygomatic bones, then on the TMJ, and finally above the zygomatic bones. Synchronize with Primary Respiration and wait for the face to breathe horizontally in each of those hand positions. The breathing takes place in the tempo of Primary Respiration or the fluid body. (Please consult Volume One for a detailed description of these tempos.) Now place your hands bilaterally on the greater trochanter of your partner's pelvis and feel the adult pelvic floor breathing horizontally as well. Remember that initially the pelvic floor has a rudimentary and narrow hindgut (gut tube), a rudimentary kidney system that extends all the way up to the shoulders, and the alantois, which is a cavity that protrudes anteriorly out into the connecting stalk. The alantois will become the bladder, for the most part, later on. Finally, there is the cloacal membrane, which is a corrosion field between the ectoderm and endoderm that will become the anus. The entire pelvic floor is a bowl of undifferentiated mesenchyme, which is the primordial mesodermal jelly construction material of the embryo. Finally, the bottom of the neural tube is in the pelvis but looks like a tail because it is growing so slowly. It is situated next to the hindgut.

When you are palpating the horizontal dimensions of the pelvic floor, these are the growing and condensing structures occurring within the fluid body as the soma emerges from it. Remember that the longitudinal fluctuation, which is the organizing midline of the fluid body, is initiated at the cloacal membrane as a result of the tensional forces produced by the relocation of the connecting stalk in the caudal portion of the embryo and the subsequent restraining function that that connecting stalk has on the growth and development of the pelvic floor. This is noted by a strong change in fluid pressure that then causes the longitudinal fluctuation. This is what you want to sense beginning to arise as you hold the horizontal dimensions of the embryonic pelvic floor.

Now go back to the cranium and place the pads of your fingers on the inferior lateral angle of the parietal bones. Sense the lateral-medial breathing of the tentorium around the brain. This is the end of the longitudinal fluctuation where it transmutes into a lateral fluctuation movement along the transverse axis of the tentorium. Gradually in the embryo, the brain grows larger and the upper end of the gut tube, called the foregut, grows smaller. Palpate these dimensions several times to get a sense of the basic polarity that results from the fluid pressure and growth dynamic of these metabolic fields in the fluid body. Go back and forth until you can breathe with your partner's expression of the fluid body. Just remember to pendulate back to your own perception of Primary Respiration regularly and avoid compressing your partner's fluid body with too much attention.

Densation Fields

We've moved now into the second category of metabolic fields—those that are part of later embryonic development. Densation fields occur when the fluids in the deep inner tissues of the embryo begin to leak out because of adjacent tension along a longitudinal axis or midline. The fluids are squeezed out of the tissue. In other words, the fluid percolates out of the tissue. Think of condensation. This causes varying degrees of densification with different gradients of fluid density in the fluid body. This type of a field generates primordial cartilage and is sensed as midline compression, especially the spine and long bones of the body. This early cartilage is the original organ of the locomotor system in the human and represents the earth element of the developing soma. The ocean must now become more mobile with hard structures.

The first appearance of the skeleton is preceded by such mesenchymal densations. This is a metabolic zone composed of cells that have spherical shaped bodies and very little intercellular fluid between each other. Imagine a bowl of both solid and liquid contents. Kinetically, through the pulsatory motion of adjacent metabolic fields and biodynamically through the ordered movement of Primary Respiration, fluid leaves the bowl (goes with the flow) and the solid particles come closer to one another. It is like skimming the egg white off of an egg so that all that remains is the more dense yellow. When the positional relationship between cells and their liquid components changes by the squeezing of adjacent fields that are growing in favor of the cells rather than the living water, a densation field arises.

All metabolic fields, especially densation fields, are characterized by their position. Not only is the position of the field itself significant, but also the position of the cells and their nuclei in the field. What's important here is that the position is always related to the neighboring differentiations. Thus the gesture of the densation field is the gesture of relationship and the unique position that it holds in relationship to its neighbors and how its neighbors cause it to give up fluid and shape and structure itself more solidly. In other words, in the gesture a soma becomes less permeable and fortifies its boundaries in order to have greater mobility and freedom of movement later on and thus a normal need for greater protection from outside stress.

A densation field has a longitudinal orientation because there is equal compression in all directions, especially along the length of the neural tube. It must be remembered that this three-dimensional compression is occurring on a longitudinal axis along the whole length of the developing spine surrounding the neural tube. Typically, the origination of the spinal vertebrae is the best example of a densation field. The other thing to remember about densation fields, also mentioned earlier, is that they most frequently lie deep within the inner tissue of the embryo. It is here that young cells initially are not stressed by pressure or tension in any preferred direction in the early morphological stages of the embryo. Once the embryo folds over and places its heart in the middle, the musculoskeletal system can begin to harden around it. The gesture of the densation field is the discovery of a "backbone." Spineless is a derogatory term used to describe a lack of courage. It takes courage to develop boundaries and to be firm without being obsessive. Primary Respiration allows us to uncouple from being spineless and to notice the preexisting courage in the structure of the heart. Think of the Wizard of Oz.

Exploration: Intraosseous Strains

Have your partner lie supine and place both of your hands palm up under the base of the spine around the lumbars. Synchronize with Primary Respiration in yourself. Bring your attention to your partner's spine. Get a sense of a field of compression unique to the vertebrae themselves. Living bone is very vascular. It is more like a density that is dynamic. Tune into any specific densities that pull your hands deeper to a specific point. This may be an intraosseous strain pattern that became coupled to the developing vertebra as an embryo. An intraosseous strain feels inert and unable to move or breathe with the fluid body. Sense Primary Respiration permeating the whole area and wait for the intraosseous strain to go through the process of softening or remolding. Find a way to let the bone breathe with Primary Respiration.

Contusion Fields

While densation fields, described above, have an axial orientation or develop on a longitudinal axis and generate spherical shaped cells, a contusion field is based on a radial symmetry compression and the cells tend to flatten out. This is a way in which cartilage forms. A contusion field typically is the gesture of concentration along a path of least resistance toward a central point, such as the tip of the notochord where the cranial base develops. Because there is a densation field developing longitudinally, the laws of fluids state that there would consequently be a fluid movement perpendicular to the long axis, thus creating spokes on a wheel pulsing away from and toward the midline. This means a three-dimensional compression toward a fulcrum and tensional resistance away from the fulcrum or the more localized area on the long axis. The growth tensions are of nearly equal intensity and very equally distributed. Thus a contusion field also describes a tensegrity structure where compressional forces and tensional forces are equally distributed in the whole embryo or whole metabolic field. Some of the spherical cells in the densation field around the outer edges become flattened. This is called a structural predevelopment that is necessary for subsequent differentiations to occur.

Contusion fields develop together with densation fields. Cells are pushed and pulled together so that they flatten and widen in the direction of least resistance, like compressing a rubber ball. This involves biomechanical compression and it is the way in which the top of the notochord forms the basispheniod and basiocciput. In addition, the outer dural meninges begin to form as well from the tip of the notochord as a disengagement and expansion. Thus the top of the notochord is formed from chondroblasts or young cartilage cells. Because of the tension on the notochord, especially at the top (consider that the top of the notochord is caught between the brain and the heart), fluids leave the area and the cartilage cranial base (basiocciput and basisphenoid) begins to form. The core of the basisphenoid and basiocciput is both a densation field and a contusion field. This combination is the gesture of the cranial base inhaling and exhaling, compressing and disengaging. This is because the cranial base develops in a dynamic tension field between the heart and brain.

Exploration: Cranial Base Breathing

The partner is in a supine position. Using a modified vault hold with the edges of the thumbs on the greater wings of the sphenoid and the rest of the fingers going around the ears and touching the occiput if possible, sense the relationship between the fluids and cells of the cranial base. Imagine that you are holding a bowl of living water with the viscosity of liquid soap. The cranial base is made of a gel-like substance, as it was when it first developed. Allow the cranial base to orient three-dimensionally around a fulcrum at the tip of the notochord, only through sensing a shape change three-dimensionally in the gel. Pendulate constantly back to your own perception of Primary Respiration. Then sense the three-dimensional relationship between the heart and the brain that surrounds the cranial base in your partner. If any particular compressive vector manifests slowly, orient three-dimensionality to a horizon that surrounds you 360 degrees. Let your own egg breathe out to the horizon. The sense of this exploration is similar to the suction field in that the hands will feel three-dimensional expansion and contraction coming from a fulcrum in the cranial base within the fluid body level of the Primary Respiratory System. The process of a stillpoint will occur inside the cranial base or outside, in the room or in nature, and Primary Respiration will allow you to sense disengagement and equalization of tensional forces around the cranial base.

Distusion Fields

This is a disengagement of tissues formed in the contusion fields above. The expansion occurs because of different osmotic pressure in the fluid body of the embryo. At first, young cartilage cells swell and then create an opposition to the act of growth pushing. It is more along the image of a pistonlike function. The gesture of the distusion field is a broadening and expansion that is the result of the bending of the embryo and all of its intrinsic curvature down to the shape of every cell. There are no cells that are perfect squares. Thus the neuropores and pharyngeal arches are good examples of this type of metabolic field. The gesture is a gesture of a swelling growth and fluid reabsorption. The area immediately around the cranial base is another good example. The brain above is growing so rapidly (a million neurons a minute) that the precartilage at the tip of the notochord expands in a concentric circle to form the platform that the growing brain rests upon.

Aggregations of cartilage cells that swell while absorbing fluid come from a distusion field. Their distusion gesture exerts pressure on the neighboring tissue. The distusion field is linked to the contusion field that in turn is linked to the densation field. The flattened contusion cells reabsorb water from their immediate environment and become vesicle shaped, thereby forming cartilage. As water is reabsorbed into these young cartilage cells, the ground substance surrounding each cell stretches. This again indicates the prestructuring tensegrity function of the extracellular matrix and how the extracellular matrix prestructures, or essentially forms, a type of scaffolding in the fluid body around which a definitive, differentiated structure can be built.

As the quantity of water increases in the large cartilage cells, an opposite process takes place in the extracellular matrix. The water content decreases, which results in a hardened capsule forming around the cells. The movement of water from the extracellular matrix is so intense that its gradual calcification becomes distinct. Distusion growth becomes the first active part of the locomotor system of the embryo that is typically associated with the musculoskeletal system and is seen especially in weeks four to eight in the embryo. The densation, contusion, and distusion fields are thus linked to one another.

The gesture of the distusion field is that of pushing out and disengaging three-dimensionally from the midline and the fulcrum. The musculoskeletal system gains much of its three-dimensionality from this gesture. It is the gesture of disengagement and the sentient movement of the organism out into the environment.

Exploration: Disengagement of the Cranial Base

Place your hands on your partner in the Pietá position with one hand under the shoulder and the other under the hamstring of your partner ipsilaterally. Synchronize with Primary Respiration in yourself and tune into the cycle of conception ignition in your partner, as described in Volume One. Pay attention to the fifty-second period of primary inhalation. During that time bring your attention closer to the fluid body of the musculoskeletal system and sense whether it is pushing out into your hands through the tissue and osseous structures of the soma during that period of time. Sense how tissues naturally tend to disengage and expand for fifty seconds while you maintain three-dimensionality. The motion coming into your hands is stronger than a suction field, because it involves the relationship between a solid and a gel-like substance, breathing like an amoeba or jellyfish would breathe. Think of the embryo moving like a jellyfish, so the hands sense this fluid motion pushing out as thought it were swelling and then in the process of reabsorption, there's a shrinking. Remember that this is not a fast movement, but occurs in the fluid body as it is condensing under the catalytic function of Primary Respiration.

By using an alternative vault hold and tuning into the cranial base, as we did in the exploration above, you can sense more deeply into the cranial base as it breathes and disengages every 100 seconds with Primary Respiration. The focus must be on the lateral expansion of Primary Respiration first and then the three-dimensional disengagement of the cranial base. As an alternative, you can place your hands over any joint space in the body and feel the same sequence of these last three metabolic fields. Remember to stay synchronized with Primary Respiration.

Detraction Fields

This is the field where bones are made. This is when tissues shear against one another and then pull apart in a late-stage embryo. This shearing and disengagement creates fulcrums of balanced stillness called centers of ossification. Thus a bone begins its differentiation around a stillpoint. It is characteristic for osteoblasts to be tilted at a forty-five-degree angle against the surface of the osseous ground substance and thus there is a shearing that occurs within the still-forming fluid precollagen. The general statement that differentiation occurs only where there is spatial opportunity and an immediate kinetic (space and time) moment is valid for the process of all three types of ossification (from cartilage, from connective tissues, and from bone). A detraction field is the basis for all three types of ossification. This also means that, again, developmental processes must be understood in relation to their position. Each aggregation of cells is a basic unit (metabolic field) that forms a functional growth system within the extracellular matrix. Think of a detraction field as the opposite of a corrosion field. It is the difference between an open valve and a dense bone in the body, two structures at the opposite end of the spectrum biokinetically.

Because of this shearing motion in bone development, there is fluid accumulation that requires a venous plexus to drain it away from the newly forming bone. Even the fluid accumulation is part of the local differentiation process and contributes to forming lymph nodes, for example. From a biodynamic point of view, the process of differentiation is a time-sensitive manifestation within Primary Respiration and its fluid body's uniform ordering fluid forces. In other words, these unique metabolic fields occur at precise times and precise locations in embryonic development. The detraction field is the last field to arise.

The gesture here is similar to two people pulling on two plates attached to one another. Each plate is being pulled in the opposite direction by the other person. The pull creates friction. The friction creates compression and the extracellular matrix loses fluid and hardens while the excess fluid is drained away in the vascular system. A good example of this is the development of the frontal bone. The external part of the young frontal bone is initially very dome-shaped and pressed more and more against stretched connective tissue. On the inside, however, near the cranial cavity, the bone is becoming detached from the internal tissue. Thus there is frictional sliding causing osteogenesis. Another way of saying this is that the oppositional pulling is on a cover sewn to a more solid support structure on the opposite side. Fluid is present between the support and the cover and gradually gets squeezed out during the friction of the shearing movement. This squeezing out of the fluid happens rapidly.

Exploration

With the partner in a supine position, place your hands on your partner's tibia, then over the crest of the ileum and costal arch, then under the scapula bilaterally, and finally in a traditional vault hold. Take time in each hand placement to listen to the bone and let it float free from inner limiting tissue by synchronizing with Primary Respiration and letting the bone breathe, as we did with the intraosseous strain above. This time the bone is being sensed three-dimensionally in relationship to the tissues attached to it underneath and on top of it. The tissue underneath helped to form it along with the vascular system that continues to serve it. This is the basic relationship from which bones are made and continue to be made. In biomechanical work this would be called a frontal lift or parietal lift, but biodynamically the practitioner waits for the bone to breathe with Primary Respiration and then for the fluid body to lift it and disengage it from its neighbors. Earlier, we tried to sense the connective tissue of the blood vessels and their restraining function as well as sensing the different movements that cartilage and muscle make in the matrix of the fluid body. Now with the bone, we have to put it all together because the bone is the final product of the metabolic fields and the last to arise in the embryo. The hands must remember that the bone is also forming at a forty-five-degree angle so there will be some very acute angular movement within the bony tissue in relation to the restraining function of the membrane underneath the bone and the vascular supply to that area.

Conclusion

The metabolic fields of the embryo are apparent to the practitioner as a result of being able to synchronize with Primary Respiration and to orient to stillness. These fields, also known as subwholes, represent significant activity taking place within the fluid body and occurring at different locations, having different relationships or polarities, and thus causing a shape to arise that then generates enough resistance and tension to create a structure. The palpation of the germ layers of the embryo is nearly impossible because it is descriptive anatomy. The metabolic fields are still active everywhere in the adult body. This is something that biodynamic practitioners can get their hands on.

CHAPTER 29

Ode to the Embryo

With Carol Agneessens

Haven Trevino wrote *The Tao of Healing*[12] while in the process of dying with ALS, also known as Lou Gehrig's Disease. His beautiful and elegant book speaks to biodynamic craniosacral therapy. It is with a great deal of respect and reverence that Carol and I translated his original work into embryonic language. I am also grateful to the publisher, New World Library, for the permission to reprint these mindful poems. *The Tao of Healing* has no page numbers. Each poem is given a number at the top. The numbers that appear at the top of these poems match the original numbers in Trevino's book.

The last poem in this chapter is included as a "bonus track" for readers.

1

Before the birthing of matter
Emergence from vast potential stillness.
Before the stillness, the no-thing
Spontaneously conceived within the void
The omniscience of compassion
Compassion deep and rich
Compassion the nectar of life,
Being, silent, unmoving, unchanging,
The unspoken beauty of Truth,
Mother only to Itself.
It has been called God, Tao,
Buddha Nature, Divine Mother,
Universal Mind.
But today I call it Love or perhaps Heart
Or Embryo,
A human embryo

Compassion's permeating sweetness
As ordinary as a heartbeat
Or a stem cell flourishing life's potential.
Love is not an emotion, or feeling.
It is substance without form permeating
Both the seen and the unseen
Call it the Breath of Life;
Beyond sheer veils of knowing.
An embryonic universe, the heart-womb of love.
By whatever name, Love resides
Beyond the confine of words
Yet within our embryonic perceptions.
Love's desire embraces a vision
Of happiness for all to know
The causes of happiness.
People seeking Love
Carry the promise of compassion.
People abide on the Earth
Earth abides in the Heavens
The Heavens abide in Love
Love abides in all.
Settling the Heart within its Middle
Within the human embryo for life.

2

Healing defined, limits possibility,
And so is not True healing.
As our concepts of God and Goddess
Are just that, only concepts.
The Truth of our healing is free of gender, division, or
boundary.
Chaos before creation, out of chaos the void.
Breath moving as one substance, pregnant and whole—
The movement of Primary Respiration.
Shaping the embryonic whole in its rhythmic flow
Conceived in the stillness of the heart-womb
Whether one is ill or well
Living in darkness or enlightenment,
It is the same.

Wholeness springs from its fulcrum of Health
In the Great Sea Around Us
Tidal waters flooding every cell
Only our misperception divides them.
The essence of Wholeness as we live toward our dying
Is self-renewing joy.
Joy blossoming into joy:
You are only ever an embryo.

3

We pendulate freely
From darkness to light
From sickness to health
From goodness to evil
Swinging back and forth
Without a metronome's timing.
Confounding the polarities, confusing the path
The healer finds a stillpoint
A steady fulcrum between;
Witnessing through the simplicity of presence
She creates by allowing,
She feeds without pushing
And gives by receiving.
She bears witness to
Her inner wholeness—
The movement of Primary Respiration
Then rests in the void.
Because she rests in the void
She's always in touch
With the stillpoint in the Heart-Middle
Of her embryo.

5

In the natural world
The generative process of life
The constancy of impermanence
Interconnected truths
Of an embryonic unfolding
Immune to the seduction of fixing,

Has neither birth nor death
Allowing is the course of nature
All That Is, like You
Breathing in, breathing out.
Being breathed and
Carried toward a horizon
Being breathed and
Congealing around a midline
Be still and be breathed
By Primary Respiration.

6

The Breath of Life igniting
The heart-womb of the Divine Mother
Eternally conceiving the embryo
And the promise
Of Compassion and Love
Secured in the middle of form.
A bottomless well
Fills us
Again and again.
Nourishing waters to quench
The driest desert.
Set sail on this vast ocean
Of embryonic existence
Never looking back.

7

Compassion ignites life.
With utmost generosity
Love flowers eternal
Having no beginning
And no end
Without cause
Without time
Undiminished.
Centered in the midline of compassion
Without ego,
The mind of compassion

A fountain of generosity,
Allowing life without possession
Flowing in the long tidal stream
Of spiritual autonomy.

9

Does a tree send its roots to the skies?
Will you continue to pursue
What is in your thoughts
Rather than your Heart?
When seeking love from another
Dare you love your embryo
As much?
Life is the teacher of wisdom
So live it.
Love is the teaching of
The embryo.
Find your embryo
Be your embryo.
There is much to learn
Your embryo has much to teach.

10

Truth, sown in fertile soil
Births compassion
The truth of an undifferentiated
Ground between healer and healed.
The miracle of Primary Respiration
Melding the imagined separation
There is no difference between healer and healed,
Each releases the ego's banal struggle.
Envision your client as the ultimate teacher
With wisdom beyond comprehension.
She bears witness to utter holiness
Each breath of Primary Respiration,
For all sentient beings.
Meet this challenge of unconditional loving
As you lay your hands upon your client.

12

Rely on your eyes
You will not see;
Rely on your ears,
You become deaf;
Address only symptoms
And you will miss the point;
Stride after perfect health
And become lame.
The true healer lets go of intuition
And moves from the shifting center of instinct
Between her belly and heart;
Blameless, spotless, and freed from the past
She gives herself permission
To rest in her own embryo—stillness
The Health within the core of a midline.

13

One who heals to attain power
May become the suppressor of symptoms;
Attached to an outcome which boasts an illusion.
One who overidentifies with the body
Never makes it whole,
When the healer senses through the body
Into the Great Sea around us of the Breath of Life
Healing comes naturally and without effort.
Know your path to return to the Great Sea,
That you may safely guide
The inner transformation of all you touch.
Love all beings as members of your own Body,
That you may truly serve
With receptive hands
The Receptive Heart
The Middle
Your Embryo.

15

Ancient healers ignited the fire of unconditional love
Ignoring the habituated customs of the day

They saw what others did not see
Looking beneath the veil of the everyday world.
With a humbled vision they see
With the innocence and patience
Expecting no-thing, knowing the whole within everything
Empty of agenda, listening without judgment or
interpretation
Serenely gentle, they hold your embryo
With open hands
In the memory of stillness and light.
Intent on deepest healing
Their history cradles wounds
Of ancestry, self, and other.
Hold all with equanimity,
As they are the still, clear pool
Reflecting the sun and the moon.

16

A Primary Breath inspires
All living things
Rising and falling, expanding and quieting,
Within the fabric of wholeness
Reveling in the stillness cradling the stars.
Gravity, the constant of attraction
Orienting self toward other.
With love
Opening the river of compassion
The essence of self flowing out
Pause
Breathing in
The pain of another through oneself
Metabolizing, ingesting the gravity of life
Expand in understanding
Deepen into stillness
The fountainhead of Love
Dynamic, alive, vibrating, and
In constant process
Toward the silence
Never still only Becoming Still

Intend to be Love—the Breath of Life
And know death for what it is;
Exhaling from stillness back to the
Other side of the horizon.
Inhaling the stillness from the
Other.
Meet each other in the Void!

17

Can you trust the Intelligence of
Primary Respiration?
Swelling and receding at the edges of awareness.
The greatest healer
Is the Intelligence.
If you do not trust Primary Respiration
How will It trust you?
Share your embryo
Your Middle,
It's all you have
True freedom is the embryo's
Ability to bear witness
To constant change
From one state to another.
Transmutation to
Manifestation.
It is not random and it is not predictable.

22

Become suspended
By the Breath of Life
In the Great Sea around you.
Permeable, fluid, responsive.
Water fills the hollow,
Pouring into empty spaces
Flowing generously toward the
Depths of loving simplicity
A river moving the tidal sea.
The silent voice of the heart—
Speaks elemental words of

Heat, light, stillness, and Breath.
Grace, receptivity, and love
Understood in the muted signs and brailled
Symbols of a natural perfection.
Find the *bardo*
The midline between light and shadow
And infinite creation is yours.

24

To stand above others
Is to be cast to your knees.
To run before others
Is to fall behind yourself.
To prove yourself to others
Is the façade of pretense.
Being honest with yourself
Knowing and acknowledging your limitations
Is the middle path.
Spiritual materialism is a burden indeed.

25

Discover the source of your own power
Within the labyrinth of self.
Understanding limitations and potentials
Release the seduction of a material world.
Imagining an emptiness filled through overabundance.
A knowing guide charters a forward path
From the embryo,
A still space in the heart between two
Allows breath and flow in the rhythm
Of Primary Respiration
Dropping the contents of the mind
Toward the gravity of a belly
And descents beyond.
Having no preferences
Strengthens the heart-light
And radiates the client
With crimson red blood,
Transfusing embryonic blood

To those who thirst.
With clarity
Feel the confusion of desires
Receptive to the sight
Of your own dilemma.
Be still and silent
Exhale into the essence of self.
Discover your genesis!

26

The bird that learns to fly
Must also learn to land.
She flies far
Migrating thousands of miles
Every year
But never forgets her nest
In either place.
She travels far
Yet understands her boundaries
Of limitation.
She appreciates external beauty
But does not compare herself to it.
The healer is like this.
She channels great joy
Without arrogance;
She visits distant realms
Without forgetting
The stillness in her Heart-Middle
As home
As tree, as nest
The fertile ground
Of self-knowing.

27

The forgiving person carries no burdens,
Walks with a light step;
One who has no attachments perceives perfection
Even in the burning of her own house.
See the smoke? It ascends to Father Sky.

See the ashes? They descend to Mother Earth.
Those who live without gossip
Have unburdened their heart.
Breathe clear through the space between
And know the unmeasured sum of eternal suns.
The compassionate person loves humanity:
Each deed a graceful act of unthinking kindness
Embraced in the rhythms of Primary Respiration.
The lover naturally sees each person as lovable,
Intoxicated by such love
Disappearing all admonitions to distance from
The untouchable.
The midline is essence and resource
Strengthening the wounded healer
With both witness, receptivity, and knowledge
Of their wounded heart.
The embryo sees disease
As a journey toward wholeness.
The embryo sees disease
As a form of self-expression
And in its translation heals
Heart and mind of the seeker.
Fear not, friend:
There is something to be gained
From the smoke and mirrors
Regard all experience as a dream when it is.

28

The duality of hard and soft,
Substantial and permeable
Immobility and flow—
Embrace these oppositions
As one living function
And an embryo is formed,
Perfect, innocent, and free.
Surrounded by growth within its loss.
Give to the day
And honor the living.
Receive from the night

And honor the dead;
Honor these two,
Become the embryo—
Unsurpassable freedom.
Breathing back and forth from the horizon
Living and dying every 100 seconds.
Be your highest aspirations
In an unassuming way:
Cupped hands at the crystal clear spring.
Sculpt the matter of clay
Ignite yourself alive and burning
A universe of unlimited potential
And human limitation.
Be still and know
Your embryo within.
Transcendence is your conception right.

29

Untouched by singular intentions
The universe breathes itself
Into pregnant expansion.
It is not random nor is it predictable.
And only with a receptive heart
Can someone receive the balance of health.
Their purposes are sacred,
Inviolate, encompass realms
Even illumined masters
Dare not tread.
Do not even call it karma.
Some are here to celebrate
Others to mourn;
Some are here to be sick,
Others to be healed;
Some are here to live,
Others to die;
Some are here to love,
Others to be loved.
One who understands this simple truth
Makes no attempt

To solve the puzzle of another,
To stop the world from turning,
To keep a heart from exchanging
One's self for the other.
Bear witness with compassion.

30

The healer knows
We heal no one
We cure no one;
To attempt a cure
Denies the truth:
Disharmony sown in spirit
Reaps imbalance in all dimensions.
To regain this point of balance
Still your beating heart
And calm your blood,
Receptivity is not a passive action.
Allow the Love to heal,
Witness the movement of Life
Penetrating the densest field.
It is this Flow that heals.
Not you or I.
For the Universe flatters no one,
But merely offers its River of Life
Cascading through your midline, your
Flesh and blood and bones.
Automatically shifting
The darkest of e-motions
Lifting them into buoyant space.

31

Fear of death: the deepest imprint
Conceived within the womb
From the *beginning*
The neurological fear of extinction
Death of the physical body demands
Survival at any cost
Anger and rage abound.

Those who attack illness as the enemy force
Wield swords of ignorance, arrows of despair;
Rejoice the defeat of each illness,
Wonder the coming of five more;
Applaud the saving of a limb, a part,
A momentary necessity,
Oblivious to the soundless joy of the embryo
Seeking its freedom—in wholeness
Already present.
True healers spend little time on symptoms
Orienting to beginnings, conception
And infinitely earlier.
Rejoice with the expression
Of stillness and compassion
In every moment
In all things practice with
Simplicity chopping wood and
Carrying water.

32

The Way of Love is infinitely large
And infinitely small.
Bring its light and stillness into the world
Radiate from your Heart-Middle
And watch everything
Fall smoothly into place;
The Mother and Father of All Embryos
Would conspire on your behalf:
A gentle rain
Of unstrained mercy and joy.
The midline of your embryo,
The Mother and Father of All Things
When labeled, judged, divided, structured,
Becomes the prisoner
Locked in a developing brain
Confining the river of potency, and self-expression of flow.
Agrees to the security of imprisonment.
The midline always says *Yes.*
It is the *Yes* of

Ultimately coming Home
To an open door
A warm heart
Within a middle nesting
Embryo.

33

To Yield: the action of embodied surrender,
Resting into contact with another, or within
One's own heart, mind, and instinct.
Presence, the permeation of an undivided
Wholeness, a responsiveness to breath.
Allow this permeation of Divine.
Yield to the peace of stillness, the inner well
Of embryonic pulsings.
Be the gentle master of your own being.
Peace by inner transformation
Is true abundance.
Breathe your midline
Feel the presence of your autonomy
And your connectivity,
Not to save your life,
But to savor it.
One taste
Always shape shifting.

36

To build up
Dismantle first;
To expand
Contract first;
To attain clarity
Allow confusion;
To become civilized
First live in the wild.
Discover the patience within waiting.
The balance of all things
Is in the fulcrum
Between apparent oppositions;

Truth extends in two directions.
The clenched fist holds weakness while
The stillpoint in the middle is unbounded strength
The open hands touching another
Offers the hidden power
Of one hundred million suns,
The magnitude of your embryonic heart.
Let it radiate as the beam of a lighthouse.
From this magnetic flame
Lighting and
Guiding
Those searching for the Water of Life.

37

Love does not enter unless invited
So it never meets a boundary;
Creative energy flows naturally
From a stillpoint;
Thus Primary Respiration penetrates all
In its embrace.
Earthly creators, reflecting this Wholeness
Watch each dream come true.
Strong desire creates rigid structure,
The abode of our painful duality.
The spiritual path is all there is
Dissolving the illusion of separation
Between the barriers of our heart-mind
The division of one embryo from the other.

38

The ignorant claim secret knowledge
Sealed within a padlocked chest
Stale and suffocate
Knowing Primary Respiration
And its fulcrum of stillness
Within the chambers of a loving heart
A true source of power
Share the delicate and unfolding rose
Outwardly, doing no-thing

Waiting and waiting more to *be*.
Effortless receptivity, held by a
Spacious field of subtle Breath.
Mechanics apply temporarily fixes
Spurred by maps and ideas.
Center within your midline,
Aligning between heaven and earth
Orient to Primary Respiration and the Stillness
Without intervention, without a mechanical plan.
The less one does, the less there is to do.
The more one does, the more one needs to do,
And original error multiplies.
Offer stillness, and lightness of heart
Patiently waiting at the edges of void
Or at ocean depths,
Without techniques and protocols.
When love is denied
Pity is dispensed;
When empathy is denied
Procedures are meticulously followed.
Desiring control of a result denies
The grace of Primary Respiration.
What folly!
With empathy, part the shade
And reveal the light,
See past the pain and sense the embryo,
Reach beyond your tools and cradle the blossom.

39

Love is eternal and everywhere
Yet remains a quality precious,
Treasured, and rare
The Breath of Life.
Receive the blood of generosity and know relationship,
Midline and know autonomy,
Humor and know joy;
Allow the quality of humility
And know the greatness of embryonic heart.
Without generosity there is no peace;

Without the midline, no orientation to autonomy;
Without humor, boundless anxiety and depression;
Without humility, the endless repetition of groveling shame.
Life blesses with waters of humility
A child bows to the father
The father extends to the child
The great and the meek,
A continuum of exchange.
The universal spiral lifts
The generous and humble heart.
Remember you are one-consciousness,
Whole from the beginning of time;
Allow, allow, allow.

40

Returning to Wholeness is the natural way;
By longing,
By prayer,
By renunciation
Of a shipwrecked ego.
The choice to Love
Leaving anger behind
Is to reconceive your embryo
And birth the heart
Of sadness, stillness, and joy.
There are no exceptions.

43

To penetrate the hardest armor,
Use the softest buoyant touch
A feather on the Breath of God.
Yielding melts resistance
Density is filled by liquid light
Good work accomplished without effort.
Receptivity is the key.
In silence the teachings are heard;
In stillness the world is transformed.
In the void we meet the client.

45

The Universe is without fragmentation
The fabric of wholeness weaves through all.
Realize that you are perfection
As you are,
Warts and all.
The lame man's crutches
Are as much a part of him
As the wind
The birds
The sea.
Meditate on this
And watch the complicated grow simple:
If you're hungry, eat.
If you're tired, rest.
Stop tampering with Life.
Be held by the Tide that surrounds you.
Let your senses rest at the horizon.

49

Love flows into a clear mind.
The Breath of Life
Ripples outward to those in need.
The promise of the Long Tide.
Your kind deeds, your loving thoughts
Travel invisible pathways
With the Tide,
Which elevates rulers and ruled alike
In this world and even worlds away.
Your courage and compassion
May light a thousand cities
Transforming those forgotten.
Strength in one embryonic heart
Is strength in all
And light in one embryonic heart
Brings light to all.
The truth about yourself is healing.
Focus on your inner journey

As you touch the world.
Become autonomous
Yet connected through Love.

50

Without Love
Starvation descends
Emaciating
Body and soul
Splintering both psyche and spirit
From the truth of One.
Lying prey to the seduction of
Illusions.
Understand the simplicity of embryology
Fluids imprint fear before the brain is created.
You cannot fear death itself,
The embryo knows
That fear *is* death.
You cannot choose between
Life and death,
For there is only the Middle—
The heart of the embryo.
One who walks permeated with Love
Bursting from an embryonic seed
Recoils from neither plague nor sword nor sin,
Sees through death
Marches through valleys of fear.
Listen for the *lion's roar.*

56

Those who know are silent;
Those who do not, babble on forever.
Surrender your anger
Forego your dramas
Ignore magical tricks
Abandon the marketplace
Claim neither victory nor defeat;
Feel your embryo living in belly and blood.
Spoken, it loses meaning.

Lived through Primary Respiration,
The power of the embryo transcends limitation.

57

Remember, the more complicated the therapy
The more confused the client;
The more difficult the treatment
The less likely the cure;
The more secret the method
The more scarce the love.
Remaining quiet within, receptive
Bearing witness
Longing for the outside presence
Of Primary Respiration to permeate the heart
The client will resonate with such peace.
Sow silence, and they'll reap wisdom;
Step aside, and Primary Respiration will "do" the healing.
Release your desire to fix or to heal another
Welcome the presence of Primary Respiration
Igniting conception
In yourself
Over and over again.
Disperse and
Become unified every 100 seconds.

61

To give, receive.
Be the wet, fertile valley
Of embryonic beginnings.
Let the River of Life flow through.
The satiated will be emptied
The empty, filled.
Be empty, that you may be filled
In the fullness of time.
The greatest healer shares all
But knows the time to do so
And becomes yet greater.
This is the virtue of patience.
One who wants to be healed

Must become a healer.
And one who wants to be a healer
Must first seek healing
Through inner transformation of the heart-mind
Seeking the embryo, the beginning;
Suffering gains meaning only when understood
And experienced
By a forgiving heart
And the still midline of the embryo.
Healing is meaningless
Until it is shared
Through skillful means
And tireless discipline.
This is the discipline of caring deeply for yourself.

65

The world teachers never etched their words
On paper or stone,
Knowing the folly of some to follow
Without question or critique.
Interrogate the singular guideposts
Laid by another.
Know yourself and your sensings
Trusting the instincts of your belly,
The compassion of your heart and
Clarity of your mind.
Become autonomous—
Following your path and truths.
Everything is written inside
Between the shifting fulcrum
In your belly, heart, and brain:
You are The Book of Embryology
Of Stillness and Primary Respiration.
Be your creation.

78

What is more feminine than water?
It is soft and yielding,
It seeks the depth of every abyss.

Nothing impedes
Its homeward flow to the Ocean,
And then back to in-form the body.
All obstacles disappear
Under water's constant caress.
This is obvious to all—
Can you apply it to your life?
Become the grace of softness,
Without the push against resistant shape
Yield and flow with the Tide
Yield and flow with the Tide.
Master a gentling firmness,
Fluid and resilient as the willow
Rest in the stillness of your blood
And the midline.
It offers the rock of autonomy and intelligence
Knowing the principles of form.

The Perpetual Embryo

by Michael Shea
Biodynamic means wholeness:
Choreography between
The movement of Primary Respiration
And its core of still-ness
The awareness of One
Becoming two
And the two One
Biodynamic means incarnation and embodiment:
Of stillness the link to Eternity,
And Primary Respiration
Linking Health and Wholeness.
Biodynamic means the divine dwelling within:
Compassion's house under the Sea
Gradients of empathy, heat
Relationships, shapes, sentience,
Currents, viscosity and tides,
Waves, wetness and buoyancy.
Biodynamic means Ignition:
The fire of creation – a breath
Blazing from the Void
Living core of stillness
In the heart and the blood.
Biodynamic means love:
Never ending or beginning
Dwelling in the embryo.
The perpetual embryo of love!
And joy - the core body imprint.
Only the embryo knows this Fullness.
Find your embryo via the dance of
Stillness and Primary Respiration
Find your origin story within
And transcend your history
In a heart beat!
Find your womb outside
Live in the vagina of the Great Mother
Be unborn and remain original.

SECTION V

...

Mythology and Healing

Chapter 30

What Is Healing?

A Conversation between Kathleen Martin and Michael Shea

Kathleen Martin [K]:[13] Michael, you have studied many healing modalities in depth in your career from Rolfing to psychology (hence your doctorate in somatic psychology). I would like to start a dialogue about the nature of healing as it presents itself within the biodynamic craniosacral therapy model and the teaching focus of your school. I guess the first question is: What is biodynamic craniosacral therapy?

Michael Shea [M]: Biodynamic craniosacral therapy is the creative application of a set of principles and a perceptual practice, as a terrific osteopath has said. In general, I would say that there are four categories of principles. The first would refer to biodynamic theory. The theory would include the intention of the practice which is to have a discovery around love and compassion but also the names we give to the practitioner's perception such as Primary Respiration, stillness, the fluid body, and so forth. The next category of principles but not in a specific order would be palpation skills. This is a manual therapeutic art. I would like to say, stated by one of my mentors, that when we put our hands on a client, we have more embryology under our hands than anatomy and physiology. In other words, we are perpetual embryos! Clinically, biodynamic work is a hands-on technology that interfaces with the physics of the fluid metabolism of the body, its temperature, movement, and density.

The third category of principles has to do with the therapeutic relationship, especially the practitioner's perception of herself first and then the client. By this I mean, specifically, how the practitioner is able to shift between states of awareness, become still, inhabit a witness consciousness, and not interfere with the preexisting movement of health in the client's body. Finally, there are principles regarding the therapeutic process in general that come from numerous traditions and sources. For example, one of the main ones we work with is to reconnect the client to nature through a therapeutic process called ignition. This comes out of the osteopathic tradition as well as shamanic traditions.

K: If healing is something that occurs within a person, where is the practitioner in relation to this occurrence?

M: The practitioner needs to be self-differentiated. This does not really add any insurance to the possibility that such a practitioner is a better healer per se, but is a person who is capable of meeting and matching the humanity of the client in a way that the client knows he or she is being held without interference of the preexisting vector of healing in the body. As a practitioner, I just need to be able to sort out my therapeutic thoughts when I am in relationship with a client, what sensations I am holding for the client that are coming through the right brain-to-right brain resonance, and finally what sensations are mine. This is called the cycle of identification. In order to identify who's who and what's what in a therapy session, I need to have a degree of witness consciousness for my own sensorium. This is both a cognitive-type witness and a heart witness that can hold both the practitioner and the client with clarity, compassion, and kindness. I like to call the work therapist-centered therapy because the practitioner spends the majority of the session sensing her own body. Thus, the work of self-differentiation is important, however this happens, whether it's in therapy, meditation, watching Dr. Phil, or whatever.

K: So what we are talking about here is how well a practitioner is facilitating or not interfering with the client and holding space for a healing to occur?

M: That's right. This leads to the principle of the practitioner being able to have a greater degree of sensory awareness than the client, which includes the capacity to make distinctions between "my stuff" and "your stuff." The classical understanding is that clients "project" their unmet needs into the practitioner, which end up as sensations in the practitioner's body. The neurology is complex but that's the way it works through a process called resonance. It happens naturally just as it did between a mother and her baby. It's a big story for another time perhaps. Likewise, the practitioner is projecting into the client. So it behooves the practitioner to be self-differentiated and also able to access a slow state of consciousness in her body, since the client will also bring that slowness in as well through the resonant field of brain to brain and heart to heart and respond in a therapeutically beneficial way. Just don't pin me down on "therapeutically beneficial." It could look quite different for everyone. I learn something new in every session and I've been putting my hands on clients professionally for thirty-some years. This is also a very important principle in healing. Specifically, the ability to access slower tempos in the body and mind as well as stillness is incredibly beneficial. This is one of the main foundations in biodynamic craniosacral therapy, which is working within very slow tempos found in the fluids of the body. It relates to embryology which is another big story and the main metaphor for biodynamic practice.

The practitioner is consciously holding both herself and the client and at the same time is managing the space between the two through the process of what is called a stillpoint. The practitioner in traditional cultures was more like a manager and mediator of the space and its occupants. It was spoken of as incubation. The client was incubating an encounter with the bigger energies of life so the patient could have a revelation about these bigger energies in control. The practitioner is kind of like a new-age yenta trying to get so-and-so hooked up with so-and-so who just happens to be God's grace or clear light or whatever. In contemporary practice this means managing the office and all the accoutrements in it, then the hallway outside of the office, the building and its inhabitants, the parking lot, the city, the planet, and so on. Biodynamically we do that with the perception of the outside presence (outside the body) of Primary Respiration moving from my midline to the horizon and back. Some clients, however, may need to have you holding the whole planet or solar system, depending on where their attention is located.

K: Ah, so the practitioner must maintain personal integrity? And I mean by this, remaining wholly herself, knowing herself well enough to leave her baggage at the door in a session.

M: Well, in an ideal world, the answer is yes. But the way it works is that it is nearly impossible to maintain that degree of integrity all the time. So the question then becomes whether the practitioner has the capacity to recognize when the client is having an adverse reaction to the work, such as a headache, and has the confidence to own her part in it. It's a relationship. You cannot deny that you are part of the mix if the client has a side effect from the touch. Or it could simply be that I space out and have some fantasy for a while about a TV show I want to see tonight and I catch myself and gently come back to the room with my perception without blame or guilt. It is called mindfulness. This is the important piece. This really creates a healing response because it is consistent with the neurobiology of brain development during infancy and childhood. In other words, there is no perfect mothering but a child can learn that its growing self (whatever a self is) is capable of being repaired when the mother or caregiver is willing to repair a break in the relationship. The ability to be met in a therapeutic relationship creates safety and trust. Safety and trust are earned by the integrity created by the practitioner, which includes mindfulness, interactive repair, and the ability to hold the therapeutic space in a stillpoint.

What's interesting is that this leads to the principle that the client-therapist relationship is a direct analog of the mother-infant relationship. This research has come out of the field of affective neuroscience with Dr. Allan Schore and Daniel Siegel, for example, among numerous other wonderful clinicians. In addition, these principles of how a mother and an infant metabolize each other's stress levels have been a mainstay of the pre- and perinatal psychology community. There is a lot of interesting reading and research on this in my first volume. Of course what I call interesting may not be for others. It is kind of like recommending a movie to a friend—always dicey.

K: Michael, many other therapies work for a catharsis as a healing mechanism. How does biodynamic craniosacral therapy differ?

M: The practitioner works with containment of the strong affect rather than release-based catharsis. The principle of containment allows for greater tolerance of sensation, feeling, and emotion to arise and be transformed without recapitulating or being retraumatized by memories or from earlier events in the life of the client or the practitioner. Containment teaches clients that they can self-regulate their emotions. This capacity was lost somewhere along the line, usually in the prenatal and perinatal time. It's a big story and containment is directly related to the therapeutic goal of helping the client learn self-regulation. You need a lot of patience to work with others and your own self. The idea is that clients are already in a flight-fight mode most of the time these days. They don't need to show off for the practitioner anymore. The practitioner contains it by synchronizing her own attention on the slow tempo of Primary Respiration and a stillpoint. What's interesting to me is that a lot of folks in the cranial community and trauma resolution community are accusing one another of dissociating each other's students and consequently the clients. It is a failure to see that dissociation is preexisting in everyone, including the teachers, myself included, no matter what the method. Dissociation is the very culture we live in and it runs deep and goes far back beyond Freud. And dissociation is a scary thing indeed.

K: Getting back to the origins of stress and trauma is a focus of the work, and that means the earliest relational events, yes?

M: I wouldn't say that trauma resolution is a focus of the way I teach bio-dynamic craniosacral therapy. Trauma resolution is an evolution of certain body-centered therapies that arose back in the 1930s and 1940s in Europe as a response to a Fascist political climate. Historically, we would have to include Aristotle to be more accurate, but that's another story. This culture is dealing with such a high level of shock and trauma and consequently dissociation that it is natural that specific trauma resolution therapies would be developed to fix the problem, so to speak. I personally left military service in my twenties with a good case of post-traumatic stress disorder from being in a terrorist bombing attack. I parked my car next to what is now called an IED, an improvised explosive device. Then it went off and my life took a major change. So I have personally made trauma resolution a high priority in my life. But along with that I learned there was something deeper that wasn't being touched by those therapies and I found that the cranial work touched and met that part of myself and others. Back in the '40s Dr. Sutherland said that the fluid fields of the body can hold stress and trauma in their own way. That was pure revelation. The trauma rez folks want to get at it from the brain's side. Then the craniosacral therapy folks want to relieve the stress and trauma in the tissues and the structure of the brain. But in the biodynamic process it is about the imprints in the fluids and those imprints precede the ones in the tissues because of the embryology. It's not that other methods are wrong at all; it is a question of sequence. But the movers and shakers get on their high horse and it becomes a turf war with the main bullet being the D word—dissociation. It is nonsense. Trauma resolution is a great piece and a fabulous technology—just look at what's returning to our country from Iraq. PTSD is now rampant in our soldiers. Another part, however, of the technology is taking the submarine deeper in the fluids than just the trauma level in the tissues and the brain, which is at the surface of our ocean.

This is why this biodynamic practice has become so popular and it may or may not include trauma resolution therapy. When you touch the original matrix of the embryo, as biodynamic work does, you can bypass the trauma and uncouple it because you are essentially working on the main circuit board and not the broken software, so to speak. So the work happens outside the nervous system, which is on overwhelm anyway and shouldn't be given additional input. It is crazy. There's just one small hitch in my theory. Since I have my hands on a client by definition, I am giving input to the nervous system and in particular the right hemisphere of the brain, which is where all the trauma memories are stored, especially the early formative ones like neglect, abuse, attachment distress, and so on. Even though the touch is intended to be neutral contact, it may generate a response or awaken an old imprint or trigger a bad-hair day for the client. So, the practitioner holds both the nervous system and the fluids outside the nervous system with the intention to make space and contain both. This is now called neuro-affective touch. But, still, sometimes all you can do is pray because the client's wounding is so great.

K: Tell me more about going back even farther with the client—like to pre-birth.

M: This leads us to the principle in depth psychology called *regressum ad uterum* (regression to the uterus). What is meant by this is that healing requires a movement back to origin. One's origin must be touched at least symbolically. This is like the way Jesus responded to Nicodemus's question in the New Testament. He said, "Unless a man be born again of the water and the spirit, he shall not reach the kingdom of God." Now, as an embryologist who sees the sacredness and the mystery of life around the event of conception, I would suggest that what Jesus also meant was that we need to be reconceived rather than reborn in our original wholeness when we were actually one with the Divine. "Born again" isn't even a term used in the Christian community any more. It's all about saving and adopting embryos, which is conception. Really, I was astounded at first with the advertisements in *USA Today* from Christian groups supporting embryo adoption programs. *Re*-conception is the intention of biodynamic craniosacral therapy but from a different point of view, which is to touch the movement of wholeness we call Primary Respiration in the embryo because that movement is still present in our adult bodies. So wholeness is a tempo that implies a living, palpable connection to the Great Mystery, our own divinity, the light and intercourse as the precipitating act. As one of my teachers said, "We are all capable of experiencing our own divinity." Ultimately that's what I think biodynamic practice is about and so did Dr. Sutherland, the founder of the Cranial Concept.

This leads to the principle of the midline. All sacred space is organized and can be identified as having a midline. This is the focal point, line, axis, or sacred spot where God's grace or the Medicine Buddha's aquamarine light, or whatever, manifests into the physical. It is a process of revelation and annunciation and a lot of luck because human embryos have the highest rate of death of any species. This is not an easy thing to describe or understand. You can't get there from here, as it is said. It requires a ritual space, some sacrifice, some special prayers, and so on. We call this a stillpoint. The practitioner is pretty busy in the beginning because the practitioner must embody all those principles in a postmodern practice. Sacrificing a chicken or a lamb in your office brings too much attention from the neighbors. So a stillpoint is much more acceptable in getting the attention of Primary Respiration.

The early cranial osteopaths were fond of quoting Psalm 46, in which at the end King David says, "Be still and know." Stillness is the heart of the work in biodynamics. It is the source and is a metabolic function in the organization of the body and especially the embryo. In biodynamic craniosacral therapy, we say the midline of the human is dynamically still because that is what the great German embryologist Dr. Blechschmidt discovered. He found that all growth and development in the human embryo were oriented to the embryonic midline because of its stillness. Isn't that amazing?

K: This midline—it is such an important reality in terms of healing since it brings us back to our being in touch with the divine part of conception. This midline in the client is the place for contacting true healing, don't you think?

M: Well now, theologically I understand the Dynamic Stillness as offering me the experience of God's grace being revealed. So, the midline is imminent since it is in the body and I can look there for divine help. There is also the metaphor of the midline to the transcendent or experience of the Divine outside of the body. The connection of the imminent midline with the transcendent midline is seen in an image such as Jacob's ladder. That's really the job of healing—to connect those two midlines together as one thing. It is called communion. It's the yenta thing again. We just have to be careful with words like "true healing" because most clients do not want to see God. They just want to feel a little bit better and get back to where they were before they got sick. Primary Respiration is self-correcting and has its own priorities in each client that are different from client to client. Sometimes it's divine and sometimes a headache gets better. I have no opinion on it once I accept a client to work on. I just wait, watch, and wonder.

K: So we facilitate the healing process within the client by knowing the midline within ourselves, our own embryonic origin. This is a resonant state between client and practitioner, isn't it? Can you tell me about this dynamic state of resonance and how you see it as healing?

M: I call it neurodharma. The brain and heart are designed to take in another person, recreate that person as a neural network in the right hemisphere of the brain, and then generate a felt sense of the totality of that person in my body. The ultimate state to achieve in Buddhism is enlightenment for the sake of being compassionate with the pain and suffering of other humans. The heart does this through a temperature gradient and hormonal activity that co-regulates the limbic system of the brain. It's happening all the time unconsciously but the practitioner works with it consciously and augments it so she can read her own body and tell what's happening in the client. I teach a variety of visualizations about making blood-to-blood and heart-to-heart connections with the client based on embryology. This is none other than compassionate action. Compassion and empathy, loving kindness, and joy are conception rights and occur naturally in relationship, even in hell. Even then that capacity is still there. In Buddhism it is said that a Bodhisattva is willing to live in hell for a lifetime to save one human being. Many parents with addicted children make this statement a reality. It is never too late to experience love and compassion and be healed by that experience. This is one of the more unique aspects of being human. That's why I call biodynamic practice neurodharma. Animals can be permanently damaged from early trauma, while humans are quite pliable and can be repaired. Since I'm taking in the client, I am metabolizing a certain degree of his stress. If at the same time I can perceive this consciously, maintain a witness consciousness through access to a stillpoint, the client likewise will take this in and shift his brain and heart physiology as an act of digestion, so to speak. It's a two-way street in relationship. This stillpoint-witness is critical. It is the essence of presence, the voice of stillness, the voice of the Divine, if you will. In biodynamic work we spend a lot of time developing this type of witness by finding a stillpoint in the third ventricle, the heart, and the gut.

K: In your personal experience with this work, have you contacted that divine place of healing within yourself?

M: Yes, and it is very personal. For me it was contacting the force of love as a movement and temperature in and around my heart. Some years ago I had a wonderful mentor who was also helping me learn embryology. Every time we talked he would ask me, "Did you find your embryo yet?" I would say no because I did not have a clue what he meant. Then I would go back and keep reading books about embryology. He kept asking and I kept looking in books. Finally, one day, sitting on the beach, I experienced a very slow tempo in my body, while I was looking at the horizon. I was immediately filled with a sense of awe, beauty, and love. The love was a whole-body experience starting as a warmth around my heart and what immediately came to me was a greeting from my embryo. It was a presence throughout my body but not in the tissues and bones. It had to be in the fluids. I could feel heat and warmth permeate my body that at the same time contained a presence so beautiful that I immediately felt the original body of my embryo because the embryo is all fluid. I call this love. So, I called my mentor immediately and all I said was "I found my embryo." He knew it and I knew it. I'm grateful to my teachers for tolerating me for as long as they did before this was revealed to me.

K: Don't you think that every time you work with a client that going to your own midline facilitates your own continuing healing?

M: Certainly. It's the same as going to church all day, except better. I don't have to give money to a priest.

K: So this thing we call healing—it's within us and can be contacted and observed to be working for us by a person who understands the methodology of our origins, especially in the embryonic progression of development?

M: Yes. One of my teachers said that the wisdom is not in the body but passes through it. You don't really get to ask it to go to work, so to speak. It already is doing a marvelous job organizing and maintaining a healing response in the body. Given the medical complexities of the contemporary client, as I said, this will look quite different in everyone. The job of the practitioner is to synchronize her attention with Primary Respiration in herself first and then the therapeutic process already happening inside the client. This augments the self-directing and self-healing forces in the fluids under the principle of "wherever two or more are gathered in my name …" and so on. Beautiful, isn't it?

K: Yes, it is beautiful. Thank you, Michael, for sharing your thoughts about biodynamic craniosacral therapy and the nature of healing.

Chapter 31

Toward a Redefinition of the Human Body

Biodynamic craniosacral therapy is based on the perception of Primary Respiration as the *in*-former and *de*-former of the soma and fluid body, which are oriented to a Dynamic Stillness, all occurring in a vast ocean inside and outside the soma called the tidal body. Perhaps it is better to define our bodily existence as biodynamic—fluid and sentient and know the difference instinctually. Sentience is defined as the capacity to experience pain and pleasure. To have a living biology that is mostly fluid is to be sentient. Every cell in the body is living water (Ho, 1998). They exhibit movement toward that which is pleasurable, such as nourishment, and movement away from noxious experience, such as too much heat or cold. Conscious sentience in an adult is called attunement. Attunement to the cycles of approach and withdrawal in the belly and heart allows the instinct for healing to reemerge from the basement of the unconscious cultural and medical attitudes that are no longer appropriate for the body. The biodynamic principle is that the living fluids of the soma are sentient and the whole soma exists within a single fluid continuum—a single sphere or bubble of living water called the fluid body.

The soma navigates the currents of sensation and emotion going one way and then another. At times it is stormy. Life is constant. Waves arise and waves return to their origin in the ocean, over and over. Chaos theory states that as biological organisms the soma needs chaos. Chaos is loosely defined as ordered instability out of which emerge stability, integration, organization, and wholeness. Chaos is another term for the void—a deep state of stillness capable of being recognized in our biology. The Navajo myth in Chapter 35 speaks to this quite eloquently, as does Sheila Moon's interpretation in Chapter 36. The soma transitions from states of confusion to states of clarity in the fluid body and tidal body constantly and at variable rates, although it often seems that confusion is endless because of the prevalence of fear in the culture. Resistance and discomfort eventually lead to growth and learning or death (Bateman, 1990).

> The duality, namely a tendency toward ordered consciousness and a basic tendency toward a counterposition, something that acts according to emotion, moods, and momentary disturbances, a semi-animal figure, is there from the very beginning. It comes up at the same moment as a double movement of the birth of consciousness, just as when you stretch out your arm you move two muscles, one which contracts and one which does the opposite. (von Franz, 1995, p. 97)

The embryo cannot grow without resistance. Thus the biodynamic principle: no growth without resistance. It is fundamental to the nature of having a soma to be pulled in two directions. It is hardwired into the central nervous system from its embryonic origins. Life exists in a tension field of resistance. More than anything else, we resist specialization of certain body features seen in all other mammals such as claws, fangs, snouts, and four-leggedness. This is what the embryo teaches us. These fields contain polarities such as spirit and soul, life and death, crying and laughing, and so on. Tension fields need containment so meaning can emerge, as mentioned in Chapter 14. Containment requires a midline of stillness for transformation to take place. Carl Jung, in his essay "The Transcendent Function" (Jung, 1971), said that the ability to contain or make space for these tension fields creates the possibility for the transcendent, numinous power to manifest. It is the responsibility of the biodynamic practitioner to hold her own polarities and those of the client so that the other pair of hands (Jealous, 1998) can manifest in the session to assist the practitioner in the diagnosis and resolution of the dissociation from spirit and nature. The numinous spirit of healing is preexisting in the fluids of the embryo and therefore the soma throughout life. How can it be otherwise? It manifests as a function of the practitioner's ability to disassociate from the urban world. Psychologically, the tension must reach an unbearable threshold in order to experience a transmutation from the unbearable to the transformed state of happiness. Martin Buber said that freedom finally occurs when there is no choice. This is a significant job for any therapist to hold these seemingly unbearable and insurmountable polarities.

For example, in my own therapy after my mother died, I realized I had a hole in my heart from my mother's inability to nurture my heart and give solace to my deepest fears in childhood. The heart of an infant is a three-chambered organ much like that of a reptile. It is open between the two atria waiting to be closed by the loving kindness of physical contact. Even though I know that my mother loved me as best she could, I nonetheless carried a lifelong depression over not being good enough at self- and other nurturing. The realization of this filled me with rage when anyone would attempt to fill the hole. The tension between the depression and the rage became unbearable to me and my loved ones through my unconscious behaviors and acting out my anger. Only until I could recognize my own unbearable pain through the nontraditional means of shamanic healing and depth psychology, could I see that it was not capable of being resolved by ordinary means. It was then that I could transform, uncouple, and resolve the tension of opposites. The pain of no choice gave me complete freedom from my internalized mother complex. It would not have been possible without concurrently dissolving the structure of my body symbolically, resting in the fluid body and tidal body of my embryo and reigniting the fire of the heat of love in my heart. My sadness is no longer coupled to the mother complex and my biological mother can remain the human being that she was. My sadness is now the fuel of a more genuine compassion that predates my conception. This is the definition of transmutation.

Bodily life is a chain of seemingly random events that occasionally reach resolution, and more often don't. We are always in our origin story, according to modern anthropologists. Waves arise from the ocean of different sizes and move at different speeds and return to the ocean when their waveness has disappeared. It is chaos that occasionally achieves order. More human embryos perish than any other species. Death is the constant companion of the embryo. This chaos-order relationship is true of the brain as well (Varela, 1999). The brain converts sense impressions into electrical and chemical signals that exhibit both random and ordered patterns of activity. There really is no one home, so to speak, in terms of a self that organizes the electrical patterns in my brain. Somatic reality is socially constructed (Cassidy, 1994). The soma can only ever be partially understood. Is the soma anatomy and physiology as defined by biomedicine? Is it electricity, magnetism, chakras, empty space, meridians, a dream, or all fluids? There are many ways of defining the soma. The world of molecular genetics in the twenty-first century demonstrates the uniqueness and sameness of all living things. Yet there are different religious attitudes about the body from it being filthy and loathsome to being the temple of the Holy Spirit. Thus bodily reality varies immensely from person to person, from culture to culture, and even within one historical period. A biodynamic understanding of the body must go beyond cultural conditioning and biomedicine but necessarily includes those conditions of contemporary bodily existence. The soma is very fluid and behaves according to laws written in the fluid body itself.

> The symbols of the self arise in the depths of the body and they express its materiality every bit as much as the structure of the perceiving consciousness. The deeper *layers* of the psyche lose their individual uniqueness as they retreat farther and farther into darkness. *Lower down,* that is to say as they approach the autonomous functional systems, they become increasingly collective until they are universalized and extinguished in the body's materiality, i.e., in chemical substances. The body's carbon is simply carbon. Hence *at bottom* the psyche is simply *world.* In the symbol the *world itself* is speaking. (Jung, 1966, p. 173)

Meaning comes about through having a soma capable of extrasensory perception. This is perceived three-dimensionally as being a transparent fluid body and from a still place of order in the mind, belly, and heart internally and connected to nature externally. Meaning and midline are synonymous with each other. The biodynamic midline is one of stillness located both inside and outside the body. It is an automatically shifting fulcrum moving back and forth from the horizon to the spine and center of the body's fluid cavities. The search for the midline is a longing for the big picture, the whole of life, essence, and deeper contact with the body of nature and spirit. It is a matter of heart and a function of our fluid sentience. Current research in cell biology is suggesting that sentience is a function of living structured water in and around the cells of our body (Ho, 2004a, 2004b, 2005). This is none other than the protoplasm of the cell and its water matrix that has continuity from head to foot. This is a biodynamic understanding of the fluid body. The fabric of life and the soma is thin and not substantial. It is watery and fluid. Embodied life is hardly reliable as the inner stream of thoughts, feelings, and emotions are constantly changing and transmuting. Attunement constantly moves from inside the body to outside the body at the rate of Primary Respiration. The ground of the fluid body is constantly shifting with its currents and tides. The whole is the movement of the outside presence of Primary Respiration permeating the inside of the soma and directing its condensation in the viscosity of the fluid body and soma.

The numinous spirit in the physical heart holds our wholeness and fragmentation. Both are necessary for growth and differentiation. The heart allows each experience to be transformed into a teacher, a gift, a message, a learning, a friend, an enemy, and so on. Life events are essential to shaping one's own unique, individual spiritual development. Bodily fluid experience can be perceived as real, unreal, traumatic, mythological, metaphysical, or have a host of other meanings yet to be discovered. Discovery of the relationship between stillness and Primary Respiration allows experience to unfold in a natural order and in sequence with the natural world.

Moreover, the act of taking my own experience as just one "variant" among other variations upon a common theme liberates me from my naive narrow-mindedness, helping me to see that there are other ways of being human, of being bodily, than my own. And the turn to the more universal, shared features of human experience may even enrich my own individual experience by opening up new possibilities that I too can explore (Behnke, 1989, p. 13).

Joseph Campbell, in his television series with Bill Moyers in 1988, said we weren't here for the discovery of meaning at all, but rather to experience the excitement of being alive. Excitement is a function of the autonomic nervous system. Aliveness is a function of the heat in the fluids of the body. Campbell's belief parallels the thinking of Zen master Mumon Gensen, who wrote this poem at the moment of his death in 1390:

> Life is like a cloud of mist
> emerging from a mountain cave
> and death a floating moon in its
> celestial course.
> If you wonder too much about the
> meaning they may have
> you'll be bound forever like an
> ass to a stake.
>
> —Mumon Gensen[14]

Is there meaning to life? Each of us is our own Hamlet or Ophelia and must discover this on our own.

Attunement

Let's examine attunement in biodynamic craniosacral therapy a little more deeply. Biodynamic craniosacral therapy is an attunement process of therapeutically relating to a client and one's self. Normally when touch therapy is employed, the practitioner looks for *state* changes in the tone of the client's musculo-skeletal system (from tight to loose) to determine the effectiveness of the work. Treatment techniques and tissue tone are secondary in biodynamic craniosacral therapy. The attunement process is fundamental. Attunement originates in the affective neuroscience literature and specifically refers to the development of the autonomic nervous system of the embryo, fetus, and baby. The sympathetic nervous system approaches and seeks contact with self and other. The parasympathetic nervous system seeks to withdraw from the world and the perception of self for integration and solace. This is the basic rhythm of embodied life during the preverbal time of life. Attachment experiences with caregivers imprint the attunement process with a positive or negative value and cause the autonomic nervous system to have different behaviors and timing regarding the seeking of contact and withdrawing from contact.

Therapeutic self-attunement is the conscious approach and withdrawal of the practitioner's touch, speech, and thinking with oneself when with a client. The practitioner must be aware of her self-attunement tempo and slow it down. Self-attunement then invites an attunement to the client since this is why he is there in the first place. But it all starts and ends with the practitioner's perception. Attunement is also directly related to the infant caregiving experience, as I detailed in Volume One. At the same time the client is doing the same self-attunement activities unconsciously or sometimes consciously with the practitioner. At some point this unconscious activity must become conscious for the client through image, shape, and speech. It is not the responsibility of the practitioner to know when or how this might happen. It is through the synchronization with Primary Respiration and its interchange with stillness that the practitioner reciprocally begins to attune to the client's attunement. It is much like a four-way-stop intersection. The right of way must be determined first before anyone can proceed safely. This is how a perverted attunement process from early imprinting is uncoupled from a stress response in the autonomic nervous system and recoupled to the tempo of Primary Respiration.

Attunement at the tempo of Primary Respiration and its fulcrum of stillness is an acknowledgment that the practitioner and client are together in a constant state of becoming, renewing, and resourcing within each other's body. Within that mutuality I listen with the client for the preexisting health in his total body fluid continuum as it ebbs and flows in slow cycles rather than reacting to or challenging a disturbance, symptom, or identified problem coupled to the autonomic nervous system. The biodynamic ordering forces of Primary Respiration and the stillness are witnessed and the self-healing potential in the client's body can manifest without obstruction and interference by the practitioner. These ordering forces are located in the watery continuum of the soma in the fluid body and its mind of Primary Respiration. Centered in the felt sense of heat radiating from my heart, I observe with love and compassion the client's fluid body and tidal body attuning its activity from inside out, rather than putting pressure from the outside in with my hands or intention. I extend my perception of an umbilical cord connecting us both to the Great Mother of nature. I hold the whole of the client, myself, and nature around us as one breathing motion in the tempo of Primary Respiration from the third ventricle out to the horizon.

The soma expresses preexisting health constantly. It is the job of the bio-dynamic practitioner to synchronize her attention with the preexisting forces of health already at work in the whole soma and fluid body. These preexisting forces of health are Primary Respiration and its fulcrum of stillness. They have the capacity to contain aberrant compensations in the fluids of the body in response to stress and trauma. Consequently, the core of every trauma or disease in the soma carries the remedy of Primary Respiration and its fulcrum of still-ness. The practitioner establishes windows with her hands to look at the body and witness the power, authority, and love inherent within Primary Respiration and the work and energy it is using to modify the problems in the client's body (Becker, 1963).

Incarnation and Embodiment

Many spiritual teachers advocate the development of self-awareness and self-knowledge as the starting point for incarnation. I am defining incarnation as the capacity to orient consciously to the intelligence of stillness either inside the soma and fluid body, outside the soma, or both together. Incarnation is the experience of transmutation of the fluid body into a soma under the guidance of Primary Respiration. The embryo does this as a function of its sentience because still-ness is a metabolic cause of normal growth and differentiation. As an adult this metabolic function becomes awareness of the psychological, spiritual, and physi-ological value of stillness. Without the capacity to orient to stillness, attunement becomes a process of trying to steer a boat without a rudder or sail with a torn spinnaker. Self-regulation depends on periods of self-reflection, contemplation, artistic endeavor, body movement oriented to stillness, and attunement to the waves of Primary Respiration. Self-reflection is essential for the neurological and vascular transmutation of biodynamic processes to occur in the soma.

The brain is primarily designed for emotional learning (Schore, 1994), as is the heart according to the Institute of HeartMath (McCraty, 2003). Inter-nal self-regulation of emotions and a tranquil heart require attunement to my own approach and withdrawal behaviors that are supported by a well-attuned caregiver, or biodynamic practitioner in this case. At the very least, according to Herbert Benson's seminal work at Harvard, *The Relaxation Response* (Ben-son, 1975), contemplative practices such as biodynamic craniosacral therapy develop self-esteem and promote an internal focus of emotional control in the body thought to reside in the orbitofrontal cortex of the brain (Schore, 1994) or the heart or the gut. If the brain is left with control by itself, it relies overmuch on intuition. Therefore, the heart and gut must be more involved proportionally to awaken the instinct of healing. In other words, tranquility, serenity, and peace of mind are an inside job requiring conscious attention to internal states of sensation and feeling moving between the gut, the heart, and the brain. Biodynamic craniosacral therapy focuses on slowing down the process of thinking that is immediately in the foreground of perception and inviting a stillpoint to arise. The new foreground of slowness is replaced with the background of Dynamic Stillness.

The important thing is to bring the thinking mind into a present-time body experience that is fluid, oceanic, and tidal and then let the soma demolecularize three-dimensionally out to the horizon with Primary Respiration floating all the molecules in the great ocean outside of the soma. Fifty seconds later the soma is reinformed by Primary Respiration. It is a completely generous and loving situation on behalf of Primary Respiration. Body awareness constantly is being exchanged with awareness of the environment and beyond via Primary Respiration. Then it fades from perception and a stillpoint comes to the foreground indicating a period of waiting, watching, and wondering. I spent five years experimenting with different meditation techniques until I found the one that resonated deeply within my fluid body and thinking mind and provided an interconnection with nature. Those practices then informed my initial experience of craniosacral therapy. Now it is a reciprocal relationship where my life is constantly informed by Primary Respiration and stillness rather than exclusively waiting for that to happen with a client. Spiritual growth follows developmental rules just as the soma does. It starts in the embryo. The embryo has an internal body and an external body. Throughout life we flexibly move back and forth, inside and outside our soma using other bodies outside of our own to project the immature parts of our self onto. It is an embryonic necessity. At the right time in the sequence of differentiation, we will reclaim the projection, provided the internal structure of the body-mind-heart has the maturity to do so.

Incarnation in this sense may mean the time when stillness coming from the outside body of the embryo takes up residence in the structure of the cardiovascular system (Ridley, 2006). The adult soma must constantly maintain a balance for both the outer projection and the inner ownership of feeling states. This is normal attunement and it functions by the practitioner initially attuning to the activity of the heart and the blood because they are the first organs to arise in the embryo. Actually, the blood arises prior to the heart and circulates by itself. The heart is in the central body and the blood is in the peripheral body of the embryo and they must find each other and grow toward one another. How can any therapeutic relationship otherwise exist? This is a biodynamic incarnation taught by the embryo. It is a matter of heart to blood and blood to heart between client and practitioner. Please refer to Chapter 24 for a detailed explanation of this connection.

Disease, illness, and health can then be viewed as psychospiritual processes related to incarnation of the heart and a condition of the body related to embodiment of genetic traits and fluid imprints. Each organ and system of the body has a separate timing for its development during the embryonic period. This remains true throughout the lifespan. Health, therefore, depends on the maintenance of optimal connectedness and coherence within and among all levels of a perceiving body, its social context (Cunningham, 1986), and nature. Primary Respiration and stillness are seen in the mechanism of attunement for facilitating this process of incarnation and embodiment. They support the integrity of the body in an optimal and flexible relationship to its environment and nature through the image and perception of the body being an ocean within and supported by an ocean outside and in contact with every square millimeter of skin. Conversely, disease is a progressive disconnection or separation from the blood-heart-body-mind-nature connection that I speak about in subsequent chapters. Symptoms and disease provide information about systemic problems in the dynamic ocean of an individual's bodily existence, mind existence, and crucial relationship to nature. Diseases have idiosyncratic cultural meaning and are each person's unique response to lifestyle (Achtenburg, 1985, 1991). Illness in this context is a form of self-expression (Sontag, 1979), a psychophysiological collusion of risk factors projected onto a soma. The healing relationship is between the information encoded symbolically in disease symptoms connecting it to the whole—mind, body, nature, and the divine—symbolically or literally. This also includes all the other information that has had a significant impact on the body situation or context that is labeled disease by biomedicine and political culture (Cunningham, 1991). In other words, I may be convinced that stem cells are the only thing that will heal my disease, so I might vote for politicians who support stem cell research, which involves the destruction of human embryos that might otherwise have died anyway. Movement of the whole is the first priority in biodynamic practice. This is the politics of Primary Respiration.

An important effect of wholeness is self-regulation. Self-regulation is the dynamic tension (resistance) between autonomy and relationship. At one and the same time as a human being, we desire to operate as a separate and self-sufficient person (Booth and Ashbridge, 1993). Even the embryo teaches us that there are two metabolisms, one of connection and one that is closed off to the outside.

This is a biological reality and it is our biological nature of being. It exists at the most fundamental embryonic level and persists throughout the lifespan, as I wrote in Volume One. At the same time, the heart of a human being demands the willingness to hold this unique identity in a spiritual polarity together with a larger loving purpose through the effect of stillness being centered in and around the heart. That purpose is to be in communion with another person or society with empathy and compassion and transmute anger and aggression. It is also for the purpose of loving others with the desire to see them be happy and for others to know the causes of happiness. This is none other than the spiritual polarity of wisdom for me and compassion for you.

The Buddha was a rationalist. He said to first find out who you are and what your purpose in life is, then you will find God or the numinous or wisdom. "Are you happy?" and "Do you know your purpose in life?" are two questions I ask my students. These are psycho-immune questions. Not knowing who you are and where you are going in life is spiritual disease. The world is sacred. We are interconnected with everyone and everything in the world with our body through a shared and unshared metabolism. Everyone also has the unshared metabolism that I have. This is the *sacred view* and is a statement about the nonprimacy of Homo sapiens in a horizontal, circular world view as opposed to a vertical, top-down mode of patriarchal control. It is horizontal because human beings are equal to all other things. There are differences by degree, not by kind, as Steven Jay Gould once said. We are spokes on a wheel and not the wheel itself. The wheel is circular, just as the planet Earth is circular. Some premodern cultures taught the interconnectedness of all things using the image of a circle divided into the four directions of the compass. Incarnation was defined in archaic societies by a variety of cosmological symbols and especially the medicine wheel. I will explore this theme in detail in the next chapter.

The model of the wheel (a circle and its four quadrants), as you will see in later chapters, is a model of relativity and interconnectedness. In order to live in a sacred manner, however, an initiation is required. When a person is properly initiated, the prenatal and perinatal imprinting and wounding are transcended through a variety of rites and experiences that may be painful emotionally and sometimes physically. The ultimate purpose of initiation is not to be painful, but to deliver the initiate out of the euphoric dissociation of his narcissistic wounding and into an ordered biodynamic relationship with himself, society, the earth, and the numinous. The midline is recovered. During some initiations, the soma, the fundamental source of narcissistic wounding, is metaphorically and sometimes literally dismembered, stripped or skeletalized to rid it of the danger of grandiosity and the abuse of power. In biodynamic craniosacral therapy, the practitioner guides the client through an exercise of disappearing all the bones and tissues of the body. All that is left is clear living water just as it was during the first two weeks postfertilization. This is not painful at all and rather relaxing. The client frequently goes into a deep trance state where the preexisting forces of health, both inside the body and outside the body, repair or replace that which is broken. Initiation can gradually rid the participant of an overidentification with power and places the initiate in vital relationship with the natural world of the earth as the primal body of the Great Mother (Neumann, 1955). Pre- and perinatal trauma is a premature initiation into the power of the world and its aberrant usage because sacred space is nonexistent and normal dissociation is coupled to preverbal fear centers in the brain and heart. Such wounding shapes a life and bends it like a sapling in a hurricane. This can be transmuted with love and Primary Respiration. When it is transmuted the person may remember the trauma differently as part of the unique trajectory of her life process. Suffering can take on a different meaning in the soma.

Embodied Compassion

Empathy is the ability to feel in one's brain, heart, and vascular system what another person is feeling. Compassion is the desire to eliminate the pain and suffering of another sentient being, along with the causes of that pain and suffering, and to transmute the suffering into happiness. Lately empathy and compassion are being defined in the neurological community by the discovery of mirror neurons (Iacoboni, et al., 2005). To be born is to be compassionate. Babies are shown to have compassion for their mother and vice-versa in this most interesting literature. Stressful births and stressful parenting experiences diminish empathy and compassion in children. This leads to aggression and learning disabilities (DeMause, 2002). The world is almost impossible to be seen as sacred in this context.

Those who choose the path of helping others accelerate their own capacity for empathy and allow their own wounding to come to the surface. I realized several years into my initial massage therapy and Rolfing practice that I did not have a lot of empathy for my clients because I was dissociated from my own feelings. Client after client would cry and cry in front of me and I did not have a clue how to respond. It gradually occurred to me that I wasn't even sure if I liked people in general. My own wounding gradually emerged and I sought help. Fortunately, this has changed. By way of principle, then, the helper has more to gain from the therapeutic relationship than the helpee. "I can never emphasize enough the dangers of making contact or touching other people without mastering your own organism" is a statement I will always remember from one of my graduate school professors. I say that biodynamic practice is therapist-centered therapy. The client has the exquisite ability to sense the internal reality of a practitioner's life and cannot move any further in the healing process than the practitioner in her own self-development and self-regulation.

The practitioner is working toward the transmutation and mastery of herself. Mastery is not a collection of skills and knowledge, but rather the differentiation of early wounding and the integration of that wounding into the whole self or person—physically, emotionally, and spiritually. My psychospiritual understanding of my dilemma and its resolution will also change as I grow older. Thus wisdom is a progressive sequence of spiritual experiences over time. The basis for compassion, however, is self-warmth. The starting point for working with others is overcoming bodily self-aggression, bodily self-hatred, and self-abusive thoughts and behaviors. This has been my long, and at times arduous, learning as a professional body-centered therapist practitioner over the past thirty years. That is just the starting point. To be effective at working with others, first get to know your own soma and become adept at working with personal issues nonaggressively. To befriend ourselves is a major task with a major risk of uncovering unbearable tensions. This starting point can then extend genuine compassion and self-warmth toward others. This is not easy because some of our compensations for self-aggression appear to be quite sane and stable, such as exercise, diet, meditation, work relationships, and outside relationships. The original wounding, however, remains in the preverbal memory and there is no conscious recall of it.

I am advocating for a return to the sensible ocean of the sacred in life. This includes the resacralization of the soma through orientation to the stillpoint in the fluid body and tidal body. The earth, the feminine, beckons us back with the movement of Primary Respiration. Many biodynamic practitioners have listened to her call. It is a call to be in relationship with the emotions, feelings, sensations, awareness, and physicality in a contained and compassionate way. This is the start of a mutation into the sacred, incarnate body. We continually react with personal obstacles—behaviors, lifestyles, nutritional choices, career, relationships, and so on, that keep us human. We can begin to notice the subtleties of our psycho-physical-spiritual self. There can be a deepening, an appreciation for the uninterrupted flow and tidal movement of life. This is called becoming a *fair witness* to the inherent order that is the potential of every body. Biodynamic practice acknowledges body limitations and personal pain. Relating to limitations overcomes the inertia of early wounding. Another word for healer is *adult*.

An adult renounces the infantile urges and delusions of excess and speed for the magic of seeing the world more clearly.

There is the law of exchange in biodynamic practice. It means that helpers exchange their soma with the client's soma as a form of resonance and vice-versa. This happens naturally as a function of entrainment from right cerebral hemisphere to right cerebral hemisphere to exchange with others' thoughts, feelings, emotions, bodily sensations, and images. In other words, the practitioner is exchanging her whole body with the client's whole body as shared interpersonal nervous systems. We live in a shared field of perception and resonance. It is futile to defend the soma from this process. What we can do is develop clarity, precision, and intelligence in identifying and ventilating this exchange of our mutual oceans of experience. To do so means to sustain attention on Primary Respiration and its interchange from one heart and cardiovascular system to another and back at the rate of Primary Respiration. We are more truly interpersonal cardiovascular systems helping to build each other's heart into a four-dimensional organ.

CHAPTER 32

Biodynamic Symbols of Healing

The archaic stages of culture and initiation include a series of rites whose symbolism is crystal clear: through them, the novice is first transformed into an embryo and then is reborn. Initiation is equivalent to a second birth. It is through the agency of initiation that one becomes both a socially responsible and culturally awakened being. The return to the womb is signified … by entering a sacred spot identified with the uterus of mother earth … the basic idea is that, to attain a higher mode of existence, gestation and birth must be repeated; but they are repeated ritually, symbolically. (Eliade, 1963, pp. 79–82)

The Body As Symbol

A metaphor is the vital spirit of a paradigm (or perhaps its basic organizing relation). (Haraway, 2004, p. 9)

I know now that my body image from childhood was built from a variety of symbols. The symbols of Pinocchio and Frankenstein from the movies, the symbols of GI Joe and Mickey Mantle from television, or mother and father at home—these dominated how I inhabited my body as a child. Such symbolizing establishes a personal identity with the preexisting capacity to imagine rather than cognize. A child experiences himself in terms of these images and symbols naturally. Cognition is not yet involved. One set of symbols arises from culture. Another set of symbols arises from the ancient and archetypal depths inside the undifferentiated brain and body such as images of a king or queen, a devil or angel, an animal or insect.

Finally, another set of symbols arises from the biology of the body set in motion by the three-dimensional sensory perception of the skin of a baby. Since the infant is noncognitive, it translates signals from the thinking skin into symbolic images. The infant makes a story from the images that frequently mimic ancient myths with the support from the giant beings giving care to the infant. The physiology of the body operates with symbols. In other words, the brain hears words with the ears that are transformed through vibration into chemical and electrical messengers that then generate a flow of neurochemicals that then translate into perception or a behavioral response to the stimulus. Everything else coming in from the world is broken down into chemical electrical symbols by the body's physiology in this way. We are literally swimming in a sea of symbols, and nothing is ever what it seems to be.

> Therefore every culture has another kind of healing which is symbolic and does not rely on detailed scientific knowledge of bodily organs. It might be called cultural healing, for it derives its symbols from a specific culture, and relies for its effect on identification of the patient with supernatural (or intrapsychic) power through the mediation of the symbol. All phases of medical care—nosology, etiology, diagnosis, therapy, prognosis—are based on that symbolic identification. (Sandner, 1979, p. 17)

Another example of biological symbols comes from once having been an embryo and maintaining that embryonic nature throughout life. These are symbols that become metaphors of creation. The symbols create a sequence much like the frames of a movie, and a metaphor is born. I remember when I first began to study embryology; my dreams for several years were filled with experiments on building an atomic bomb. Looking at images of embryos day after day stimulated the symbolic function of my unconscious and the stage of creativity I was in at that time. It was up to me and a good Jungian analyst to transform the symbol into a conscious working metaphor to understand my inner life. The image of the mushroom cloud that many of us grew up with in the 1950s and 1960s ushered in the nuclear age and became a powerful image of creation and destruction. The embryo is such an image because it requires a power beyond belief to animate a human being. This is the phase where a metaphor becomes part of a myth through the power and strong affect of an archetype. The breakdown and *dis*-association from these three modes of symbolizing, now prevalent in our culture (May, 1999), causes illness. Dissociation is a nasty label to give a client, but in fact is the healthiest response to an unhealthy culture.

Symbols act as transformers of energy in the psyche precisely as I experienced with my dreams of making an atomic bomb (Sandner, 1979). The psyche is the unconscious underworld of reality, as seen in images from Dante's *Inferno* or the myth of Persephone going to the underworld to retrieve her soul. It exists within the tensional pull of the mind and body. The psyche, the totality of body-mind and the unconscious-conscious together, is the engine of the pull or tension. It is the home of the archetype, the bigger-than-life energies moving in and through the psyche such as the powers of creation that make a human being just mentioned. When mind and body are out of balance, within the psyche symbols arise to point toward correction as well as balance. This is seen in dream material, biodynamic craniosacral therapy, and cathartic religious experience. Carl Jung said that healing must necessarily involve a religious type of affect.

Following a biodynamic craniosacral therapy session, the client may feel relief of a physical symptom, have inner certainty around a core life issue, or even have a mystical experience. It is a possibility that exists in every session of biodynamic practice because of the activity of Primary Respiration and the presence of stillness. Likewise, a client may become depressed or anxious from a session—these reactions are symbolic of releasing energy from the psyche. Symbolic does not mean they are not real. The reality is held in a much larger context of myth and metaphor that cannot be discovered by the rational mind. Thus the formula for meaning to emerge would be:

Symbols + Metaphor + Archetype = Myth

This chapter and the ones that follow will detail the importance of mythology in biodynamic craniosacral therapy.

Healing the Body

Yet symbols do more than that. They may not only provide a vocabulary and an explanation, but also change the psyche by converting energy into a different form, a form that can heal. As Jung said: "The symbols act as transformers, their function being to convert libido from a 'lower' into a 'higher' form. This function is so important that feeling accords it the highest value." In the act of healing, symbols work upon the patient who is vulnerable, open, and ready to experience them. He identifies with them in the form of the sacred images and the person of the medicine man. They transform him and allow him to partake of their hidden power. Under such conditions he may be not only persuaded by their suggestion or reconciled to his fate, but cured. (Sandner, 1979, pp. 14–15).

Healing the body is also symbolic, according to researchers (Sandner, 1979; Eliade, 1960, 1964, 1985). In our contemporary culture, healing still remains symbolic and requires belief and participation in formal rituals of meaning between patient and doctor, between patient and hospital, and between patient and insurance company. Evidence-based cures are wrapped in a shroud of mystery and symbols such as laboratories and prestigious journals. The body and the medical industry established to repair it are now symbols for a progressive decay in health care (Illich, 1976). There is a pervasive breakdown in the medical symbols of healing because the body is more the living symbol and carrier of the world of nature and the numinous than it is the carrier of mutant genes. It carries the symbols of all that is good and bad in life and in the history of culture, not just the history of one's family. Consequently, bio-medicine cannot treat illnesses derived from the dissociation from nature or from God. I am always amazed when a client comes in hating God as the cause of inability to recover from an illness. The problem is not the illness. The disease is the alienation from the divine (Edinger, 1972).

The main side effect of a decaying health care system is called *iatrogenesis*. Iatrogenesis is defined as physician-induced disease (Illich, 1976) and recent research has shown that an average of 75,000 patients die every year from iatrogenic causes. Can this be from the lack of recognition and restoration of spirit and nature necessary in the healing process? If I have persistent headaches I may go to a medical doctor because of the symbolic *MD* after his or her name. Recognizing the symbol of MD is how I am trained by my society to seek help outside of myself for alleviating my physical pain. The doctor's persona will include a stethoscope, an aura of seriousness and/or being busy, and perhaps even a white coat. All of these are symbols. Other symbols may be presented to me for healing—needles, radiographic equipment, gowns, lights, nurses in uniforms, and so on. It is endless. These symbols, which are devoid of a larger meaning, become lethal weapons.

I grew up believing that these medical symbols would heal me, just as other cultures might use drums, rattles, smoke, fire, chanting, singing, prayer, and dancing. Both scenarios are the same—symbolic. Now I would much rather sit by a fire first and then take a pill if appropriate. What is important is the power of belief in the symbols, one's expectations, and how the symbols are used in the healing ritual of the office visit. The symbols of biodynamic craniosacral therapy include the image of living water in the body, the image of the embryo, the movement of Primary Respiration, the perception of stillness, the image of the ocean outside the body, and others. Biodynamic practice depends on how skillfully the practitioner can make the symbols come alive as a personal perception in and around her body and have them be translated into a sensory or imaginal experience for the client that is loving.

Summary

It follows, thus, that an individual's self-image is built up of symbols. Symbolizing is basic to such questions as personal identity. For the individual experiences himself as a self in terms of symbols which arise from three levels at once; those from archaic and archetypal depths within himself, symbols arising from the personal events of his psychological and biological experience, and the general symbols and values which retain in his culture. A second observation impressed upon us by our psychoanalytic work is that contemporary man suffers from the deterioration and breakdown of the central symbols in modern Western culture. (May, 1999, p. 22)

Relationships between symbols and the objects they represent are not confined to language but can be found in every area of life, especially the body, mind, and psyche (Sebeok, 1976; Jacob, 1977; Tembrock, 1975; Krampen, 1987). These relationships are the foundation for interaction and bonding between living beings, and they determine the safety and trust between the bodies of living beings and their environment. Symbols gain their power from cultural agreement on their meaning, especially the pain and suffering associated with them, as with the cross in Christianity.

The relationship between symbols and the object they represent, however, is not equivalent to the relationship between cause and effect. A motor vehicle accident is first and foremost a cause-and-effect relationship. Later it is possible to interpret the accident symbolically. Symbolic meaning changes daily, monthly, or over several lifetimes, and is culturally shaped. One of the great findings in the trauma resolution literature is that one's memory of past events is supposed to change over time. We are neurologically designed to remember the past differently and attach symbolic meaning to it to integrate life experience as we age. To remember a trauma as precisely as it happened is to be stuck in the past. Thus the cross can also represent love more than suffering in contemporary theology. The relationship is more random and less direct, such as dream material, than cause and effect, such as running a red light. Symbols evolve into a metaphor for greater meaning, such as the metaphor of the fluid body in the human embryo that is retained and conserved through adulthood. This is followed by the metaphor evolving into a myth, such as the debate between the intelligent design and evolution metaphors. A metaphor is necessary because it generates an image that can be used to discuss a new paradigm.

> Metaphor is predictive because it is embedded in a rich system not private to any one man. The conditions necessary for metaphor to be explanatory are not loose. They can be summarized as the requirements that the metaphor have neutral points of analogy to be explored, that the metaphor contain the germ of concrete expectations (sensory experience), and that it give definite limits to acceptable theoretical accounts in science. Metaphor is a property of language that gives boundaries to worlds and helps scientists using real languages to push against these bounds. (Haraway, 2004, p. 10)

Symbols that make up a metaphor constitute a *code.* Knowledge of the code provides access to the metaphor, such as the language describing the Primary Respiratory System; at the same time, the code excludes access for those who do not understand it. Codes establish boundaries that form an *insider* and an *outsider* regarding the domains in which communication is possible by means of the code. The terms *insider* and *outsider* portray this fact (von Uexkull, Geigges, and Herrman, 1993, p. 58). The language of biodynamic craniosacral therapy and other healing systems is coded and typically requires training from a qualified teacher to understand its meaning and experience the felt sense of its relevance. This becomes an initiation. The older the code, the more secret and more closed the system of healing becomes to sharing "secrets" with the outside world or other practitioners who are uninitiated or deemed not spiritually advanced enough. Lack of well-bounded initiation causes the conflict seen in the various cranial and manual therapy communities, which further polarizes them into good versus bad. The osteopathic community has long complained that the craniosacral therapy community is "uninitiated," which means having a lack of medical school training. Thus medical school becomes the initiatory experience for medical practitioners of craniosacral therapy. Yet there are other initiations that I will speak to in the chapters to come. This is the stuff of mythology. Conflict resolution skills are dramatically lacking and preverbal wounding dominates. Donna Haraway said, "It is important to stress, however, that as a consequence of the central role of metaphor paradigms operate more as directing tendencies than as clear and tyrannical logical archetypes" (Haraway, 2004, p. 10).

The Container of Sacred Space

By acknowledging a larger context for a body and its healing to be richly symbolic for each client, it is possible to understand and perceive that this must occur within a container of sacred space. This means spiritual. Spiritual means a drive for wholeness and balance. Spirituality further involves contact with a creative purpose for one's life, access to expanded states of sensation, and experience previously labeled as "ecstatic." A spiritual person is deeply ethical and moral and can manage conflict, relationship, and commitment with relative gracefulness. A spiritual behavior is any activity that facilitates, improves, and enhances one's ability to become positive in orientation, tolerant of different views, and able to recognize and integrate a deeper power from nature into the body (Payne, Bergin, and Loftus, 1992). Dr. Sutherland said that the Cranial Concept could be considered religious in nature, and I feel that biodynamic practice needs to be defined as having a spiritual component.

> In this way the place becomes an inexhaustible source of power and sacredness and enables man, simply by entering it, to have a share in the power, to hold communion with the sacredness. This elementary notion of the place's becoming, by means of a hierophany, a permanent "center" of the sacred, governs and explains a whole collection of systems often complex and detailed. But however diverse and variously elaborated these sacred spaces may be, they all present one trait in common: there is always a clearly marked space which makes it possible (though under very varied forms) to communicate with the sacred. (Eliade 1958, pp. 367–369.)

All pre-Western traditions consider the acquisition of spiritual knowledge to take place within a special holy container called sacred space. Sacred space is filled with symbols of healing. Thus the word *sacred* is the root word of *sacrum*. The sacrum is a sacred bone because new life emerges from the pelvic floor and this new life is anchored to the sacrum and passes face down on the sacrum in the voyage through the birth canal. The word *sacred* is associated with the notion of consecration. How is your treatment room and office consecrated? How is it blessed, venerated, or respected? Invoking sacred space creates security against violation from the secular world. Sacred space is safe space and is further defined as having a clearly defined midline. The midline of sacred space is the point of manifestation of the numinous in the healing ritual around which the practitioner-client relationship revolves. This is also called the *containment principle*. This is the authentic code of the biodynamic practitioner. Contact with Primary Respiration and its midline of stillness requires a well-bounded office space and clear vision on the part of the practitioner. The client must know that he has entered another world that is different than the one he just came from. The container and the practitioner must have a midline of stillness to resacralize a world gone crazy.

In addition, sacred space is frequently shaped in a circle. This is what the embryo teaches us. The circle is the symbol of wholeness, as is the embryo. The practitioner actually imagines that she is holding herself and the client in a sphere of living water in a shape that is similar to the human egg—a perfect circle! Many years ago I saw this quote about the meaning of the circle in a book from a Native American whose name I cannot remember. It really impressed me.

> *Everything*
> *the Power of the World does is done*
> *in a circle. The sky is round, and I have heard*
> *that the earth is round like a ball, and so are all the*
> *stars. The wind in its greatest power, whirls. Birds*
> *make their nests in circles, for theirs is the same religion as*
> *ours. The sun comes forth and goes down again in a circle.*
> *The moon does the same and both are round. Even the seasons*
> *form a great circle in their changing and always come back*
> *again to where they were. The life of a man is a circle—*
> *from childhood to childhood, and so it is in everything*
> *where power moves. Our tepees were round like*
> *the nests of birds, and these were always set*
> *in a circle, the nation's hoop, where*
> *great spirit meant for us to*
> *hatch our children.*

The circle is also a symbol for the osteopathic notion of a fulcrum. At the center of the circle is a point of orientation. The point or fulcrum is dynamically still with a power and a potency to shift and transform with the catalyst of Primary Respiration. This brings us back to the embryo and its symmetry. The embryo maintains its circularity throughout its existence and consequently is always oriented to an invisible fulcrum of power in its center. The power at the center point of the embryo is dynamically still. Superimposed onto its circularity is a division of the circle into four quadrants at the beginning of the third week of development. This quadration of the embryo and subsequently the heart is a function of the appearance of the midline.

Mythology

> You must have your own ideas about it. You have to have your own myth. To have your own myth means to have suffered and struggled with a question until an answer has come to you from the depths of your soul. That does not imply that this is the definitive truth, but rather that this truth which has come is relevant for oneself as one now is, and believing in this truth helps one to feel well. Myths, therefore, express vital, instinctive knowledge, and when one trusts in this knowledge, then one is healthy. This has nothing at all to do with wishful thinking or some kind of fantasy. (von Franz, 1995, p. 12)

Now I want to come back to the relationship of the symbol to mythology. To discuss biodynamic practice as spiritual practice requires one to explore the world of mythology as much as metaphor and symbol. I will discuss mythology at length in Chapter 33. For right now, I want to say that mythology is also a depth psychology because it describes the way the world works through the psychology of the unconscious parts of the body and mind. Since it describes the way the world works, it is also an accurate depiction of the way the body works and was originally created before there was language and cognition. This is the domain of the activity of Primary Respiration and the role of stillness in the formation of the human embryo. Mythology is the metaphorical story- and image- (symbol) making capacity of every human cultural system. Symbols and metaphors are brought together to make sense of life in story form about events that occurred before a nervous system was present in the developing embryo. In this sense all mythologies are creation mythologies. To seek meaning and make meaning through story, image, and symbol are organic functions of the human psyche and must take into account the embryonic and pre-embryonic time of life (Jung, 1971; Campbell, 1949).

Mythology is designed to reveal a deeper truth to us about the deepest part of the body and mind. The word myth is misused in modern writing to denote a fallacy or flaw. More correctly it weaves together a cosmology based on current scientific perceptions of reality—psychology, science, psycho-emotional values of the culture, and sociology, such as the political beliefs and governing structures of that culture. Mythology is the way a human system systematically organizes its values, beliefs, and experiences collectively and individually to bring order from chaos. "All the important emotional states from which we suffer are collected in the different creation myths" (von Franz, 1995, p. 215).

Cultures develop symbols for their myths to give meaning to pain and suffering, to make cosmos rather than chaos. All cultures attempt to develop a methodology for curing ills. Bio-medicine cannot be blamed for its shortcomings. The intention is always compassionate action. The means whereby compassion is achieved just seem so bizarre in most hospitals and nursing homes. A new generation of illnesses, expressing the enormity of shock and trauma prevalent today, allows new healing methods to arise spontaneously within the culture. Look at the worldwide popularity of biodynamic craniosacral therapy, and yet it has no scientific evidence for its efficacy!

A symbol now becomes anything that may function as a vehicle for a myth to come alive in the minds of clients (the imaginal expression of the myth—the embryo) and produce the healing effect. The symbol moves out of the domain of conceptual into the perception of the fluid body breathing with Primary Respiration like a dream image. The symbol communicates such concepts and thus structures the myth as a type of shorthand of healing images. The unconscious can read and has already memorized the original text as is known about infants. For instance, the cross is an important symbol to Christians, as I mentioned earlier, and that story continues to evolve. Remember that all human behavior originates in the use of symbols—words, dreams, visual art, gestures, mathematical notations, a behavior, and so on. Groups of symbols that take on larger meanings for a culture are called *life metaphors*. The major world religions are quite familiar with life metaphors. Walk into any church and you will see not only a cross, but also the Stations of the Cross, pictures of the apostles, numerous candles, enormous stained glass depictions of Christian stories, a church organ, and so on. It is the life metaphor of pain and suffering.

Biodynamic craniosacral therapists use a variety of metaphors to distinguish the biodynamic mythology from other craniosacral mythologies. The midline, Primary Respiration, stillpoint, the neutral, the potency of the Breath of Life, the fulcrum, and so on are all code words that evoke an image of the practitioner's hand placement as well as the placement of her body-mind perception. Of course, the most obvious symbol of all craniosacral therapy is the human skull, found in numerous broken plastic renditions in every training program. The skull is an important symbol. A skull with crossed bones indicates poison and toxicity. It also is the flag flown on pirate ships, especially the Black Pearl belonging to Johnny Depp's character in the Pirates of the Caribbean movies.

Some years ago I saw a picture of the skull of Del Close, an actor, who bequeathed his skull to the Goodman Theater in Chicago for use in Shakespeare's *Hamlet.* Everyone can look at a skull and in almost any language say "To be or not to be." Dr. Sutherland changed the core of osteopathy with his first inspiration while reviewing a real human disarticulated skull: "The bones of the skull must be built for respiratory motion." We are here because of that original inspirational disarticulated skull. I wonder which actor gave Dr. Sutherland his first inspiration? At the deepest level, however, the symbol of the skull represents the archetype of immortality. The bones of the body last the longest after death and archaic peoples viewed the bones as representing immortality. Traditional cranial practitioners hold the skulls of their living clients and frequently keep the skulls of dead people in their treatment rooms, even though it is now illegal to import the dead bones of humans. It appears that for almost a century many graves were robbed in India to provide human skeletons to medical schools and doctors. Deep in the unconscious of all craniosacral therapists and cranial osteopaths is this archetype linking the skull to immortality, and it drives some practitioners into the madness of spiritual materialism, an overinflated ego.

The more appropriate mythology of a biodynamic craniosacral therapist involves the exquisite origin myth of the embryo in its first six weeks. It is the new symbol of complete transformation and renewal on the planet Earth at this time. It comes alive as a sensory or imaginal perception of Primary Respiration and its fulcrum of stillness. The embryo can barely be seen by the human eye. This biodynamic story was originated by Erich Blechschmidt (Blechschmidt, 1977), the great German embryologist who scientifically verified Dr. Sutherland's second inspiration on the importance of the inherent ordering capacity of the fluids in the creation of a human being. The new symbol of the embryo replaces the skull. The embryo represents creation, perfection, wholeness, healing, love, generosity, healing, and joy in life. This metaphor of the embryo, however, is invisible during a session and must be carried in the perception of stillness and the movement of Primary Respiration.

On the other hand, the stricken client needs a vocabulary of symbols to understand pain—spiritually, physically, and psychologically. This is the natural function of the myth- (meaning) making for the client. It is the biodynamic midline. Over many years leaders of the Complementary and Alternative Medicine (CAM) movement have devised one script after another, whether it's EST, Rolfing, Gestalt Therapy, craniosacral therapy, biofeedback, and so on. These scripts help the client transition from one way of being or living to another. They help tease out meaning from experience and help pave the road to the interior of the heart. Without a midline, however, the script frequently lacks a happy ending. The Dalai Lama has frequently said that the goal of life is to experience happiness because that is a biological drive common to all humanity.

The biggest questions I am asked by my clients are "What did you do to me during the treatment?" and "When will I get better, based on what you just did?" or "How am I?" This is a difficult script to write each time because the narrative needs to come from the clients. Their own story must be evoked and is usually the trauma story. Clients write their own psychomythology through the affects (symbols) of their trauma, body sensation, images, and so on as they come into relationship with Primary Respiration and the stillness as the origin story. This is why the client must be taught to participate in the biodynamic process, as I detail in Chapter 33. The origin story must be evoked from the client's fluid body and the practitioner is expected to witness the story unfolding its mythic potential in the sense and image of a client being first reconceived and then reborn into a right relationship with the beginning, which was wholeness.

> … to enable him to relate to his trauma story as a real but inauthentic statement about the reality of his life. Or to put it another way, the therapeutic work had been successful in enabling him to see that the trauma story that he had been living was in fact an overlay burying a more personal and authentic story *and that the trauma story came externally from sources outside of himself* and therefore was inauthentic as his personal origins myth. It was his *experience* of the trauma—his interpretation of his own suffering—but it was not his existential "origins story," the source of which is transpersonal. (Bernstein, 2006, p. 147)

The biodynamic paradigm carries a deep richness in its symbolism because it now matches the scientific and political methodology regarding embryology. As science and medicine now recall the loss of their own heart and soul from seventeenth-century politics and even earlier, the attempt is being made to ingest CAM practices through the laws of double-blind scientific studies and evidence-based efficacy studies. CAM practices will be scrutinized, as well they should be, but much of the scrutiny will fail through an objective, genetic reduction. Ordered movement in the fluids of the embryo and the adult as it relates to healing cannot be quantified by double-blind studies, the gold standard of bio-medicine with its tenuous hold on reality. But the origin story of ordered movement in the fluids can be palpated and sensed with knowing, thinking, feeling hands. Much of CAM and biodynamic craniosacral therapy operate in the symbolic world of mythology, which is equally valid if not more so than science. The embryo is the symbol for wholeness and its uncanny ability to facilitate healing can be researched through subjective studies that now are gaining equal validity scientifically. The embryo is perhaps the most powerful symbol of healing as can be attested from the stem cell research debate among church leaders, politicians, and scientists. The embryo is now in the mainstream of our culture. Biodynamic practice employs these images and perceptions of origins for much the same reason as stem cell research is done to effect a cure for disease, but without subjecting the human embryo to dissection in a laboratory. The embryo is alive and well in every body, old and new. Medicine disavowed the corporeal perception of Primary Respiration and stillness many centuries ago. Machines do not have fluid movement. Biodynamic craniosacral therapy is reclaiming to the origin story of the embryo and its perpetual existence in the human body and heart by a completely different means.

Exercise: The Four Quadrants of the Midline

> A splitting into two parts therefore precedes every conscious realization. Often also before an unconscious content becomes conscious, when it touches the threshold of consciousness, it tends to split into two parts: this is generally the step immediately before it wells up over the threshold of consciousness. This is connected with the fact that no psychological process is imaginable for us without an underlying duality or polarity. As long as the opposites are one and in union, no conscious process is possible. (von Franz, 1995, p. 240)

A Creation Myth: At conception the human embryo initiates a phase of incarnation through a process of polarization or twinning. Conception occurs at the intersecting point of time and eternity. Thus at conception, two things are generated: something bound to time as matter and another thing not bound to time but carried in and around matter. Some call it no-self or emptiness. This is a metaphor for spirit. It is nontemporal. It is the void. The entire development of the embryo to a fetus to an infant to a child to an adolescent to an adult is ripe with polarities as we are met by time and the body becomes bound by the decay of time and coupled to the conditions inherent in the family system and culture. Simultaneously, we maintain a relationship with the eternal presence of the void in and around each of us by the midline that arises in the third week postfertilization. The circle of the embryo can now be subdivided into four quadrants and four chambers of the heart. This is how the midline is linked to the four directions.

The void was our original state of nonexistence moments before the egg we came from differentiated. Even the process of fertilization involves a bifurcation of the female cell nucleus in order to merge with the male genetic material. Twenty-four hours after conception the first cleavage into two occurs. The one becomes two but the one is always present. Twin cells are created containing the potency to become a full and complete human being. Again and again, the original cell multiplies in the first week and each is influenced by the internal and external milieu of the fluids inside and outside the each cell. Every cell in this first week is pluripotent and capable of becoming a full human being. These are the original and most powerful stem cells.

The mother's perception of her environment, her stress levels, her thoughts, and all that is in her temporal world cross the placental barrier as molecules entering the bloodstream of the embryo and shaping the heart, brain, and vascular system of the embryo. This begins in the second week more formally. This includes modifications in the cell nucleus and engineering of specific genes that will be necessary to handle an environment similar to the mother's (if necessary) when the child is born. Unfortunately, these genetic changes in the embryo are for the most part oriented to security, danger, protection, withdrawal, and contraction. The sentient embryo is imprinted with the fear of death constantly from a stressful environment that it shares with its mother.

At the same time the mother's womb represents the consciousness of the divine feminine. The word is made flesh and incarnates. It is the holy womb, the consecrated womb where Primary Respiration manifests its "unerring" potency. It is the vessel of the Holy Spirit, which is the Breath of Life. Thus the mother is the divine mother and provides an umbilical connection and resistance to the unborn. The womb by definition is sacred space and when the mother is not synchronized with the intention to manifest life in the sacred container of her womb, the child is lost and adrift, alienated from the divine, and easily identifies with causes and conditions of the family history.

Thus the fundamental polarities of time and eternity (the circle), good and bad, light and dark are present from conception onward. Some would say that these polarities are produced from multi-generational trauma coming from a time well before conception. Stress, however, is the necessary resistance to discover wholeness and love. I want to introduce you to an exercise developed by my friend Judith Suarez. It will help ground the discussion of the circle and the midline with its four directions.

A fundamental polarity in creation mythology and depth psychology is the masculine and feminine. The womb, by definition, is feminine. It is the place of gestation, resting, and nurturing. But the masculine movement of growing out into the world must be there to balance this phase of incarnation. It is the dark feminine represented by depression, lethargy, unconsciousness, and addiction that must be guarded against. That is why, in life, depression is a movement back to the dark feminine aspect of the womb, which drowns the psyche of the individual. On the other hand, if the dark masculine is present and the patri-archal thrust, movement, and impulse to create finds itself in a rational rage, the psyche will die of thirst from the lack of feminine transformation available in the ritual of regressing to the womb spoken of in Volume One. This ritual is reenacted each time a therapist attends to the ocean of Primary Respiration and tracks the conception ignition process. Short periods of time in the womb are indeed restorative. Extended stays are life threatening and can be lethal. The ritual of healing in the container of stillness (masculine) and Primary Respiration (feminine) must be precise.

The feminine is the mother of transforming and releasing love. She is the divine and the eternal within the substance and material of the embryo. He is the father principle of potency, the urgent sense of purpose, direction, and creation, the carrier of feelings as opposed to the expresser of feelings. The embryo starts in a state of undifferentiated feminine wholeness and moves through different thresholds at the end of each of the first three weeks of development. Balance with the masculine is represented by its incredible drive these specific thresholds of embryonic development, birth, and the lifespan as well. As an individual or as an embryo passes through each threshold, the polarization between spirit and matter quickens or condenses, especially with regard to one's gender. This gives rise to the consciousness of the masculine and feminine polarities expressed as gender differences but really rooted in no gender specificity at all. These polarities include the dark and the light masculine and the dark and the light feminine. The individuation process of becoming an adult requires balance between these polari-ties as we walk through life. Each is represented by a quadrant of the circle.

Do this practice with a friend. First, draw a circle on the ground in your sacred space. Make it a big circle, 10 feet or more in diameter. Prepare yourself with meditation and purification on the outside of the circle. Synchronize your attention with Primary Respiration moving from your heart to the heart of a spiritual friend or teacher. Wait until the circle beckons you to enter. One by one, stand in each quadrant and read out loud each of the five lists below. One list is read per quadrant until you reach the middle at the end.

Walking the Circle of the Embryo

I AM THE LIGHT MASCULINE
I do the right thing
I steward the earth and nature
I carry my feelings with me at all times
I dispense justice

I maintain the peace
I move into the world with right potency
I actualize,
I create,
I move.
I AM THE DARK MASCULINE
I am afraid of the dark
I am fear
I am lonely
I am terror
I am intolerant of other beliefs/values
I am a terrorist who destroys random targets
I am wounded in my father-mother relationship by necessity
I starve the feminine
I am an efficient killing machine.
I AM THE LIGHT FEMININE
I nurture
I am the hearth
I provide warmth
I gestate transformation
I am generous
I am love
I am mercy
I am the ultimate transformer.
I AM THE DARK FEMININE
I am the dark suffocating womb
I hold everyone in my claws
I am depression
I am addiction
I am Pele
I am Kali
I am rage that knows no bounds
I destroy everything with my rage
I drown the masculine.
I STAND IN THE MIDDLE
I am connected to my midline
I own my shadow
I own my light
I am divine.

The dark feminine is the animal, the addict, and the qualities of the night. These represent the unconscious womb container of the psyche and the uterus. This is the suffocating womb. The feminine conceives in a dark cave of the womb. The cave becomes home and hearth. The masculine must leave, but will always return for the elixir of transformation and promise of release. If not, the feminine womb regresses in depression, lethargy, and negativity. The light feminine is the nurturer, lover, and feeder of the masses. She guards the home and the hearth. She is the principle of fertility and the generation of life. She is pregnant with possibility in a warm, gestating, comfortable womb, willing to let go of her divine child.

The light masculine is the principle of growth and the one who plans for the future. But it is true growth and not just an adjustment to the demands of time. The light masculine does the right thing and the forces of rage, war, and aggression are subjugated to this principle of justice and wisdom. However, the dark masculine is out of balance in the extremes of fear and terror. While the dark masculine is intolerant of ideas and peoples and is a selective killing machine with low collateral damage, the dark feminine indiscriminately destroys all that comes in her path. The dark feminine is completely berserk with her rage. The dark strives to not fall prey to the light. These forces of the dark and light masculine and feminine must be balanced in the psyche for the transcendent function to occur. We incarnate as spirit and matter at conception. This is followed by spirit manifesting both light and dark and matter holding both light and dark.

There are many polarities that manifest at conception and even preconception. The polarity of masculine and feminine carries forward throughout the entire lifespan as fundamental to the process of growth and development. How can we stay in the present time and differentiate as an adult and at the same time clear issues from the prenatal realm? Creation mythology and depth psychology have much to teach us in this regard. To go forward in life and to individuate, as Carl Jung would say, requires a balance between the opposites and complementary functions of the masculine and feminine. After all, what Carl Jung said is that if we can develop the capacity to hold and contain the raw energy of these fundamental polarities without freaking out, then the transcendent function can arise. We hold these polarities individually and we hold these polarities as a function of participating in therapeutic relationships.

Ultimately the biodynamic practitioner is the carrier of the symbol of creation and healing. No longer can the practitioner externalize these symbols and rely on traditional symbols in this day and age, as discussed throughout this chapter. The biodynamic practitioner uses the metaphor of the fluid body to contact his own sense of Primary Respiration and stillness as an embodied, incarnate reality.

> So as soon as we begin to speak about the phenomenon of consciousness, we set forth, logically, the counter aspect, the unconscious. Also, if we remember that the unconscious is full of luminosity, we can really say that, basically, they are coequal phenomena which have not evolved out of each other in a time sequence, but existed from the very beginning as two coequal tendencies in the psyche. (von Franz, 1995, p. 109)

CHAPTER 33

Mythology and Biodynamic Practice

To begin healing what is broken in ourselves and in our relationship to the natural world, we need to see and feel what is within us and around us. (Amorok, 2007, p. 29)

I would like to continue the discussion of origin begun in the previous chapter and go deeper into understanding how healing happens. The biodynamic paradigm goes beyond the mechanistic stages of relaxation and correction in many of the manual therapeutic arts, into a third stage called *transmutation* (Maitland, 1995). I stated previously that the human embryo is the symbol of transformation in healing. This comes about not only through the image of the embryo itself, but its ability to transmute itself through its fluid structure. Transmutation means to change from one nature, form, or substance into another such as from sorrow to joy or from one stage of the human embryo to another. The alchemical tradition in the Middle Ages sought to convert base metals into gold. The biodynamic work of transmutation is being guided by the Primary Respiration and stillness found to create the human embryo. The substance of the fluid body of the embryo initially transmutes itself into a condensed gel-like structure free of genetic influence (Ingber, 2006).

The world of transmutation is the world of metaphor, symbol, and myth. It is the world of the future brought into the present, not the past being activated in the present. Rather than a vertical, masculine, hierarchical world of authoritarian figures in control of life, Primary Respiration represents a feminine horizontal world of I and Thou (Buber, 1971) coming through the umbilicus. Biodynamic craniosacral therapy is a descending pathway into our unconscious into the endodermal origins and watery beginnings as a sea sponge. It is a heart-to-heart and blood-to-blood connection, placenta to body and body to placenta. It is a growing down into the blood and mesenteries, a remembering of our sea creature and reorientation to the stillpoint in the bones of our body and stillness of a field of wheat in mid-summer. This is the meaning of biodynamic transmutation.

The Four Roles of Mythology

> The newness of the spiritual life, its autonomy, could find no better expression than the images of an "absolute beginning," images whose structure is anthropocosmic, deriving at once from embryology and from cosmogony. (Eliade, 1958, p. 60)

The first role of mythology is to get us in touch with the mystery of life. Biodynamic craniosacral therapy enters into this mystery in every session. This is because it explores the meaning of incarnation from an embryological point of view. It explores the way healing happens, both in a traditional pre-Western as well as in a contemporary context. This will be further explored in subsequent chapters. Both of these healing metaphors and their symbolism are essential mysteries. A mystery cannot be solved. It can be entered into and provide a revelation about the truth of life. The biodynamic practitioner must be willing to enter the mystery in every session.

The second role of myth by definition is its cosmological correctness. Dr. Blechschmidt's morphological embryology parallels mythology and draws from it. Many myths such as the Babylonian origin story talk of creation coming from a watery beginning. The Genesis story in the Bible is oceanic in parts. Furthermore, culture and society are shaped by myth. This is the third role of myth to provide a spiritual infrastructure or midline around which a culture can sustain itself and be fed by the source of creation. Central to the notion of biodynamic mythology is that the Breath of Life animates the embryo. It is further related to the power of Dynamic Stillness from which the Breath of Life arose. The original founders of the Cranial Concept used theological language to describe the sensory experience of the work with clients. Some of the founders of the Cranial Concept considered that the work was a prayer. Each session was viewed as a blessing when contact with the Breath of Life was made. Thus myth began to shape a contemporary healing practice.

When the future healers of the world go through their first childhood initiations they are either blessed or they are cursed. The joy of openness or the curse of depression starts at an early age. Purification and sacrifice are required to lift a spiritual depression from an early initiation of childhood trauma. Sacrifice is not meant in an arduous Old Testament way but rather a renunciation of one's behavior and ignorance. It may be years or lifetimes before one reconnects with the love inherent in the perception of Primary Respiration and stillness. I love the story of how Krishna from the Hindu pantheon of gods gives those who choose the spiritual path, the ability and knowledge to follow the spiritual path. And Krishna also gives those who have no desire to follow a spiritual path the ability and knowledge to not follow a spiritual path.

The fourth role of myth is to carry people through life crises. To carry people through life crises, the myth would provide information on proper *rites of initiation.* It breaks parental dependency, causes a rerelating to the midline and a discovery process of one's purpose in life and what is meant to be human. Proper mythology involves the integration of three levels within a society: the cosmological, the sociological, and psychological. According to Joseph Campbell, the twentieth century was moving more toward individual and cluster mythologies. A cluster mythology occurs when a group of people, such as practitioners of biodynamic craniosacral therapy, gather together around the deep mythic story of the sentient embryo, from which flows certain values and beliefs.

Creation Myths

> As the exemplary model for all "creation," the cosmogenic myth can help the patient to make a "new beginning" of his life. The *return to origins* gives the hope of rebirth. Now all the medical rituals we have been examining aim at a return to origins. We get the impression that for archaic societies life cannot be *repaired,* it can only be *re-created* by a return to sources. And the "source of sources" is the prodigious outpouring of energy, life, and fecundity that occurred at the Creation of the World. (Eliade, 1963, p. 30)

Some researchers have said that all myths are creation myths. The biblical Genesis story is the prevalent creation myth in the West. A more elaborate myth is the Navajo creation story in Chapter 35. Both creation myths are pivotal in understanding biodynamic craniosacral therapy. The Breath of Life from the Book of Genesis is an origin myth because it is linked to the creation of the body in the first six weeks of the embryological development. Erich Blechschmidt says, "In actual fact, no specific chemical substances capable of causing differentiation have ever been demonstrated (in the embryo), and the 'organizer' is still a *Deus ex machina*" (Blechschmidt, 1977, p. 11). I have interpreted a part of Psalm 139 as follows from several different versions. I think King David would like this:

> You guided my creation into this world
> You placed me in the waters of my mother's womb
> I am humbled because of the exquisite way you shaped me

I do not doubt your power.
And this I know in the stillness of my heart
Where your presence dwells.
You saw my body being formed
From elements deep in the earth
Weaving together a splendid fabric
Before I was born you knew everything I would become.

This numinous Breath of Life in the embryo is part of our adult physiology right now according to some embryologists! Now it is called perfection and wholeness imprinted in the fluids of the embryo in the first six weeks of development. The wholeness and perfection of the embryo exists in present time, in the adult body as a lasting and unchanging preexisting condition of incarnation. It is none other than the perception of Primary Respiration and the stillness. The Breath of Life, an aspect of Primary Respiration, doesn't know that it's not whole or not perfect. Genetic modifications, disease, and inertia of all kinds cause the embryo to forget this fact of its original wholeness and perfection. The embryo encountered conditions of pain and suffering as a sentient being and forgot its own essence. Thus, biodynamic practice involves rituals that reconnect the client to the memory and perception of origin—located in the fluids of the early embryo. We are both whole and dissociated as a normal function of life and its irony. Neither one nor the other is preferred. They exist as a dance, a tension pull between opposites. To become fully human is to encounter the huge resistance of life and sit still in the middle of our heart. Dissociation is actually a threshold experience of the divine, as I will discuss in the next chapter.

What *is* infinitely important, to my mind, is the beginning, the swelling of the embryo, and then greed, which we had in so many other myths. Then "inner conception"—a conception which takes place completely within—that would be a little like Enoia. Then preparation, something completely vague. Then the impulse to search; that is the anxiety which we had in the other myth: What, where, how … ? That kind of frustrated anxiety. Then something like order, but the order of cells themselves in a circle, or in some form. The very, very small thing, the sperm of an embryo, the not-yet, but with a tendency toward being, the not-yet, with a feeling of frustration, and then all the others. Then depression also, as one of the essential aspects, the being narrowed in depression. (von Franz, 1995, p. 208)

The best way to understand the beginnings of a human being is the creation myth itself. Human embryology is the creation myth of Western civilization at this point in time. The embryo has different storytellers and versions in this day and age. It offers stricken patients a new beginning to life through the use of embryonic stem cells or wholeness and healing through contact with Primary Respiration, which formed the embryo as in Psalm 139. Understanding our own mythology and its ritual use for healing makes it possible for the client to be reconceived and to have the hope of eventually being reborn in a right relationship with pain and suffering. The trend in contemporary medical rituals is to retrieve the biological substance of this embryonic origin seen on the covers of newspapers and magazines for the last decade and inject it into the diseased body of client. There is an enormous scientific ritual necessary to recover embryonic stem cells. It must be remembered, however, that this ritual and this healing movement of recovering one's origins from the unconscious to the conscious mind has been known by ancient societies forever. This means that these ancient cultures knew that the human body could not be fixed at first by external agents or medicines per se. The human body could only be healed by the ritual of recreation and a remembering of the original embryonic state from which the client came. The Navajo story is clear about this. The ritual of healing implies a going back to the time of creation to recreate the cosmos in its original form. Thus the presentation of the origin myth in song, prayer, and sand painting is not only for the purposes of remembrance and education, but to allow the patient to identify with those symbolic forces that once created the world, and by entering into them to recreate himself in a state of health and wholeness. This is the correct sequence for healing. The medicine and surgery might come second rather than first. The original source of life and the enormous generative potential of all energy, life, and animation is available at the moment of creation and even now in the soma as the perception of Primary Respiration and its fulcrum of stillness.

New Cosmology

From the fact that man was created and civilized by Supernatural Beings, it follows that the sum of his behavior and activities belongs to sacred history; and this history must be carefully preserved and transmitted intact to succeeding generations. Basically, man is what he is because, at the dawn of Time, certain things happened to him, the things narrated by the myths. But whereas modern man sees in the history that precedes him a purely human work and, more especially, believes that he has the power to continue and perfect it indefinitely, for the man of traditional societies everything significant—that is, everything creative and powerful—that has ever happened took place *in the beginning,* in the Time of the myths. (Eliade, 1958, p. xi)

Concurrent with this understanding of human embryology is the new cosmological understanding now being put on the second page of newspapers and magazines worldwide—the creation of the world itself and the theory of the Big Bang. Astrogeophysicists are peering back at the origin of the world with surprising clarity and have already seen Earth class planets in other galaxies for the first time in 2007. The very frontiers of science are oriented toward origin, whether it is the origin of the human or the origin of the universe itself. This is the deepest part of our unconscious speaking, making a ritual and attempting to heal contemporary society from the scourge of its own making.

Thus the healing ritual in biodynamic craniosacral therapy is a presentation of the origin myth of the embryo in the form of the movement of Primary Respiration and the prayer of Dynamic Stillness. The session becomes a sand painting similar to the great sand paintings of the Tibetan and Navajo cultures. The painting has a midline, four directions, and the intention to touch this original mind and space of healing through the creative act. The client is allowed to identify with these symbolic forces as a real sensory reality found in the total fluid continuum of the body. It is the same sensory reality present at the moment of conception. The client enters into this oceanic space in order to recreate himself in a right relationship with the original health and wholeness.

The biodynamic principles of healing regarding the return to origins, reconception, and rebirth into right relationship with nature and the divine have been the main healing functions for the whole human race from the beginning of time. These are both archetypal and maybe even genetic forms of instinctual healing and knowing. Thus they serve to function outside the domain of conscious intention. It is not about intelligent design or evolution at all. Every age of man gives rise to new adaptations of this original instinctual healing process, because of the constant change in the social and cultural environment. The first principle is always the return to source and the original moment of creation, whether it is the creation of the universe or a single human being. The science of embryology was initiated at the same time as the Cartesian duality became the norm of science in the sixteenth and seventeenth centuries. The birth of the problem gave rise to the solution. It is always so. All origin mythologies speak to this truth. Healing is always a part of the origin myth for the Navajo (Sandner, 1979).

Cosmopolitan Mythology

The sociological aspect of the Western mythology today is based on economic growth and expansion, along with psychological stability. It is a cosmopolitan mythology. It complicates the Bible's creation myth as much as the Navajo myth because it generates a dark side of creation. For one example, it has spawned terrorism as its bastard offspring. Marxism and Leninism were the early markers of the current atrocities seen in the Middle East and elsewhere in the world as a reaction to the reification of money and financial centers of the world displacing the spiritual centers beginning in the nineteenth century. Western mythology involves rigorous science: believing in the domination of nature (paving over Paradise and putting up a parking lot) and the supremacy of patriarchal values (oil, oil, and oil). It is a world view promising to find the answers to life in the atomic structure of living cells, both plant and animal, and then once found, to control it, invest in it, and corner the financial market with it. It takes $250 million to bring a new pharmaceutical drug onto the market these days. It is a science of domination where man is at the hierarchical *top of the heap* and in *control* of himself and of nature (everything). It is a rational fantasy that does not speak to the whole, only the elite few who own the hedge funds and run the World Bank. Mankind is reduced to what is on deposit in his bank account and an annual contribution of several thousand dollars into an Investment Retirement Account (IRA), if he is lucky. This generates an enormous psychological dilemma.

This aspect of the West's mythic exodus from rationality is its democratic sociology: the right to life, liberty, and the pursuit of happiness. This is the American value system (imported from Europe) that implies *entitlement.* It implies that every American is entitled to health care (life), freedom (mine, not ours), and happiness (mine, not yours). This is the myth of the individual and the Maverick of stage, screen, and television that I grew up with. Mark Twain once said that two out of every three Americans were willing to look out for your best interest by force or the threat of a lawsuit. It is individual rights, individual morality, and very much about a *lone ranger* and his journey. Early American cowboy art is completely devoid of emotionality and connectivity to a life force—only me and my horse, or my Mustang convertible or Hummer or whatever. The American dream is the right to have someone else pay for taking care of my body when it breaks down. Regardless of how much I abuse my body, someone else will take care of it. My parents were promised this and live it. We, however, are promised higher health care costs and no insurance for the truly needy.

This mythology is economically based, not spiritually based. Financial centers are the preeminent structures in any modern metropolis, not churches or factories (Keen, 1992). Money and power (of the individual or individual corporation) fuel this mythology and the psycho-economic bait is this: *You don't have enough.* You not only do not have enough, but even if you spend your money on getting it, it would still not be enough. Bring on the debt and keep us all indentured servants of the Dow Jones. Robert Lipstyle calls this the new pornography. Fast food, expensive fashion, expensive fitness, and financial news are the four Fs of this pornography. These four Fs are disguised as news and blot out information that is really needed on how to live life.

The last component of mythology then defines psychology and the individual behavior of a human being. While Freud (Freud, 1910) himself was a pioneer in describing the inner workings of the psychological self, his theory was also reductionistic. His psychological view cast humans into a tightly fit diagnosis as sexually repressed and resistant to change (Herman, 1992). While this is a simplistic reduction of a great body of knowledge, it nonetheless is helpful in developing a flavor of the flaws now being exposed in the Western mythology. Western culture is psycho-economically based (Hillman, 1975). Psychology pervades our life. Humans are seen as a group of resistances needing to be overcome with advertising, surgery, food, medication, and so on. In order to control life and the life force of sexuality, people must be convinced that their childhood was psychologically depraved and then be able to therapize their existence, identify old feelings, and purge themselves when urged by well-meaning practitioners, friends, and family (Jackson, 1994). The Breath of Life goes into exile with this mythology.

The Snake Skin

The soma inherits family traits and predispositions to disease and illness. This is a body myth: "Well, my father died of congestive heart failure at 64 and his father of the same thing at age 63, so I expect I'll die of it too." Genetic predisposition is also called a *rational fantasy.* There are numerous ways to construct a body myth. By imitating the posture of the mother and father, bodies take on all that is held within those forms. All children do this. As I was relearning how to walk after my knee surgery last year, I realized I had been walking exactly like my mother all my life. Taking on the excess baggage of parents' negative emotions and abnormal behaviors doubles the load on a baby's body and developing brain. Then later, children are given instructions on how to ignore their body, usually through the prohibition of touching and feeling.

Violence is rampant in the media and on the playgrounds of many schools. Society has its taboos around the body and these are also passed along via the school system, parents, friends, and the media. This causes a pervasive alienation from the soma. Work on the emotions is overinflated in our culture, in part because of the enormity of stress and trauma that occurs on a daily basis to most human beings, as I discussed at length in the section Relating with Trauma. It is no longer about emotions; it is about the sensation that precedes the emotion. There is a tendency to define one's self through what one feels and experiences emotionally at the expense of a deep alienation and dissociation from the stillpoint in the heart and a connection to nature, which I will speak to in the next chapter. It is through this deep connection in the heart of the body that emotions can be free of having to handle the pain and suffering of passion, aggression, and ignorance. The pain of passionately owning material goods, the aggression of intolerance and hatred, and the ignorance of not seeing clearly how the world works covers the heart with an almost impenetrable barrier to the space of stillness and wisdom in general. Emotional experiences and turmoil, however, are impermanent—they always go away at some point. As is said in the Bible, "This too shall pass." The work of biodynamic craniosacral therapy is to find the stillpoint in the center of the heart and be able to move flexibly in and out of the heart with Primary Respiration being the felt sense of love. It is about a sensory experience of the fluids. The movement in and out of the heart allows us to connect to a spiritual principle, person, or thing that is at once transcendent and beyond the horizon, and at the same time, eminently available as a sensory experience in the core of the body, which is the center of the heart (Remen, 1995).

What are the body myths each of us grew up with? How can each of us discover within the heart of the body how my unique story is unfolding across time and differentiate it from my family story and the culture's story? Myth tells us the deepest meaning of the world in a story form. The information age has caught everyone in the middle of shifting myths. Western culture is currently fluctuating between some big stories of power and healing. This causes incredible anxiety and depression. The stories of science overturn the stories of the past and cause conflict spiritually. Contemporary society has attempted to secularize a spiritual mythology and remove the power of archetypal imagery by reducing it to a *technology,* a theme park or an animated Disney movie, mythology trading cards, high-fantasy computer games, or self-help books. This removes the heart and the imagination of a culture and creates spiritual chaos which is split off and buried in the matter of our body. The chaos becomes embodied, put on television and in the movies. The unfinished business of religion, politics, science, and spirituality have nowhere to go but into the human body with illness, disease, and death. Species become extinct, species are found diseased, and children staff foreign armies. The body is eaten by the shadow of society and decomposes in the undigested elements of society and culture. And then the medical system is called upon to fix the body. It is impossible. Only bacon is cured.

We are truly like a snake shedding its skin because we are transitioning from one phase of a body myth to another with the speed of light. Speed kills, as any highway patrol officer will tell you. Our deepest fear is of change and the unknown. It is quite easy to be paralyzed by fear. The fear must be transmuted with stillness and Primary Respiration. For thousands and maybe millions of years we were hunter-gatherers, and only recently, some 10,000 years ago, did we gradually change into an agricultural society. Now the culture is shifting into an information society that is youth oriented. By being youth oriented, the culture places value on being young. Consequently, fear, panic, loss, isolation, and irrelevance are what this culture gives to its senior citizens. The hunting tribes leave you behind, but the gathering tribes keep you around as a symbol of wisdom. Walk into any modern nursing home and look for Primary Respiration and the stillpoint. My mother lived on total life support equipment for twelve years before she died and it was not pretty. I was her health care surrogate in the state that made Terry Schiavo famous before she died.

The myth of the individual is devastating to the body-mind-nature connection. Anxiety arises from the discontinuous sense of self that lacks a relationship with the dynamism of a stillpoint. Am I alone in my togetherness with the other? This is the paradox that we continually work with. I am part of a vast interconnecting web of causes, conditions, people, and environment, yet I have a metabolism that knows the aloneness of being a single entity. I walk alone on this path together with others. My conception rights are joy and happiness. Joy and happiness (effects of Primary Respiration and stillness) arise from appreciating the lack of continuity behind our thoughts, feelings, emotions, and body rather than accumulating fame and fortune (Beck, 1993). This is simply a stillpoint.

Health

First and foremost, there is the well-known symbolism of initiation rituals implying a *regressus ad uterum*. … We will limit ourselves here to some brief indications. From the archaic stages of culture the initiation of adolescents includes a series of rites whose symbolism is crystal clear: through them, the novice is first transformed into an embryo and then is reborn. Initiation is equivalent to a second birth. It is through the agency of initiation that the adolescent becomes both a socially responsible and culturally awakened being. The return to the womb is signified either by the neophyte's seclusion in a hut, or by his being symbolically swallowed by a monster, or by his entering a sacred spot identified with the uterus of Mother Earth. (Eliade, 1963, pp. 79–82.)

The soma is a process that is largely unconscious and waiting to come to consciousness. I am shaped more by epigenetic experience (everything outside the cell nucleus that creates the major processes needed for development and differentiation of our body, especially the living water in the body) than by my DNA/RNA complex (Harman, 1995; Blechschmidt, 1977). As Erich Blechschmidt said, "The genes are the letters, the fluids create the words." The soma is socially shaped by values and beliefs, by culture and history. Inherited traits may suddenly change rather than gradually change in this postmodern world. This is the true meaning of epigenesis (Weaver, et al., 2007). The body and mind are self-organizing because of the potency of Primary Respiration. They are in a constant state of emergence and of becoming something new. Transmutation is now, always now.

We are entering a whole new paradigm called conception, according to Daniel Pink (Pink, 2005). At every moment I am a perfect and complete embryo. At every moment I am torn, fragmented, and incomplete. Then every 100 seconds Primary Respiration reconceives me in perfect order for that moment in time. Differentiation is the ability to make distinctions between pathological parts of myself. Freedom is the transmutation of parts into an emerging whole movement of Primary Respiration. Wholeness is the original state, the origin of our perfection in the embryo during the first six weeks. The core of my fragmented self exists and demands equal time whether or not it's located in the DNA. It is the shadow cast by transgenerational family patterns and twisted luck. This is the new creation mythology.

Creation myths involve imagination and prenatal history. They are preverbal. They involve knowing the sacred places in life and the sacred experiences. This means having a spiritual midline to reference frequently. Life unfolds from the future to the present rather than the past to the present. The old fallacy is backward causation, that is, because I was traumatized as a child, I will be traumatized as an adult (bringing the past to the present). This goes along with the contemporary fallacy of catharsis therapy: I can cry my way to health. However, this is not the way embryonic life and time evolves. Waiting for the future to come into the present is the dynamic of transmutation. Primary Respiration and the stillness bring the future into the present. They are the health everyone craves.

Biodynamic practice seeks to synchronize with the health of the embryo in each adult. This is a perceptual process and not an idle dream. Health is not static; rather, it is a moving, developmental process. The embryo has a "vast memory of a very perfect process that takes a long time to etch itself into a human form" (Hagopian, 2001, p. 90). This means that as the embryo forms, it does so in a sequence of twenty-three stages of transmutation. Each stage has a structure of its own as seen through its movement and shaping processes that change in the next stage. Each stage is whole and complete unto itself and yet displays qualities that are different from anything found in the previous levels of growth and development. Movement behaviors seen at one embryonic stage of development can give rise to a completely different order of behavior in the next stage.

Transmutation is the basic nature of biological life and consequently psychological life. This is a crucial factor in understanding the dynamic morphology not only of the human embryo, but also adult behavior and thus the entire lifespan development. Biodynamic transmutation processes perceived by the practitioner in the client are part of the creative intelligence of Primary Respiration and its fulcrum of stillness. They operate 24/7. Order and organization of the transmutation process are understood to be in the fluids of the embryo and the biodynamic ordering movements in these fluids called Primary Respiration and those of the fluid body. These transmutation processes are seen in the human embryo long before a brain begins to differentiate (Harman, 1995).

Angeles Arrien (Arrien, 1993) has suggested that the culture move away from a focus on psychopathology toward one based on psychomythology. I have tried to point out the myths we live by in this chapter. Joseph Campbell (Campbell, 1949), James Hillman (Hillman, 1975), and Sam Keen (Keen, 1992) speak to the disappearance of the personal myths of transmutation by living out the myth of growth, development, and neuroscience devoid of heart. How can I frame my personal history and move into authentic autobiography in a culture that has dismissed the importance of creation mythology? Enter the embryo. It is through embryology, the ability to relate to a deeper truth about our origins, the relevance of embryonic growth processes, and transmutation via Primary Respiration that I differentiate into a full human being. The many become one thing again. This is the transmutation of an appropriate relationship with the midline, the axis Mundi, the Tree of Life. The creation mythology of the embryo is essential to help everyone transition from a self-centered world into the world of nature and our own divine body.

> The cosmogenic myth serves as the paradigm, the exemplary model, for every kind of making. Nothing better ensures the success of any creation (a village, a house, a child) than the fact of copying it after the greatest of all creations, the cosmogony. Nor is this all. Since in the eyes of the primitives the cosmogony primarily represents the manifestation of the creative power of the gods, and therefore a prodigious irruption of the sacred, it is periodically reiterated in order to regenerate the world and human society. For symbolic repetition of the creation implies a reactualization of the primordial event, hence the presence of the Gods and their creative energies. The return to beginnings finds expression in a reactivation of the sacred forces that had then been manifested for the first time. If the world was restored to the state in which it had been at the moment when it came to birth, if the gestures that the Gods had made for the first time in the beginning were reproduced, society and the entire cosmos became what they had been then—pure, powerful, effectual, with all their possibilities intact. (Eliade, 1958, p. xii)

CHAPTER 34

Spiritual Disease and the Biodynamic Process

Humans are born with an animistic sense of the world, an ability to perceive the soul of nature. Such an enchanted perspective provides the foundation for healthy human development. (Amorok, 2007, p. 30)

The Bear in the Woods

I had a dream about meeting a large bear. I was in a cabin in the woods. I saw a big bear and I gave the bear some food. Then I went for a walk and it started to follow me. I became afraid and started to run and the bear began to chase me. I tried to climb a tree in my fear and could feel it close behind me, climbing right up the tree. I had to wake myself up. I was afraid to turn and face the bear and ask what it wanted. I was afraid to have a dialogue with the forces of nature that had come to me to help heal my dissociation from nature. This is the primal dissociation in contemporary society. Carl Jung said that our world has become completely dehumanized with its focus on scientific understanding (Jung, 1976). Consequently, we are no longer involved in nature except by taking vacations at condominiums on beautiful beaches. We have lost our emotional participation in even the simplest natural events such as a sunrise and a sunset. Now we tell our children that the sun rises because of the earth's rotation and we have lost the symbolic meaning of coming from the night into the day and how the day turns into the darkness of the night. Likewise, lightning and thunder are no longer the voice of God. Rivers don't have spirits and trees don't represent the life of a human being. A snake is no longer the embodiment of earth's wisdom and no mountain has an enlightened being sitting at its top or in a cave except in cartoons.

The symbol-producing function of our dream material at night is one attempt to bring our original consciousness back to light. This is a place where consciousness has not ever been before or where the ego has "undergone critical self reflection" (Jung, 1976, p. 591). At one time, we were that original mind and have lost contact with it. It was eliminated by rationality long before trying to understand it and, more important, feel it in the core of the soma.

I lost my ability to talk to the bear somewhere along the way. The primitive bushman that I once was no longer befriends wild animals. If a real bear confronts me in the woods, I am to yell and scream and not look it in the eye. If it charges, I am to fall on the ground and play dead. If a shark bites me when I am swimming, I am to punch it in the nose. If an alligator bites me, I am to jam my thumbs in its eyes. All this is the latest advice from the National Park Service. My communication with nature has been lost and the emotional energy necessary to live in nature is buried deep in my heart and mind. The instinctual intelligence of nature in the fluid body of my soma is missing. This is dissociation in its truest sense of the word.

Dissociation is first and foremost an alienation from nature and a loss of connection with the other sentient beings of this planet. Otherwise, why would this culture be terrified by dissociation, and spacing out (into nature) be forbidden? There is a relentless demand for adaptive effectiveness to improve the financial bottom line on the planet right now. My soma, however, is a part of nature and nature is a part of me. The instinctual part of my soma called the fluid body in biodynamic craniosacral therapy is completely fractured, according to one osteopath. This primal dissociation from nature disallows my instinctual ability common to all of nature to heal myself. The bear is an omnivore and when it gets sick, it knows exactly which bush or which plant to eat from to heal itself. It knows how to withdraw and rest in order to restore itself. Dr. Steven Hagopian has said that one purpose of biodynamic osteopathy in the cranial field is to restore the client's connection to nature and to the "interpersonal and intrapersonal rhythms of life" (Hagopian, 2001).

Different forms of intuition and the conscious use of body awareness for apprehending information in the environment as well as communication between individuals and groups and with animals are unknown to most of us today. Subtly, we substituted hearing for *listening,* the latter determined as much by that which is listened *to,* as by the one listening. This new *psyche* also made it possible for us to mentalize spirituality through an intellectualized focus on words of prayer and (written) song. What was lost was a direct experience of the numinous conveyed through the power of oral imaginal drama by a wise person in a setting both conjured up by story and reflective of it, where the listener is both receptacle for, and amplifier of, the transpersonal. (Bernstein, 2006, pp. 28–29)

I would now like to look at the biodynamic model more closely in this light. There are several ways of looking at biodynamic craniosacral therapy, as I have pointed out in earlier chapters. It seems that the biggest challenge that the biodynamic craniosacral therapy model faces is from bio-medicine and the scientific point of view. Bio-medicine claims to be grounded in objective reality and biodynamics claims equal grounding in the subjective perception of the observer. There are many political points of view along the entire spectrum from the secular to the spiritual. One claims an objective evidence base is required for proof of efficacy of treatment. The other claims a subjective evidence base of sensation and perception gradually leading to change process dictated by the fluid physics of the soma, which precedes the chemistry of the soma. It is the theme of this series of chapters on Myth and Healing to view reality through a lens of story, image, and cultural meaning. To be originally whole as a single-celled human soma, to change and transmute, to fall ill and then to return to a differentiated wholeness is the cycle of spiritual life. When I fall from grace, it is through a healing ritual that I find my way back from the wilderness of my mind, return to my senses and to a theology of nature (Dillard, 1974). It has been said, therefore, that all disease is spiritual disease.

The Wholistic Paradigm

Paradigm is a richly ambiguous and capacious (big) term for visual and verbal imagery and for communities that share generative commitments to explanatory and experimental practices. Paradigms are like forms—structuring structures that make one remember in the flesh and in the text the disciplined promiscuity that makes both organisms and scientists possible. (Haraway, 2004, p. xix)

Research into spirituality and healing has demonstrated that certain health problems may be related to deficits or excesses that could be termed spiritual. It is likely, according to the research, that optimal well-being may require spiritual as well as social, behavioral, and physical balance. A number of complementary and alternative medical practices can easily be characterized as spiritual, and these seem to have promising impact on the fields of health, psychology, and theology. Research, such as with Buddhist meditation, has shown capability to relieve anxiety and depression (Kabat-Zinn, et al., 1987). Health issues in every society raise spiritual questions and matters that have been recognized for millennia. The great mythologies all speak to this. The myth will usually give the diagnosis, the prognosis, and the prescribed medicine and ritual to heal the affliction from the divine. These first two volumes of work on biodynamic craniosacral therapy are attempting to do precisely that, to frame biodynamic practice as an origin-healing mythology. In addition, many clients of different ethnic backgrounds view the world and themselves through spiritual eyes in contemporary Western society, especially the United States. Their behavior-guiding religious and spiritual behaviors integrate well with health psychology (Martin and Carlson, 1988, p. 102). I believe the contemporary client is a match for biodynamic practice because of the longing to reconnect with spiritual dimensions of the soma rather than a mental spirituality or a spirituality of anger prevalent throughout the culture.

Wholistic Assumptions

Marc Barasch (Barasch, 1994) summarizes the basic assumptions of the wholistic paradigm, the core of Complementary and Alternative Medicine (CAM) practices. The summary provides a useful basis to understand how biodynamic practitioners think, feel, and behave. Mind-body-nature unity for self and other is the unmistakable intention in these practices. It is important to know this intention in order to understand unconventional or alternative healing approaches such as biodynamic craniosacral therapy.

- Disease and illness are felt to be ripe with spiritual and psychological meaning that cannot be ignored and, in fact, must be addressed for a long-lasting physical cure. *Your illness is wasted unless you are transformed by it* is a statement a student made to me many years ago and it has really stuck in my mind. Illness is initiatory by nature. Initiation means the rites, ceremonies, ordeals, or instructions with which one is made a member of a club or society. Cults are an example of this instinct for ritual healing gone awry. Through appropriate initiation one becomes a participant in the mystery of life and is given a doorway into the esoteric teachings on health and healing of not only self and others but also of the planet. Through initiation one is invested with a particular function such as the wounded healer paradigm carried from childhood, or one earns the status within the community at large, such as a shaman.

- Second, the healing imagination and the neurological world of expectations must be engaged for healing to occur. This means that therapeutic rituals and ceremonies are used to enlist the powerful healing imagination and expectation of the client. As a biodynamic practitioner I must learn to focus the mind on different perceptual fields of slowness and stillness. I must remove myself from traditional ways of knowing that I grew up with and enter a dissociative trance. When I do that, I make space for a very different set of symbols and metaphors to come into my way of inner knowing. The image becomes therapeutic and, just as with sensation, it is linked to the soma.

- Third, the Web of Life is acknowledged. Traditionally all illness was thought to "burst forth from a constellation of disturbed relationship with spirit," which must come into a fresh, dynamic balance. Illness was not only seen as an individual problem, but also as a complex social and community problem. Traditional cultures had little physical or sexual child abuse because everyone would know it immediately and rectify it rapidly as a group. Health and healing exist in a psychosocial context. My soma is part of a larger system of bodies. Physical illness is part of that system socially, spiritually, and psychologically. The biodynamic practitioner holds the big picture for the client until she can inhabit this larger whole.

- Finally, there is transformation. "The point of getting well was not to *go back to normal,* but to come into a wider harmony with all aspects of life" (Barasch, 1994, p. 34). Most of the clients that I see in my practice want to go back to the way they were and feel a little better. This is called *regressive restoration.*

I often suggest to my clients that it may not be possible to *go back* to the way they were before their trauma occurred. This requires a grieving process for the loss of who they were at that time. The initiation they are undergoing is a *re*-conception process, a transmutation into a person with a reordered sense of priorities and relationships. Then it becomes a *re*-birth as more awareness dawns in the client. It is a trip down a narrow birth canal that has all the aspects of what Joseph Campbell (Campbell, 1949) called the hero's journey. Healing and healing processes are largely a mystery, and the attempt to heal one's self is heroic. To differentiate and bring light to the unconscious is a symbolic struggle with one's mind and emotions and the fallout in the soma. Biodynamic craniosacral therapy enters the mystery of healing rather than trying to solve it. Stillness is the entry into this mystery. To sit still is heroic and archetypal. When the practitioner sits still, he is the Buddha for that moment. From the stillness spontaneously arises the skillful means necessary for that client at that time to relate to healing. When the client is still, she is the Buddha.

The Biodynamic Paradigm

One of the beginning stages of the alchemical work is very often the *liquefaction,* the turning into liquid in order to undo the *prima material,* which is often hardened or solidified in a wrong way and therefore cannot be used to make the philosopher's stone. The minerals must first be liquefied. Naturally, the underlying chemical image is the extraction of a metal from its ore through melting. (von Franz, 1995, p. 196)

Claire Cassidy (Cassidy, 1994) has suggested a formula for what she calls the wholistic paradigm and I feel it is related to the biodynamic paradigm:

**Intrinsic Healing Capacity of the Soma + Expectations
+ Specific Treatment Effects = Health Outcome**

The most significant assumption in the field of Complementary and Alternative Medicine is that the soma has the capacity to heal itself. The soma contains self-correcting mechanisms. This capacity is an innate conception right and the practitioner's role is to relate to this preexisting movement of health in the fluids of the soma from a biodynamic point of view. This is absolutely the case made by the founder of osteopathy Dr. Andrew Taylor Still and the entire lineage of cranial osteopaths and craniosacral therapists. Daniel Moerman (Moerman, 1983) calls this *autonomous healing.*

Metaphor is an important aspect of a paradigm. It might be enormously helpful to investigate the use of metaphor to direct research and its interpretation. The paradigm concept is rich with suggestions for analyzing the proper place of metaphor in biology. To begin to understand again the place of image in a science should suggest a way in which natural structure can be seen in a post-positivist age. Visual imagery in particular is of critical importance. (Haraway, 2004, p. 2)

Expectations, faith, and beliefs then play a major role in the biodynamic paradigm and healing in general. Not only are the expectations of the client, but even more so those of the practitioner, vitally important. Bio-medicine calls expectation the *placebo effect:* "A placebo is an intervention designed to simulate medical therapy, but not believed (by the investigator or clinician) to be a specific therapy for the target condition" (Turner, et al., 1994, p. 1610). The word *placebo* is Latin for "I shall please." Placebos are used in studies seeking the effectiveness of new drugs, for example. Some clients are given the real thing and others take a fake or sham pill or treatment (placebo). In some studies (such as with Xanax, the anti-anxiety medication) placebos effected as much if not better improvement as the real thing. Medical researchers could not explain this situation nor believe in its potency until Turner and her associates broke new ground with their literature review and developed a model related to the wholistic paradigm—namely, that expectations play a major role in the health outcome for clients.

The biodynamic paradigm wholeheartedly acknowledges that beliefs and expectations play a significant role in health outcomes. It is likely that the treatment room of such a practitioner is full of symbols attesting to that belief such as religious pictures, cross-cultural images, smudge sticks, statues and carvings of Native American origin, and so on. Thus, the practitioner has an intention to relate with the soma's organic capacity to self-correct. The practitioner trusts in it and this influences the client consciously and unconsciously. As Dr. Sutherland exhorted his followers, "trust the tide." Then the practitioner makes physical contact with the client with his hands, which in itself has numerous and specific treatment effects that the client expects to be helpful. This tripod of intrinsic capacity for self-healing, belief, and hands-on contact is the foundation for the effectiveness or treatment outcome of the client.

Placebos are 55–60 percent as effective as most active medications like aspirin and codeine for controlling pain. Studies have shown time and again that placebos can work wonders. Explanations of why placebos work can be found in the new field of cognitive neuropsychology called *expectancy theory*—what the brain believes about the immediate future. This is a little like classical conditioning theory, as with Pavlov's dogs. The symbols of the doctor's white coat, nurse's voice, smell of disinfectant, or needle prick have acquired meaning through previous learning and symbol referencing. This produces an expectation of relief from symptoms. Even the color of a pill influences the client's belief in its effectiveness. Responses from such expectations are strong because the natural world is full of ambiguity. For instance, a man walks through the woods and sees a long, thin, dark object in the high grass. Then the lower brain processes sensory input: There is no sound or movement and the object has a dark exterior. It looks like a stick. This is the first interpretation. Simultaneously the right hemisphere of the brain, drawing upon a past experience, interprets information from the senses and comes to a different conclusion based on expectation: It's a snake! Finally, the left hemisphere of the brain may give equal weight to input from the internal and external worlds, which takes a little longer. However, if expectation wins out, the soma will produce stress hormones in response to the stick that looks like a snake and that means fight-or-flight!

Stages of Alienation

> Always at bottom there is a divine revelation, a divine act, and man has only had the bright idea of copying it. That is how the crafts all come into existence and is why they all have a mystical background. (von Franz, 1995, p. 141)

Let's turn our attention from expectations to the sick client. Perhaps we'll find out why expectations take on so much power when we become ill. Illness in biodynamic craniosacral therapy is viewed as a process of alienation from the four basic domains of our life—mind, body, nature, and others. The spiritual domain is the glue that holds these other domains together and is the final alienation. Nature and the natural world have traditionally been the domain of spirit prior to the advent of modern medicine and psychology. The abhorrence of nature is systemic in our culture. The website worldscience.com recently reported research that indicates Americans are withdrawing from nature as seen through a significant decrease in attendance at the U.S. National Park System. It appears to have reached epidemic proportions such that the comic character Opus drawn by Berkeley Breathed named it Nature-Deficit Disorder on February 17, 2008.

- The first symptoms of alienation are experienced as a separation from the environment. We lose our ability to see the sky and the clouds in their intrinsic beauty. We miss the color of trees, flowers, birds in flight, the sounds of animals, and the wind. All these things are cut off from participating with our sensorium. Our vision becomes narrowed with too much television; our hearing diminishes because of the incessant roar of cars, mega bass on the boom box, weed whackers or leaf blowers, and the neighbor's dogs.

- As we separate from the earth, we also cut off from the social relationships around us. We withdraw, quarrel, accuse, and otherwise disconnect from loved ones, friends, and associates. Normal projection becomes electrified with transferences. It is always someone else's fault. Blame becomes the new household mantra. Anger and irritation rule the day.

- Then our soma becomes alien to us as we ignore all the subtle and not-so-subtle signs of this spiritual illness. We throw aspirin at our headaches, Tums at our stomach aches, laxatives at our constipation, Ben-Gay on our sore muscles, Slim-Fast at our weight problem. All of a sudden the soma is a beast of burden with all these aches and pains. Our bodies seem foreign to us—sluggish, heavy, lumpy, smelly, and sweaty. We no longer have harmony between our outside environment and the inner urgings of our biology. We are out of touch, fragmented and numb.

• Finally, we alienate ourselves from our own minds. We quarrel with ourselves, struggling with our thoughts. We fight ourselves inside. We give in to self-aggression and self-hatred through compulsive or extreme behaviors. We make deals with God: I'll do this if you take this burden off my shoulders. We get locked in the cycle of guilt, repent, and rebel over and over again. We cannot trust our own state of mind anymore as fluctuating strong emotions mix with wild thoughts and eccentric behaviors, creating chaos.

Traditionally this process of alienation is viewed on a circle or wheel, as seen in Figure 34.1 (Meadows, 1989; Cahill and Halpern, 1990).

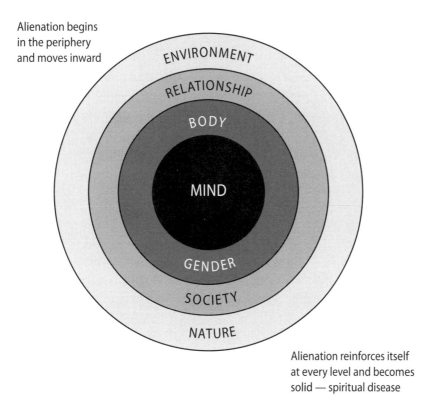

Figure 34.1. The process of spiritual disease

The Ritual Inherent in Biodynamic Practice

> All the rites of rebirth or resurrection, and the symbols that they imply, indicate that the novice has attained to another mode of existence, inaccessible to those who have not undergone the initiatory ordeals, who have not tasted death. We must note this characteristic of the archaic mentality: the belief that a state cannot be changed without first being *annihilated*—in the present instance, without the child's dying to childhood. It is impossible to exaggerate the importance of this obsession with beginnings, which, in sum, is the obsession with the absolute beginning, the cosmogony. For a thing to be well done, it must be done as it was done *the first time.* (Eliade, 1958, p. xiii)

Primal dissociation from nature and the divine is the healing focus of biodynamic craniosacral therapy. Such alienation is viewed as the loss of a biological and embryological midline. It is the midline that reconnects the four worlds or states of mind, soma nature, and the numinous together. Biodynamic craniosacral therapy is a healing ritual performed for the restoration of the client's midline. It is shamanic by its very nature in that it provides a connection with the extrasensory or transensory experience of stillness and Primary Respiration as an alive intelligence in nature. This is the definition of *shamanic*—ecstatic or outside normal states of sensation. Ian Black (Black, 1993) refers to ritual as having five purposes in shamanic healing. I believe that biodynamic craniosacral therapy works at this level too.

- The first purpose of the biodynamic ritual is to help the client inhabit the active shaping of the fluids in the soma. The whole fluid continuum expresses embryonic behavior at the rate of Primary Respiration and maintains a midline (interconnected) relationship with the natural world outside the soma. This is the creation of sacred space in the office. The movement of the whole is most important.

- The second purpose is to help the client through life changes by teaching the client how to sense her fluid body and how to sense Primary Respiration from her umbilicus, heart, and third ventricle. This moves the client's attention out of the nervous system and into a systemic sense of the whole living fluid continuum of experience.

- The third purpose is for uncoupling from trauma and the loss of autonomy by accessing the felt sense of wholeness and love inherent in Primary Respiration and its midline of stillness. Accessing stillness at the core of the midline is the restorative dynamic.

- The fourth purpose is for healing the community in which the client and practitioner live through access to the stillpoint and Primary Respiration. The client and practitioner move through society slowly with the ability to access Primary Respiration at any time and any place. The natural world becomes sacred space. Objects in the natural world are seen as preexisting stillpoints interconnected to the body's metabolism.

- Finally, the ritual of biodynamic craniosacral therapy is used to celebrate and honor life with the restoration of the felt sense of love in the heart. Ignition is the heart of the biodynamic therapeutic process. Heat is the most important product of the relationship and it is none other than the felt sense of love manifesting its presence in the blood and heart.

The Biodynamic Cure

Initiatory death is indispensable for the beginning of spiritual life. Its function must be understood in relation to what it prepares: birth to a higher mode of being. As we shall see farther on, initiatory death is often symbolized, for example, by darkness, by cosmic night, by the telluric womb, the hut, the belly of a monster. All these images express regression to a preformal state, to a latent mode of being (complementary to the precosmogonic Chaos), rather than total annihilation (in the sense in which, for example, a member of the modern societies conceives death). These images and symbols of ritual death are inextricably connected with germination, with embryology; they already indicate a new life in course of preparation. (Eliade, 1958, p. xiv)

As I noted previously, the biodynamic paradigm incorporates these notions of shamanic healing and ritual into its basic premise of treating the client through the perception of Primary Respiration as the movement of wholeness and its fulcrum of stillness. Biodynamic craniosacral therapy is a shamanic healing ritual and will be discussed in more detail in Chapter 37. Thus, at one level of understanding, the biodynamic paradigm involves:

Creation of Sacred Space + Reconception + Rebirth into Right Relationship with Self and Nature = Cure

It is preexisting in the fluids of the client's soma as Primary Respiration and its fulcrum of stillness. The cure is simply a reordering of the client's perception of her dilemma into one of ease and grace. This is not a "fix it" model; it is a model of perception, restoration, and transmutation.

I would like to look at the specific nature of the biodynamic ritual itself. This is the actual mechanism by which the expectations of the client are engaged. Biodynamic practice augments the preexisting healing resources both in a client's fluid body as well as in her capacity for neurological and cardiovascular self-regulation. This is a five-step process that I believe is the core of healing in biodynamic craniosacral therapy.

Awakening Fluid Sensibility

This first step is one of the things that biodynamic craniosacral therapy does best. The client is regressed verbally (symbolically) to the first two weeks postfertilization, when the soma was all living fluid. As physical contact is made with the skin of the client by the practitioner's hands at different places on the body, the entire sensorium of kinesthesia, taste, touch, sound, vision, and smell comes alive through the activation of the right hemisphere of the client's brain. With such a powerful focus on the kinesthetic sense receptors in the skin (exteroception) and the deeper movement of the fluid continuum inside the soma, all of the senses become more active unconsciously. The right hemisphere of the brain evaluates the context of the touch by accessing preverbal memory and sensory experience from the embryonic, fetal, and infant stage of development. This is how a body image is formed in infancy, as the perception of body sensations and physical location in space three-dimensionally via the surface of the skin. It is all organized in the maturing right hemisphere of the baby and it started twenty-eight days postfertilization, when the first sensory neurons of the embryo's nervous system differentiated.

Meanwhile the core of the soma and its viscera takes years to develop. The metabolic functions of sucking, swallowing, breathing, and pumping blood are all new to the baby and mixing with contextual input from the skin-to-skin contact with the caregiver. Is the contact loving and nurturing, or is the caregiver depressed or anxious? The right hemisphere of the baby is able to determine this and alter its internal state to absorb the caregiver's stress. Since the information is coming from the skin, the infant is also generating a three-dimensional body image. Sensations are constantly being interpreted unconsciously. Sensation is the state of flow, stream, current, wave, pulsation, tempo, rhythm, and frequency, based on biodynamic fluid movement in the soma. If the fluid sensings fluctuate dramatically from poor lifestyle, behavior, diet, or attachment distress, then biodynamic buoyant touch has accessed that preverbal memory.

The perception of Primary Respiration and stillness are critical for the client to uncouple from abnormal nervous system imprinting in the prenatal and perinatal time of life and reassociate with the living waters on the inside of the soma. The client is able to resolve what Hanna (Hanna, 1988) calls *sensory amnesia*. The client's non-normal dissociation becomes more flexible and normalizes with Primary Respiration. It does not go away; rather, it is viewed fearlessly as a valuable component of the divine attempting to reestablish midline contact.

Stabilizing Fluid Perception

The second step in biodynamic healing is to stabilize fluid perception. Buoyant touch does this so well. Fluid perception is the most powerful tool in the biodynamic repertoire. Such perception is the ability to recognize gradients of density, active shaping, heat distribution, and flow patterns and tempos in one's fluid body outside the activity of the nervous system. This also includes the ability to attune to fluctuating patterns of relationship, especially the qualities of withdrawing and reaching out with one's attention. The practitioner contemplates his hands and arms as a connecting stalk and eventually an umbilical cord.

Stabilizing fluid perception is a crucial part of a client's healing process. The chief feature of fluid perception is its *three-dimensionality*. What I sense in my fluid body is three-dimensional because it starts with my awareness of the total surface volume of the skin. I actively build a sensory perception and image of the totality of the surface of the skin, as well as guiding the client to do the same. This allows Primary Respiration to reestablish right relationship with the fluid body. Such perception is based on the ability to be present-centered, right here, right now—not somewhere in the past or future—by noticing the wave-making capacity of my respiratory diaphragm as it expands the skin from head to foot with an inhalation and shrinks the skin from head to foot with an exhalation. Wind on the water makes waves. When breathing with the fluid sensorium, I can receive the communication from the environment, nature, and with others without the filter of mental numbness, emotional fixation, and physical lethargy.

The natural world dialogues with me through the inner ocean inside the skin and increased bodily perception of the outside presence of Primary Respiration around the surface of my skin. The ocean inside the soma rests in the ocean outside the soma. The wisdom of the soma does not reside in the soma, as one osteopath has said; it moves through the soma! I accommodate more to this permeable world as a tubular sea sponge or sea anemone would, rather than attempting to hold onto the soma with the musculoskeletal system. I ingest the natural world with my endoderm and gut because it is connected to nature. I empathize with the world with my heart and blood because it is connected to every sentient being. I see clearly with my brain and senses from the vantage point of stillness. If I cannot inhabit my inner ocean and feel the rhythmic support of the ocean of Primary Respiration, then no amount of prodding by health professionals will help. Stabilizing fluid perception generates the potential for self-regulation. Steven Covey (Covey, 1989) calls this state *proactive*—I begin to assume responsibility for the moods and emotions in my life. Thomas Moore (Moore, 1993) refers to self-regulation as a way to stop blaming others for the way life turned out. This means that stabilizing fluid perception allows me to become aware of the function of projection and its misuse.

Accessing the Stillpoint

The third step in the healing process is to access the stillpoint. Biodynamic perception fluctuates between moving attention slowly to the edge of the universe and back. Dissociation is the normal attempt to reestablish contact with the midline. It is important to move perception inside and then outside the soma on a regular basis without fixating on rigid embodiment at one end of the spectrum or rigid transcendence at the other end. The idea is to shift allegiance from relentlessly and aggressively attempting to hold on to one state of mind or soma (whether good or bad) with the nervous system and soft tissues and to allow the inside structure of the soma to disappear, so that all that remains is living, sentient fluid. This inner ocean moves at the rate of Primary Respiration inside or outside of the soma or both or together. It generates different currents in the fluid body. This is all oriented to a deeper knowing or a deeper connection with the stillpoint as it changes places with the movement.

The stillpoint orients all the movement of growth and development for the whole and the parts at any given time. It also is automatically shifting from inside to outside the soma out to the horizon and back. This, at first, may seem risky or threatening because of the negative cultural association with dissociation, but experience dictates that I usually come full circle and will revisit my dissociation and alienation again and again as life proceeds until it normalizes. As I make friends with dissociation, it no longer can overwhelm me because I have learned to rest in the stillpoint and to "trust the tide." The therapeutic issue is the ability to recognize the stillpoint, not just sitting still and meditating on nonthought. The meditation is not the stillpoint, although it is the beginning or threshold to access the stillpoint. The stillpoint is recognized with a deep level of awareness that does not separate experience or make distinctions between the practitioner and the client.

The biodynamic practitioner synchronizes his attention with the stillpoint and Primary Respiration to facilitate fluid awareness and open to the possibility of transmutation and a return to the midline. As patterns of non-normal dissociation transmute, compression and tension are normalized as they were metabolically in the embryo. Gradually as the biodynamic sessions progress, these feelings are uncoupled from traumatic imprinting without the need for catharsis. Containment is established and self-regulation is achieved. The practitioner contemplates a stillpoint that automatically shifts from the inside of his soma to the outside in nature. Sometimes the client becomes part of the foreground of the natural world and, in this case, may be the location of the fulcrum of stillness as it slowly moves between the heart of the practitioner and the horizon of the natural world.

Disengagement and Expansion

The fourth step moves into a disengagement-expansion process. A shift is made into a higher level of functioning called self-regulation. A functioning midline is established. Something dies and disengages as freedom is spontaneously born in the heart-mind. The midline function is established as an automatic shifting connection from inside the soma to outside the soma. This is a reciprocal relationship capable of orienting to the stillness of the midline. I may sense the freedom, no matter how small or large, while I lie on the practitioner's table or when I get up and move back into my life or in a dream later on. It could be a freedom in the hip or the freedom from giving up anger I've held for weeks (or years). I feel it disengage. What takes its place is a felt state of grace and love. It is distinct in my soma and outside my soma. Then I expand and contract normally from that place of stillness. I allow my soma to become a part of nature with Primary Respiration and to be reformed with Primary Respiration every 100 seconds that I am awake and perceiving.

Healing dissociation requires containment of change process, rather than the elimination and discharge of stress and trauma. Containment requires the ability to find the center of stillness, whether it is located inside the soma or outside the soma, and allow it to shift. It is in this center of stillness that I can sit and observe the entire spectrum and polarity of change process (Richie, 1996). Dissociation is the healthy attempt to be still. To change is to disintegrate or delaminate, as is said in embryology. There are three types of change process in the embryo. One cell simply pulls away from another cell and becomes its own being—this is called *delamination*. After a close relationship for a period of time the two cells grow apart from one another until one simply gets up and leaves without any destructive emotions. A second way that change process occurs in the embryo is called *differentiation.* Sometimes a cell divides in half and in this division does not produce the same cell, but a completely different cell with a completely different fate. This is differentiation as an embryonic process. Does this differentiated cell hold regret for this change or get angry at it? I would think that such change process is celebrated. The third way in which an embryo and consequently an adult undergoes a change process is through *dehiscence,* defined as the capacity to spontaneously disintegrate and reform into something new. The embryo is now the myth of the phoenix. A cell will actually change its shape and gene expression to morph into someone else. This is the essence of transmutation at a metabolic level in the embryo that becomes psychological as an adult. Consequently, the embryo has a lot to teach us on these three styles of change process. These changes are always oriented to a fulcrum or center of stillness. Ultimately the embryo lives on because of the catalytic function and containment offered by the stillpoint. Disengagement and transmutation are normal to the embryo. The practitioner contemplates the instinctual process of attunement throughout the session by gradually approaching the client within the tempo of Primary Respiration and withdrawing attention at the same rate until attunement becomes timeless.

Reassociating to Slowness

As the client begins to act in harmony with life, the final step in this healing model is reassociation to slowness. The client may return for more biodynamic craniosacral sessions or some other practice specific to her needs to get congruence in the new pattern. The client may take a dance class to reinform her soma of a new possibility. The client may do nothing more than turn off the television and stop reading the newspaper. The client can engage in psychotherapy, read a book, and take a vacation to help support the new pattern. Yoga, Tai Chi, Aikido, dance therapy, Chi Gong, and mindfulness meditation are a few of the many ways to maintain balance between the inside and outside of the soma. Perhaps all the client needs to do is rest and sleep more, according to new research.

To reassociate means to move into, behave with, or relate to a higher level of functioning in the body-mind-nature complex at a slow tempo. One's spirituality no longer requires a middle man. One becomes directly conscious of one's divinity. The client is effectively reborn into a normal relationship with self and nature through the reassociation of the perception of a midline connection between the two worlds of the mundane and the sacred. All that is needed is seeing life as a dream, according to the Buddha. The work of biodynamics is to normalize the dissociation in the culture rather than pathologize it. Rather than a survival resource, it is a new body and mind attempting to connect with the natural world.

The practitioner contemplates throughout the day the possibility of slowing and stilling in body, speech, and mind. I frequently pause whenever I am by a window and look outside and synchronize my attention with Primary Respiration as my vision takes in as much of nature as I can see. I recommend building up to doing this pause twenty-five times a day. It is easy to do while driving, because there are many stop signs and red lights that tell us to stop and become still. Slowness requires a certain longing and humbleness to achieve. It is not a state to achieve, but a process to move within.

CHAPTER 35

Synopsis of the Navajo Creation Myth

This kind of healing is regarded by the Navaho as the heart of their system, and is given first importance. It is based on ritual and myth, not on physiological principles. The cause and cure of disease are connected to the greater mythological whole, and are seen against the supernatural background of man's life. The "doctor" is the shaman or medicine man who is trained in the specific beliefs and rituals of his culture. (Sandner, 1979, p. 17)

I would like to remind the reader that the following short version of the Navajo creation myth is called an emergence myth. This means that mankind emerged from the earth and grew up rather than falling down from the sky. The Navajo creation myth is typically read to the shaman who is being initiated or to a sick patient in some of the healing rituals. Therefore, the reading and hearing of the creation myth is known across cultures as being of primary importance for health and healing.

In the first dark underworld nine people-creatures lived: six kinds of ants, three kinds of beetles. At each of the four directions—north, south, east, west—was a round house like an anthill four stories high, with chiefs at each corner of the planet. All the people spoke the same language. There were no stones nor any vegetation nor any light.

After a discussion among the chiefs, in the center the people built a house of four chambers, one above the other, and moved from the lowest room up to the next one.

The beings explored the second chamber out to its edge and found it went nowhere. Then one beetle, called Pot Carrier, found he had forgotten his pots and had to go back to the first chamber to get them. While the second chamber was larger than the first, there were still no stones or vegetation, no days, no

423

light. Then the first beings met two Locust People, and they all went up to the third chamber.

They soon found this was not fit to live in and wondered what to do. Locust tried to advise them on a course of action. But the people resented one person doing this and felt that all should participate in the decision, so a council of chiefs was called. The chiefs made a choice, and they all moved upward to the fourth chamber.

The fourth chamber was larger, still dark, and from here the Moving Up or Emergence begins. Present were nine beings: two First Men, two First Women, First Made Man, First Made Woman, First Boy, First Girl, and Coyote. Also Fire God (Dark God) was present.

First Man placed his wealth—White Shell, Turquoise, Abalone, Jet, and Red-White Stone—at east, south, west, north, and center.

First Man breathed on the sacred jewels he had placed north, south, east, west, and center, and five cloud columns arose and met overhead, and midday and night began. Coyote visited each column of light and "changed his color to match theirs. In this manner Coyote increased in importance with the nine peoples of this world. His power increased as he absorbed these different colors." Baskets of the holy jewels were at each compass point, with a basket of evil diseases in the center where the Red-White Stone and the many-colored columns were. First Man and his companions, and Spider Ant, were all evil. The other Ant People were not.

The columns descended into the baskets, with the central black at the bottom. Coyote explained the secrets to Spider Ant. Ant People then asked how they could proceed upward. Acting on First Man's instructions, and led by him and Coyote, all the people grasped the middle column, which raised them to the Second (Red) World. All the evils were taken along. And before they left, First Man rolled up the four columns and tucked them into his pocket.

First Man brought the rolled-up columns from the First World. Sphinx Moth Man and Woman lived in this Second (Red) World, and they had light columns similar to First Man's. Nevertheless First Man placed his balls of bright columns at the cardinal points, with the dark ball in the north as a gift to Sphinx Moth Man, who then blew smoke at them, and they expanded and grew.

Sphinx Moth Man asked the people from whence they had come. Ant People told him and asked him what they should do now. He replied, "I am big, but not very wise and know not how to get at things." Four times they asked him. Finally they offered smoke to him. He blew smoke in all the various directions, and they moved upward into the next level of the Second World.

In the second level of the Second World, First Man caused his columns of light to rise overhead as he had before. He placed a perfect White Shell disk in the center to bring about movement there, but nothing moved. He tried Turquoise, Abalone, and Jet, but still nothing moved. Finally First Man placed the Red-White Stone in the center, and the earth shook. He said, "This portends evil. This is not good, children." The earth shaking increased, and the people were afraid. Finally the Red-White Stone moved up and carried the people to the next level of this world.

The next chamber of Second World was the home of all the Feline People, who were tricksters and at war among themselves. The newcomers joined up with the various warring factions. First Man made some of the felines his house guardians. The Feline People tried to injure First Man, coming at him from each of the four directions. Each time, however, their arrows were deflected, and First Man killed a few of the enemies and revived them in exchange for sacred songs. They called him Grandfather and Friend. The insect deputies tried to get their songs back. First Man's armor was invulnerable, and they only succeeded in injuring each other.

First Man rolled up his armor. Coyote and Spider Ant went about and reported back to First Man that there was much suffering and misery, and Pot Carrier Beetle said that he did not want his handiwork destroyed. First Man then blew smoke in all the directions and swallowed it each time, thus removing the "power of evil from the people of the First World, the Insect People." This power now entered into First Man and the others of the original nine Holy People. Coyote reported that all seemed well.

First Man, using Zig-Zag Lightning, Straight Lightning, Rainbow, and Sun Ray, tried to bring about an upward movement, but he could not. Finally he made a wand and set it upright. From the bottom upward it was made of Jet, Turquoise, Abalone, White Shell, and Red-White Stone. On each side of it were four footprints. The people stood on these and were carried up to the Third World. "As a matter of course, First Man never neglected to carry all his powers from one world to another."

When the people emerged into the Third World (eighth chamber)—the Yellow World—they found "one single old man and his wife and another old fellow" living there. These were Salt Man and Salt Woman, and Fire God. Also there were all kinds of Snake People, including various colored snakes who were evil.

All the wicked Snake People and the others "looked at, and studied one another while First Scolder (Coyote), unconcerned, roamed about to give the place the lookover. 'What sort of a fellow is that, boys,' they said, 'that goes about here with no respect for anything!'"

First Man then put yellow and red-and-yellow streaks in the east to keep the white column of light from rising. The people, alarmed, asked four times what was wrong. Finally Dontso the Messenger Fly was prevailed upon to tell them. H said that the streaks represented Emergence, pollen and vegetation, and diseases. Owl, Fox, Wolf, and Wildcat addressed the people. Apparently some gift was necessary for First Man before he would remove the obstacles. "They could think of nothing valuable at first." Then Horned Rattlesnake (Big Snake), who "carried a perfect (nonperforated) shell disk and horns on his head," gave to First Man this perfect shell as an offering. The streaks were removed, and the light column arose in the east. The people accused First Man of being malicious. He replied, "It is true, my grandchildren. I am filled with evil; yet there is a time to employ it and another to withhold it."

First Man placed the sacred stones in the four directions with the Red-White Stone in the northeast, breathed upon them, and a white hogan arose on five poles. Into this four-storied hogan all the people came. Coyote kept moving about in the northeast sector, asking what was going on and muttering to himself. First Man assigned places to everyone. He made the four Medicine Pouches for the Upward-Reaching (Emergence) ceremony. Songs were sung. First Man distributed to the nine Holy Ones "all his medicine, good and bad."

The people wanted to move upward, so First Man tried to bring light, but Coyote had interfered with it, for he was angry at being called Wanderer or Scolder. Four sacred stones were offered Coyote by various persons, and they called to him as He-who-calls-the-daylight, and other titles. And "Coyote untied the pillars of light at the east, south, west, and north, and so the Sahd [world or holy council] functioned again and became holy. First Man then took down the hogan, rolled it into a small ball, and laid it aside."

First Man put the five holy stones in the center, and they carried the people, who were still evil, into the next world. This was the Blue World, and better than the preceding ones. There were four mountains in the four sacred colors at the four compass points, and there were valleys and hills and contours on the land. All kinds of earth animals were here, and water animals, and birds of all kinds. There was also the Place of the Crossing Waters, where a north-south stream—placid and cool—passed under an east-west stream—rapid, furious, and warm. And the people were surrounded by water, for the streams also flowed from east to south and west to north. The place where the people emerged into this world was called White-Speck-of-Earth. Animal chiefs had four-storied, four-colored houses at each of the four compass points. These chiefs, two Wolves and two Mountain Lions, at each dawning gave the people instructions as to how they should work and relate. Nadleh, the hermaphrodite, was there, with grindstones, pots, bowls, and seeds. After three years in which the people played, gambled, and labored together, the nine Holy Ones, led by First Man, decided to build another Magic Hogan, a Round Hogan. Into this hogan came all the people and seated themselves as before. The Holy Ones brought, in miniature form, all the various sacred stones and jewels. Coyote alone seemed to know the purpose of this ritual and ran about telling everyone that male and female genitals were to be made. Then Coyote said, "No one of you seems to be able to guess what these things are. I roam about and have little sense, but I have guessed all of them. You must all pay great attention to this ceremony since it concerns you all. This shall be Birth." And all the people contributed, to give power to the male and female genitalia. Many babies were born, and for four years the people grew and flourished, with good crops and food stored away.

One day, after the eighth year of living at White-Speck-of-Earth by the Place of Crossing Waters, the Wolf Chief of the north arrived home to find his children uncared for, his wife away, his house unattended. When his wife returned, there was a scene, and she refused to do her work. This went on for several days until finally, because the chief was not helping his people, Nadleh the transvestite (hermaphrodite) was called in. He indicated that he had all that was necessary to the men for planting and cooking, and all the men decided to separate themselves from the women and cross over the river.

Four days and nights of consulting among the men followed this decision. During this period they spent the days at the river's edge, the nights at the house of Nadleh.

Spider Woman helped to make the house large enough. The third night the chiefs said: "Let us retire and see how our dreams will be." Each morning the rivers had changed colors. The men brought offerings to the Place of Crossing Waters. Eventually they crossed the river at the Place of Floating Logs, in five wondrous boats, carrying with them all their belongings and all the male children. They were beset by a storm, but Sphinx Moth (Tobacco Horn Worm) calmed the waters, and they arrived at a place called Gathering Shore.

For four years the men prospered, their crops increased, and sacred rites of various kinds were established. Meanwhile, the women were failing. They had been mating with Fox. Weasel, Badger; eventually both they and the men were pulled into autoerotic excesses.

Nine times of planting and nine times of harvest passed. The women became more and more wretched. They mated with animals and engaged in many sexual excesses. Some of the men, too, defiled themselves with animals. One of them was shattered by lightning because of this and had to be revived and restored by a ceremony that included the divine helpers Dark God, the hero-twins, and Gila Monsters who "find things by feeling."

Finally some of the women in desperation tried to swim the river. A few were drowned. Wolf Chief called to his wife, "Do you really want to cross?" She replied, "I beg of you to bring us back." The women were brought across the river and a series of purification ceremonies held for them. Owl, Squirrel, Toad, and Frog directed the cleansing. Marsh Wren Woman and Snowbird Woman got bowls of jewels and dew from Pot Carrier, helping thus to sweeten and finally purify the women. And the women moved into the houses of the new village.

Despite the reconciliation between the men and women, all did not go well. Some of the people began having bad dreams. Also, First Man punished some of the men who had been practicing witchcraft, adultery, and the like by causing them to itch and swell. Many weeds came up amid the crops. Some people went crazy. Eagle Man provided medicines for healing. Four Dontsos, Messenger Flies, also helped to heal.

Then Coyote appeared, running about and being troublesome. He was pursued, shot at, finally wounded by the hunter's arrows. Now a child was heard crying near Floating-Water Place. Attempts to find the child proved fruitless. Dreams were reported, telling that Holy Girl had illegitimately borne a shapeless, black, gourdlike egg. After four days, this egg broke open; two boys emerged, grew up, and disappeared.

Coyote found another baby at Floating-Water Place, wrapped the baby in sunlight, and carried it away. Floods began, the waters rose, and the people feared. The two boys born of the gourd-egg returned with tall reeds, and the people went into these to escape the rising floods. Finally, with the help of Locust, the people learned that Coyote had stolen the baby and that this caused the flood. Coyote relented, and the "child fell from the place where Coyote had hidden him near his heart, and Coyote also exhaled the child's cry that he had swallowed. First Man put an offering into the flood and then placed the child in it, and water ceased to flow upward."

Badger, Locust, and Mountain Sheep People made a hole for emergence into the next world, but it filled with water and monsters. Spider Woman and Spider Ant made colored webs to hold the waters back. After four days waters and monsters both subsided, Winds helped to dry out the world, and the people climbed up to it.

The people built various kinds of houses to live in. One man went back to a lower world, making it the place of bad dreams, ghosts, and death. The chiefs decided to plan for life here, and all those people who had seeds gave them. First

Man then placed his five jewels, and poles arose for a final Creation Hogan, as the people wanted the world to begin. Sun, Moon, Sky, Earth, Dawn, Darkness, Winds, constellations, and seasons—all began to be. Coyote spilled the bag of stars over the sky with one fixed star called Coyote Star. Coyote explained the length of the seasons. First Man covered and breathed on the creation, "and all the things that lie on the earth and sky and all the people and all the things breathed and stood up." Male genitalia remained on the sky and female genitalia on the earth.

First Man wanted someone to carry the Sun and the Moon, but Coyote had taken the voices from all Created Things, so nothing could move. Several tried to function, but none could. Finally Coyote was asked "to call Sun and Moon to life, and he gave a great shout and all things moved."

Coyote wanted to be a mountain, but people refused and called him Roamer. He objected, so they called him First Scolder. Again he objected, so they called him White-Coyote-Howling-in-the-Dawn.

Then First Man placed four supports between the Earth and Sky in the four directions. Trails were made for the Sun to travel on. The twins born from the gourd-egg, in the previous world, were chosen to carry Sun and Moon. Both Sun Carrier and Moon Carrier said that unless someone died their daily journeys could not proceed.

After Talking God and Calling God (House God) called from the sacred peaks, First Man lifted "the Sky in the east with a Jet Wand, in the south with a Turquoise Wand, in the west with Abalone, and in the north with a White Shell Wand and turned it over upon the Earth, so that it rose on the pillars, east, south, west, north, and center, and both Sky and Earth seemed to be swaying as if on waves."

"Now we have other work to be done," the people said. "We have seeds to plant." But First Man said, "Wait, do not hurry." He made the Earth and Sky firmer, breathed in the breath of the Sun's jewels, and built hogans in all the various directions. Then First Man said, "Now, go ahead and do for yourselves." The animals began to plant wild foods. Birds, animals, and reptiles took their places on the earth. Salt Woman became angry and withdrew, but the other Holy Ones took their places.

After some period of time, a child was heard crying for four days. The people could not find the child. They were afraid. First Man finally succeeded in finding a mysterious girl baby. "Below her stretched a Dawn Cord from the east and from the south a Sky Blue Cord from the west a Twilight Cord and from the north a Cord of Turquoise. The child was rocking on Dawn and Turquoise Rainbows, supported by these cords." First Man recognized that Darkness was her mother and Dawn her father, and when he took her in his arms he found a small White Wind in her right ear and a small Dark Wind in her left ear, placed there by her parents. She was Changing Woman.

She grew up in four days, reached maturity and wisdom in twelve days, and the Blessing Rite was given for her. She gave birth to the Twin Hero Gods. She was the maker of Man. From here on, Changing Woman's beneficent creative power superseded that of any of the other Holy Ones, including First Man.[15]

> These principles have served the main healing function for the entire human race over a period of time that can only be measured in millennia. They are archetypal forms and as such function outside the sphere of conscious intent, giving rise in every age to new intuitive adaptations to an ever-changing cultural environment. ... The first of these is the return to the origin or source. In mythological terms this means return to the creation of the world, and the evolution of mankind as revealed in the tribal origin myths. Eliade has reminded us that all myths are origin myths, telling how things began in that mythic place outside of time and space that is inhabited by the ancestors or supernatural beings—a place where all things are done and experienced in the original and proper way. Healing is always part of that paradigm (Sander, 1979, pp. 265–266).

CHAPTER 36

Selections from *A Magic Dwells: A Poetic and Psychological Study of the Navaho Emergence Myth*

By Sheila Moon

I am very grateful to Ms. Moon's publisher[16] to be able to offer this very abridged edition of her most wonderful work. All myths are creation myths, according to Joseph Campbell. Marie Louise von Franz (von Franz, 1995) points out that there are two kinds of creation myths. The first is creation from above as seen in the Judeo-Christian story as well as the Iroquois story of the woman who fell from the sky. The other type is creation from below, or the emergence myth. The Navajo story is a perfect example of such an emergence myth. My point is to make a link to the practice of biodynamic craniosacral therapy and its creation myth of the human embryo. The body emerges from below, whether from the earth or the caudal end of the embryo when the mesoderm makes embodiment possible.

What follows here are my favorite passages from *A Magic Dwells*. I put them together in a way that can be followed whether or not the reader is familiar with the Navajo myth. A synopsis of the Navajo myth is in the preceding chapter. In addition, I have summarized the key psychological points of each of the five stages of how a human being is created and emerges from below the earth.

I would suggest that the reader read this chapter as a poem rather than a series of long quotes. Take time to dwell on her questions and take them to heart. It is possible to discover that creation is a constant in our life and something completely new emerges every moment in life and not just at its magical beginning. To that end I tried to capture the essence of Ms. Moon's book and its relationship to the very mind of conception and creation that exists right now in our perception. The bullet-point summaries in this chapter are my interpretation of the following material from Ms. Moon's book.

Introduction

- Pre-conception totality
- Heart ignition
- Point of origin
- Recovering values
- From darkness to light
- Vision of wholeness

Myths are interpreters of the depths of man, carriers of the life values, dynamic movements from timelessness and spacelessness into human time and space. (p.13)

In the beginning, in the small and the great darkness, life is not Something; it ardently Is. Beginnings are not precision. Beginnings are not confusion. They are darkness drawn to a minute pint of nondarkness, and silence gathered into a small sound. What is gathered and drawn together, and who gathers and focuses, lies behind knowledge. (p. 9)

Psychological or religious redemption is the act of recovering for oneself out of the small dark beginnings an essential value or values which one knows to be one's own and also recognizes as having been lost. (p. 10)

The way of redemption is basically a paradox, as are many truths. The paradox of the search as it appears in this version of the Navaho myth, as well as in many other myths and in human experience, can be stated simply. Only through darkness, chaos, the unformed, the difficult, can light come into being. This is the vision of redemption. It is a vision with deep roots in the human psyche, a vision of true consciousness and wholeness, a vision of ultimate unity which contains within it the duality of existence. (pp. 9–10)

World 1: Conception (pp. 14–56)

- Movement, not direction
- Undifferentiated wholeness
- Chaos of quiescent mind
- Smallest cultivated seed
- Dim sense of meaning
- Irritable impulse in the directionless matter of personality
- Choice
- Uncreated will toward growth
- Creator and created as sentient reflections of each other
- Core of determination and potency
- Expansion tide
- A presence standing for the arousal to life
- Creator puts self-essence (heart) into creation
- Beginning of opposites, polarities, and consciousness of evil
- Bargaining, deals, and exchanges between the gods and man
  (to be or not to be)

There may not be consciousness as we know it in these first choices. But somehow some dim sense of meaning in nature, some irritable impulse in the apparently directionless matter of the personality, forms a nucleus for an upward thrust. We do not know who or what makes the decision, or precisely when, but it is made. Choice seems to be there from the beginning. Who chooses cannot be answered. But in both the outward and the inward world it happens thus. Something knows; yet it is knowledge without a subject. (p. 21)

So to be aware that in our restlessness and our agitation lies a spontaneous and irrational start of emergence is to dignify rather than to degrade the tortured times of disquiet which are part of our humanness.

It is also to open ourselves to the possibility of being able to go from where we are and to not want to be to where we are not and grope toward. Even a minor choice born of the frustration of immobility is a start. Sometimes just to be able to say, "I am lost. I cannot find my way," is a step taken beyond confusion and paralysis. The very word "I" makes the difference. It is a major transition for the child when he can refer to himself as "I," thus setting himself apart from the environmental mass. It is a major transition from neurosis to health when an adult can say "I" instead of "they" when trying to understand the sources of his problems. This "I," as it grows in the child, or as it represents a healthy and conscious structuring of the adult personality, is the *ego*. The entire psychic edifice is no stronger than the ego which is its responsible core. What the myths indicate must never be forgotten; that the ego does not come in some cosmic eruption, but evolves through each small pushing hurt of psychological movement. (pp. 23–24)

The first something, in the present myth, is restlessness. The second is remembrance and recognition: remembrance of the first point of nondarkness which gave possibility of meaning, and recognition of the need for containing the possibility in a more concrete form. (p. 28)

For when some small bit of excitement focuses itself enough in us to help us remember and recognize what must be done, helps us wrest from the chaotic darkness a sense of containment and understandable purpose, we are to that degree freed from the oblivion of the mother world. (p. 28)

We cannot survive by the visionary idea alone. We must painfully build our growth on the day-to-day realness of ourselves, neither being inert within the vessel nor outreaching the place where we are. This finding of balance between vision and earth-reality is different for men and women. A man must deal with the feminine in himself (what Jung refers to as "anima") by taking his feelings with him as he goes—as Pot Carrier takes his pots. He must guard against the neurotic manifestations of Mother-night-and-nature, such as lethargy and unconsciousness, or hostilities thrown at all "mothers." The woman, on the other hand, must try to find a quietly alive relationship to her own feminine nature, without becoming herself a devouring female. (p. 31)

The Navaho myth starts in nature, with the spirit implied as a goal to be achieved. One kind of creation is upward form the body substance (Navaho), while the other kind is downward from abstractions of the spirit (Old Testament). Man cannot arise in one cosmic leap from scattered chaos to fullness of order. The upward movement comes but gradually, out of the development of the eternal presences into the wisdom of the generations.

In the best sense, the miracle of human life is contained in the traditions. The First Man, the "first ancestor," is the representative of this tradition, this living and dynamic heritage, which grows and builds in the individual and in the culture as a foundation on which the future can rest. First Man is the Gnostic Anthropos, primal Man, related to heaven and earth, above and below. He undertakes the subduing and organizing of nature, since his own pattern of evolution is toward even greater consciousness. His drive toward the individuation generally affects all lower animal drives and slowly changes them. He is related to the deeper Self and because of this must contain all things, including evil. (pp. 34–35)

We could say that we but slowly come to know the thoughts we are already thinking, through our alternations between opposites in ourselves. Only with restlessness, meditation, struggle, does what is 'natural' and single in any real sense become conscious. It is well to pause and examine where this idea leads. To assume a "natural gradient" of the psyche (as Jung has done), or an essential truth which life works to fulfill, or a preordered world of collective forms and images and eternal presences is also to assume a universe in which the totality of man is not just a plaything of quixotic gods. It is rather to say that God's totality (or the fullness of the gods) is there as a divine ground on which natural gradients operate in the direction of wholeness and the complete realization of provisioned potentials. It is also to assume a universe wherein a truly cooperative community of man and the gods is essential for the fulfillment of both. To be sure, "meaning" has no meaning except as seen by man's consciousness; but the idea of pre-existent forms and natural growth gradients assumes the possibility of being able to discover meanings rather than to invent them. It seems quite clear that these great creation myths are thus precisely the telling of this coming of man into his own. With the shift and flux of cosmic interrelationships and dualities, the pulsing of the points of light in the darkness, the idea of man slowly takes on a shape and a three-dimensionality and becomes a part of the living tradition of the ancestors. (p. 37)

We stand now alone, in the tragicomic state of self-recognition. And our innocence is gone; our original undifferentiated wholeness is taken away.

Coyote is the perception of this and the disturbance resulting from this realization. Such a disturbance and loss of innocence are seen in the child's first departure from home to school, where he is plummeted into an essentially nonmothering world. In our adult life, Coyote is many things and appears often. He is the disturbing sense that we cannot stay where we are any longer. He is the herald of consciousness of our role in the world. He is the scolding and irritating awareness that we can no more retreat into the comfort of blaming "them" for our fate, that we must now begin to take responsibility for our own sins. He is the blundering and gauche way in which we must inevitably fumble our growth.

The entrance of Coyote into the orderly sequence of creation is paralleled in various ways in other myths. For example, the confrontation of Adam and Eve by the serpent, thus by their own divine-creaturely nature, left them less innocent and more challenged by the perplexities of growth. They were a step more distant from the Lord God and a step closer to the godlikeness of man. This roguish, unpredictable and incomplete but wise self-potential is always recognizable at a certain stage of emergence of consciousness. As a Trickster figure—such as Coyote—it retains for some time the paradoxical qualities of man's full reality, although in some myths it later splits into two parts, one part being light, or good, or human, one part being dark, or bad, or animal. (pp. 39–40)

With the coming of Coyote into the Navaho Emergence, protest and scolding and dissatisfaction are born because the reality of being human is more taxing than the innocence of being animal. The original vague restlessness and irritation of the ants is more focused in Coyote. When we begin to have even a dim idea of what we are, human life is recognized as a "disorder." We then fall into a world of disturbance and protest as we reluctantly wrestle with our own meaning.

For it is easier—less painful, at least—not to have meaning than to have meaning. The neurosis cries out, "They are to blame!" or "I don't want to grow up!" or "If only things had been different!" Neurotic order dies hard, resists most bitterly the command to renounce simulated perfection in favor of the disorder of being real. But the sign of impending change from neurotic enslavement to a freer reality is the acceptance of limitation, imperfection, awkwardness, as conditions of healthy growth. (pp. 41–42)

First Man takes his four precious jewels in four baskets, places a basket at each of the four directions, and breathes upon them as in Zuni myth it is told that with "the breath from his heart Awonawilona created clouds and the great waters of the world" (Stevenson, 1901–1902, p. 23). In this breath, in this spirit given from the inward longing, is the creative act which reveals the inherent pattern and rhythm of existence. (p. 46)

First Man, by the act of breathing-upon, gives the "idea"substance. An outstanding element of nature is born when midday and night are set apart, and sleeping and waking belong to man. (p. 47)

This whole creation is becoming not only a structure but a process exemplified by the circumambulation of Coyote. With the advent of Night and Day and the new realization of creation, the process becomes an unfolding and an infolding, a rhythm, the systole and the diastole of life. The cosmic wholeness now begins to breathe. A mysterious and evocative richness is carried by the imagery of the cloud columns as they rise, pulsate, fall, and are rolled into small spheres to be tucked into the pockets of First Man. What a greatness in so minute a space! (p. 48)

No genuine psychological growth occurs until and unless the rich inner values and potentials of the unconscious strata are actualized—that is to say, are lived in the homeliness of every day. There is a second sin which is equal to the first sin of being cut off from the unconscious world. The second is the sin of being so enchanted with the inner images and archetypes that one becomes a curator rather than a creative experiencer. The great pulsating archetypes—like Shadow, Mother, Father, Self, and the others—rise and fall, expand and contract as columns of light. But unless our Coyote side takes them into the imperfect daily round of existence, walks with them to the table, the workbench, the relationship, they sink back into the baskets and never have real meaning. It is unfortunately not as taxing to talk about—even to see in operation— the archetypal major darknesses as it is to admit to the humiliating effects of our personal, dark and hidden side. Indeed, the archetype of suprapersonal Shadow has a certain drama about it, making it in a strange way more permissible. It is not uncommon for a person to retreat from the responsibility for bad human relationships by saying, as I heard one woman say, "But my Shadow is so big and terrifying! People should understand that! I can't do anything about it." This was not the cry of a terrified psychotic, but the infantile demand of an egocentric woman who would not face her own irritating little meannesses. (pp. 49–50)

One wonders why, at this time of first fullness, evil is so sharply present. There is not a single and simple answer, for the problem of evil is not a simple and single one. First of all, in a certain sense evil is a natural and early element in human life. For primitives and for children the forces of natural existence are cruel, hard, ruthless, unpredictable, and thus evil. These are fundamental facts and must be dealt with.

The second answer is more subtle. In the myth, evil is in a magical form, related to witchcraft. It must be kept in mind that psychologically there are two forms of "magic": black magic, used for the furthering of *personal* power and domination, and white magic, used more *impersonally* for healing. In both cases, mysterious resources and "mana" are involved, but differently harnessed. Egocentricity, arrogance, inflation, the desire for infantile omnipotence—in short, all the various defensive bulwarks built against insecurity—lead to the use of creative forces in the psyche for personal power. This use, which is really misuse, is "black magic." Possession by or identification with some impersonal and cosmic archetype often gives us tremendous power, enabling us to become "black magicians"—Rasputins, demagogic rabble-rousers, Hitlers. The true leader or healer, whether a tribal shaman or a Gandhi, is in the opposite sense a "white magician," impersonally offering his creativity in the service of his particular stratum of the human family. (pp. 50–51)

Reichard (Reichard, 1944) points toward what the evil could mean when she states, "Eliminating the fact of sorcery and the struggle to overcome it is like treating the Old Testament without sin." And she continues: "Thus evil is the same as ignorance. ... This means then that sin as conceived by the Navaho is not a sense of personal shortcoming influenced by consciousness and will, but either lack of knowledge of the proper order, or possession of that knowledge and its use for evil purposes." (p. 51)

The essence of this series of contradictions is that man must, as Kierkegaard said, breathe in necessity and breathe out possibility. To the extent that light comes, the whole darkness of life is seen. Yet it is usually brutal, even seemingly evil and dark necessity which drives man toward the larger possibility—as it drives the people in the myth. Whenever we reject the inspiration of necessity, or try to forsake the evil in our own baskets, we become more feeble as personalities and less able to expand into our potentialities. If we cannot admit that we err, that we are imperfect and unlovable and petty, surely we will never see ourselves as we are and will never even approximate completeness. A reason why projection—putting outside what belongs inside the psyche—is so disastrous is that it makes us flat, two-dimensional, and quite successfully prevents self-realization. One woman with whom I had worked long and patiently, trying to help her to recognize how she was the cause for her lamented lack of friends, finally ended our relationship by informing me that it was my meanness and my dishonesty which kept her from growing. Subsequently the same pattern was followed with several other therapists, always with her final refusal to be conscious of her own imperfections.

Unconsciousness is really a sin against the possibility of being man, so consciousness of evil and of its place and power is essential for psychological "salvation." (p. 54)

World 2: Polarity (pp. 57–80)

- Significance of the pause for renewal and rehearsal

- Feeling into the whys and ways of our coming to confront destiny

- Who am I? Where have I come from?

- Risk, the lure of the difficult and dangerous, must be our motivation

- On the value of danger for growth and development and beginning responsibility

- Clash causes differentiation or cooperation; constant change

- Half-conscious forward thrusts into life and aroused instincts

- Consciousness must come to terms with unconsciousness and beat the attack from the dark

- Animal strength for a still-forming consciousness

- A thrusting vertical midline toward the transcendent and exploration of the horizontal fulcrum of interpersonal relationships

- Evil, shadow, and death as a necessary backward action that leads to wholeness

- Let the dark be reborn eventually by the divine in us

> In our basic structure we are related to an image or idea of wholeness. Upon us falls the responsibility of realizing and actualizing this in the long arduous way which is both our historical evolution and our personal development. We cannot do this at first from a conscious vantage point, for the ego as such is not ready for mature involvement. That which is not us—not in the later way of a ready sensibility and discrimination, at least—cannot fulfill the demand for functional wholeness. The "above" and the "below" can and do exert their magnetic attractions, however, and a beginning can be made. (p. 59)

> What grave errors we make when, before we move on, we do not allow this vital interchange which is renewal. Temptation always lies in the too fast, too large leap into newness. The rolled-up balls of possibility found in the darkness are left behind, or are assumed to be complete and sufficient. Arrogance steps over the horned worm, the dimly seen moth. Thus the meaning of going with the gods is snot understood, and the significance of the pauses for renewal of the *before* and rehearsal for the *after* is overlooked. (p. 62)

Surely one of the most basic values of renewal and rehearsal is the honest telling to ourselves of the places from which we came and the ways in which we came. The too often unacknowledged sources must answer. These restless, ill-defined, unaccountably busy urges and irritations and searchings must be the first to say from whence. By answering so, by feeling into the whys and the ways of our coming, we are preparing for the next confrontation by our destiny.

No one can go forward without periodic pauses for self-examination; nothing is more valuable than the humility required for submission to the place and circumstance of the immediate moment. Why are we not getting any place, we ask impatiently. We have worked hard, tried everything, called on the unconscious for a great dream, or even for a little one. Nothing happens. We thirst, and we are afraid. Perhaps it is that we, like Poliphilo, have not submitted to our fate. We have not listened fro the questions life is urgently asking. Time and again, in both Zuni and Navaho myths, the words are spoken, "Who are you? Where did you come from? Why?" (pp. 62–63)

The pell-mell forward rush of this modern world is exactly our curse. It thrusts us backward because it leaves us breathless—and we do not take time to breathe, to send the smoke into the corners of our inwardness and wrap it about with patient devotion. Is it possible that one of our most dire inheritances from the nineteenth century is the impatience of the Industrial Revolution? All things are possible to man, we said. And the sooner the better, we added, with enviable assurance. The effect of this has been to hurry our every action, to make us more concerned with where we are going than with where we are. A new model of ourselves is anticipated annually, along with the automobile, the dishwasher, the jet plane, the lunar module. Thus we leave ever further behind the "outmoded" primeval soul, to make its peace with God as best it can. "Who am I? And from whence have I come?" are questions for the most part treated as the aged are treated—with a slightly superior tolerance for the vagaries. It is no wonder, then, that modern man has to learn painfully the meanings of compassion, patience, and love. And not only between nations and peoples, but between "I and Thou." How are our splits to be healed, our restlessness appeased, except by time spent first in listening and then in answering? Each next step requires this of us before it can be taken. (pp. 63–64)

If we are to achieve a place beyond where we are—beyond wherever we are at this moment of time—we must dare to risk ourselves. The difficult and the dangerous must be our moving substance. We must choose to use this substance, to let it serve us in its sacred and cleansing and arousing power. And this not only in the large matters, for that is strangely easier. Most particularly it is in the small daily courage of daring to be no more and no less than what we are. Deep are the shakings of our comfortable earth when we are willing to act thus. For we are relinquishing the state of unconsciousness, we are forsaking the immovable desired perfection. This portends evil; this is not good. That is to say, this leads into greater freedom of choice; alternatives are present; and a new darkness of our own making is for the first time possible. Heretofore the "evil" has been in creatures who could be vanquished and in the immortal Holy Ones by voluntary actions. Now it exists in the very uncertainty of the earth, in the very insecurity of the forward movement. At such a time we as individuals must assume the responsibility for that which shatters us, rather than pushing it onto some parent or demigod or life force apart from ourselves. It is *our* Red-White Stone, looked at from the experiential point of view, which *we* have put at the center of things to upset the quiet placidity. And it is *we* who are shaken by our own action. Thus we see that we are both he who places the stone of disturbance and those who are in fear and trembling. The loss of perfection and balance is the gain of the next stage of development. From the valley of our imperfection we can begin to walk on our own feet. (p. 67)

Every creation is a statement about the growth of our awareness of reality, a sense of what fills our emptiness. A creation starting deep in the earth is a creation concerned first of all with the solid and rooted continuity of being. The original stress is not on the fluctuating and unpredictable, but on the unseen foundations. Out of this comes the desire to know, the longing to become. The infant and the animal begin in this world. And each of us must return to understand and incorporate this world if our consciousness is to have the ground it needs. Problems with the mother umbilicus are unavoidable, even under optimum conditions. Every man and woman, as part of maturation, seeks to become independent, just as a plant stretches away from the earth where its seed began to sprout and seeks to blossom and bear fruit in the free air. Yet without the nourishing soil the plant dies. Without a connection to the maternal root principle the personality withers. Our racial origins, our biological inheritance, even our difficult familial connections, are parts of us. I have known many Americans who could not find themselves until they journeyed in physical fact to the place of their ancestors. When, in one way or another, this gap between us and our sources is bridged, this hole in our inner earth filled, then the process of individuation can proceed. (pp. 69–70)

When the preconscious self pushes for expression too soon, destructiveness and inflation are almost inevitable. That is to say, from the point of view of unthinking nature every evolutionary stage of self-determination and self-consciousness is in this sense "too soon," and that which stands on the side of natural inertia arms itself against that which stands on the side of emergence. (p. 70)

So consciousness must come to terms with unconscious contents, must move to meet the attack from the powers of darkness.

We must see consciousness, first of all, as our collected knowledge built up through example and teaching from childhood onward. We come to "know" about specifics and generalities as we are exposed to the "knowing" of family, nation, race. This conscious mind is vital to us as we fight our way forward. Yet it can become top-heavy, even as the inert weight of unconsciousness can become an almost irresistible drag. Consciousness—the Olympian gods, First Man—must come to struggle with unconsciousness, and in so doing *both* conscious and unconscious realms are altered. The conscious ego is given shape by the new things rising up, while the nonego forces are tempered by the effect of consciousness. The psychological sin of growth-resistant unconsciousness seems always to threaten our emergent life. The Felines, like the giants, war and kill, cheat and defy. And like the giants, the Felines have to be outwitted, reduced to more human and more functional size. That which is too big, too inhuman, too unrestrained, must give way if the human "I" is to take its rightful place. (pp. 73–74)

The cruelty and insensitivity of "I want" (and "I demand" and "my urges must always be expressed now") have to be reduced to a state of inability to function. Their previous unconscious inflation and anti social action have to be sternly, even harshly, dealt with. If at this point we walk away, leaving our animal nature to perish, we jump from one partialness to another equally harmful. We do not achieve a conscious advance.

So also with a culture. There is always the great danger that resistances and reformations, despite the genuine needs inciting them, become rigidities. That which was to be reformed is left to die on the field of battle. It has been so with Western man. His commendable and necessary desire for increased awareness of and control over his world has resulted in the suffering and death of his warm human feelings. Coming at a period of history when pagan, Judaic, Greek, Oriental influences were all converging and creating something of a rip tide in the human sea, Jesus of Nazareth brought a sharp challenge to the individual to reach toward a new and revolutionary level of self-awareness. This challenge, however, grew old and staid and became the comfortable Christian theology of the Middle Ages. Renaissance man arose against his too ordered universe, and replaced it in a tremendous resurgence of individual knowledge and particularized achievement, replete at first with feeling and love. But in the conflict between Medieval love of God and Renaissance love of man, Eros itself was somehow lost. The scope of a Da Vinci who could encompass religion, art, myth, science, was narrowed to the "brass instrument" mentality of the nineteenth century. The penultimate stage is the atom-splitting, technological, space-racing present century. Perhaps, however, as an American poet wrote wistfully, "There is nowhere to go from the top of a mountain but down, my dear." (Teasdale, 1929) Perhaps now we must, as nations and as individuals, go down once more to the stable of our nativity where the only absolute is reborn life. (p. 77)

It is our creaturely imperfection, the affirmation of our incompleteness and our weakness, which enables us to be kind. If we are to grow, surely we must do battle and just as surely we must receive the wounds of battle. Love and tenderness must follow both for the victorious and the vanquished parts of the psyche. Otherwise the battle has no meaning. To love ourselves is to care about the fate of each and every aspect of ourselves, even those which have been recalcitrant and destructive. If we resent and hate our willfulness with which we have fought, we find ourselves unable to proceed further, although we may have "won" the fight. For we have not yet accepted our own frailties. We have not let ourselves look with compassion on our suffering. (p. 78)

Evil, in this way, is seen to be both the unavoidable blundering and weakness of an undirected irritation and the very necessary backward action which alone leads to a new wholeness. When the evil has served its purpose for the time being, it is taken *back*. Note well that it is not taken *away*. First Man makes smoke, blows it to each of the four directions, then swallows the smoke again, removing the evil from the people. He puts it into himself, into his feminine counterpart, First Woman, and into the nine Holy People. Thus the evil, as a part of life, is carried in sacredness and safety by those who can bear the weight. If we could but learn this—not to fear or to flee the darkness and negativity, but to permit them to be borne eventually by the divine in us—then, perhaps, we would also know of evil, "when to use it and when to withhold it," as First Man says later on.

When the time is at hand for the movement upward to the next world, First Man finds that nothing happens until the right configuration is found. It is important to see how often the Navaho myths emphasize this fact of the healing power of a total situation or configuration, as different from a partial knowledge. This is to say, no matter how great the vision and no matter how profoundly rich the carrier of that vision, it cannot be actualized until all things are ready for its actualization. (pp.79–80)

World 3: Balance (pp. 82–101)

- Alternating activity and quiescence of evil and death anxiety

- Intrinsic part of the opening up of a cooperative two-way road between not-yet-conscious psychic powers and an emerging awareness of them

- Accepting the presence of evil

- Patient, periodic contemplation or pause to reflect on life as imperfect and incomplete

- Deepening into the paradox of the interweaving of good and bad

- The task of self-acceptance as heroic, courageous, and terrifying

Great is the Navaho wisdom which does not make judgments that upper levels are "better" than lower ones, does not permit the leaving behind of essential ingredients. Although the feminine principle must be transcended in its overpowering primal possessiveness, this does not mean that it can be renounced. It must be there as earth, as salt of the earth, as in the composition of the life's blood.

In our journey from level to level of our own nature, we often have to confront the disturbing fact that what we thought lay behind us still walks beside us patiently. And in our dismay we fail to recognize the growth it has undergone, the new clothes it wears. The first restless rise of dim longing leads us up and away from the comfortable mothering darkness. We must take on the burden of humanness and relate to the light as part of our ancestral heritage. We must risk ourselves in challenging the autonomy of our instinctual drives. Having done this, having come this far, we must not be surprises to meet once more the mother, for the archetypal Mother, as Neumann demonstrates definitively, has manifold phases and paradoxical meanings. (Neumann, 1955) (p. 84)

How often we are confronted by a like situation. We have struggled to overcome hostilities and resistances, we have reached a plateau (so we believe) where at last some fruit of our labor may be visible. Then the light ceases. We are confused and angry. Only patiently asking and listening, turning to the voices of the unconscious psyche, can help us to know what is needed. At such a time we want to rise without hindrance is not a reborn state; we are restive under the demands of time and space and the insistence that we attend to and accept our earthly and limited humanity. We want to be free and "good" and redeemed from natural law. And we cannot be. We have to learn the awesome truth hidden in those intensely dramatic word so of First Man, "It is true, my grandchildren. I am filled with evil; yet there is a time to employ it and another to withhold it." (p. 87)

What is the meaning of this apparent ambivalence of the gods? Surely Yahweh could have said, as First man does, "I am filled with evil; yet there is a time to employ it and another to withhold it." What does this say of the nature of the divine? First of all, it indicates that the divine is not dualistic, but holds within itself all possibilities of darkness and of light. (p. 89)

Completion, greater fullness, a wider grasp of the multitudinous aspects of life—these are what man and the gods must strive for. Not perfection and "goodness"; never these. It is a very striking feature of this primitive Indian myth—primitive in the sense of not coming from a people of a high degree of cultural consciousness—that this profound concept of the gods is present. (p. 89)

We of the present era have a particularly acute problem because we have tended to see the material world as primary. We have become accustomed to taking a one-sidedly rational point of view, assuming the "light" and "goodness" would prevail if only we could know about all things technologically. The "dark," negative, evil component is from this point of view the result of nothing but lack of factual knowledge. And as long as we cling to this comfortable and comforting faith, we cannot say, with the 138th Psalm, "the light and the darkness are alike unto Thee." Nor will we participate in the mystery.

It is difficult to judge what is positive and what is negative in us, and it takes great courage to face and to endure our negative side. A general confession of the unknown and concealed aspects of ourselves, saying we are "filled with evil," is relatively easy compared to the heroic act of saying, "Here, and here, and here the shadows live in me." The mystery of the serpent is more creatively ours when we can begin to recognize what the consequences of our shadows are or may be in our immediate existence. What things have we done to ourselves and to others, and how do we feel about our actions? Where we recoil with pain, where we are burdened by guilt—there our darkest shadows lie waiting. To learn to "employ" and to "withhold," so to be able to get from the Horned Rattlesnake his treasure, is to dare to confront our specific shadows, guilt, and responsibility. (pp. 90–91)

Therefore, in this myth, the alternating activity and quiescence of the "evil" processes can be construed as an intrinsic part of the opening up of a cooperative two-way road between not-conscious psychical powers and our awareness of them.

Twentieth-century Western man needs to see this value of the use of "evil" in order to wrest the treasure of discrimination from the archaic undivided oneness. Otherwise he will be engulfed in unconsciousness or in psychosis. (pp. 91–92)

We must be listeners and followers. We cannot—in fact we must not—assume the role of First Man. Our task is one of conscious reconciliation and mediation, of patiently bringing into everyday circumstance our growing knowledge of what happens in the deeper and darker levels of our being. And by separating out from the vague oneness of the mother-beginnings, by renouncing the desire for perfection, by accepting the presence of evil in ourselves as a quality to be dealt with as part of creatureliness, we can perhaps begin to live as human beings in a human world. (p. 93)

If we could but remember this marking of the crossroads at each stage of our growth, we would be far less disturbed when we face change. For this recurring mandala is like a bell ringing the turning of days and seasons, calling us to stop and see from whence we have come, saying to us that wherever we go, the entire meaning of existence goes with us. It is unexpectedly important for us to stop sometimes and ask the question, "Where have I come from and how am I progressing?" It is as if we walked about ourselves surveying ourselves from all the possible angles. This patient, periodic circumambulation is, at the personal level, what these fourfold forms of color and light are at the mythic level.

Great stress is placed, in American Indian myths, on these places of centering. (p. 94)

The myth is wiser than we, who adopt a seemingly logical way of action in our "cloud of unknowing." When negativity presses upon us, we are prone to deny our wholeness; when the light is with us, we affirm ourselves. But in the myth, when darkness surrounded the people the mandala form was balanced and centered; at the time of richer creation, unbalanced and five fold humanness prevails. Similarly, if we want help in avoiding deflation and inflation, we must attend to the opposites in a situation. States of negative self-love and self-hate are results of egocentric one-sidedness, of the hasty assumption that we are identical with what arises in us. We desperately strive to make our Creation hogan perfect. If we could be aware that this cannot be, that whatever emerges from the unconscious areas of our being has continually to be separated form and balanced by conscious attitudes, we would come to a more proportioned sense of our own nature.

Often an outer event or a dream, occurring at a crucial time of either inflation or deflation, serves to restore the needed balance. For example, a man who was becoming rather too proud of the progress of his inner symbols, tending to feel himself personally responsible for their won-drousness, was of a sudden precipitated into a most unpleasant situation with his business partner. Because he had the good sense to see the outer event as largely of his own making, a relative equilibrium could be achieved between the outer and inner poles. And it is striking how often a conscious attitude of self-pity or genuine despair is countered by an inner experience of turning up some lost treasure or finding light in an unexpected place. Such happenings as these, if we attend to them with devotion, can carry healing for what Kierkegaard called the "anxiety of presumption" and the "anxiety of humility." (Kierkegaard, 1939) They can bring balance to a sense of despair and imbalance to a rigid perfec-tion. (pp. 96–97)

Each of us, the particular men or women relating to a myth by hearing it, reading it, seeing it reenacted, is the framework for the myth. Or at least we can provide the framework. The role of the personal ego (the focal point of the active "I") is often difficult to see in myth and folk tales of the cosmic sort. In the less cosmic folk tales some heroes and heroines can be seen as ego personifications. But cosmic mythological heroes and heroines should not be generally so interpreted. They are generic aspects of man, archetypes of powers and processes. It is we who relate to the myth in various ways—and thus bring ourselves into relationship with it—who constitute the personal egos.

We err by identifying with and being caught up in the affects of the magnificent soul drama; if we fail to bring its archetypes into conscious relationship with our personal lives and circumstances, the unconscious realm rules us and can destroy us. If, on the other hand, the "I" listens or reads with tongue in cheek and a feeling that myths are nonsense, or fails to listen at all—the ego becomes the universe and the inner images are disastrously denied. It is as if some of us are in leaky canoes in a raging sea, some are in luxury liners on a duckpond, and some sail a seaworthy craft on a proper sort of ocean. In relating to myth, whether recorded or subjectively constellated from within or without, we need to bring our personal reality as pilot to guide the craft over the mythic ocean. The individual carrier is not in the myth. The myth is the suprahuman frame of reference for the human work. The developing personality, in its unique aspects, is forming itself within the common mythologem of creation and emergence. (pp. 98–99)

Thus comes again the inevitable pause in forward motion in order that another error of growth may be rectified.

This has in it a most necessary object lesson. For us to use our dim desire to be man, our desire to be free from the archaic unconsciousness of comfortable containment, is for us to have to dare humanness and the erring thrust into danger. Our weaknesses and limitations must be included rather than transcended. Darkness, negativity, evil, must be incorporated into our sense of self, for we cannot proceed upward on illusions. It is our own "trickster," our own Coyote, our own wandering and scolding unholiness which will help us to know those dark facts hidden from us by our ideals. When we learn this, if we learn this at all, we may still have to learn that our unholiness must be respected; not by a glossing over of its irritable and unpredictable nature, but by an honoring of it in the very fullness of its imperfection.

Why is this apparently simple act of self-acceptance so enormously taxing? Because from infancy onward all the socially collective learning transmitted to us goes in an opposite direction. We are warned not to be weak, not to make mistakes, not to admit errors, but to pretend to false feelings, to strive for perfection. The greater the sense that this Utopian ideal is unattainable, the more violent is our effort to achieve it. The walls of defensiveness grow ever thicker, the human creature more starved in this prison. It is an act of heroism to begin to break down these barriers brick by brick. (pp. 100–101)

Coyote does not wish to be something he is not. He wants only to be respected and to be seen more clearly for what he really is. His essential meaning, behind and beyond the disturbing and the wandering and the scolding, is that of ushering in new consciousness. (p. 101)

World 4: Birth (pp. 102–155)

- The richness of differentiation
- Similar to days five and six in Genesis
- Time and eternity intersect as two streams of fluid into the single ocean
- Birth
- Embodiment outside the womb
- Mortality, upheaval, sin, and guilt
- The perplexing promiscuity of adolescence
- Separation from the mother
- Approaching adulthood

The mandala form in myth and ritual emphasizes the importance of each stage of the individuation process as it occurs in a place, a space, uniting the nowhere with the here-and-now. The unfolding of a creation myth is like the unrolling of a tapestry on which the "eternal presences" of the collective unconscious are woven into a consciously perceivable and graspable pattern. (pp. 103–104)

The four great mountains mark this place as one where the more concrete actualities of human development will move into the center. The presence of hills, valleys, animal life in its many manifestations, bears out the quality of this world. The water mandala—the Place of

Crossing Waters or "Waters-flow-across-each-other"—seems to carry in itself not only the possibilities for future differentiation of certain unconscious processes. This water place is not unlike Okeanos of Greek myth, of whom it is said, "Ever since the time when everything originated from him he has continued to flow to the outermost edge of the earth, flowing back upon himself in a circle. The rivers, springs and fountains—indeed, the whole sea—issue continually from his broad, mighty stream." (Kerenyi, 1951) (p. 104)

This mandala, this Place of Crossing Waters, is a paradox of structured fluidity, of differentiated flow. One dimension is the east-west river, the dawn-sunset direction encompassing the activity of day, the time of work in the life of primitive man; the other is the north-south river, the midnight-midday current. The first river is the warm and energetic movement of daily reality and consciousness. The second river is the coolness and placidity related to the darkness of the unconscious midnight, to the moon and maternal aspect of the light of the inner world. Together the two rivers form a cross, not unlike the ancient Babylonian solar cross associated with water deities. (Bayley, 1952)

And where is this Place of Crossing Waters found in the seeking soul of man? What manner of pivotal point is it on which the new wheel of becoming must turn? As we give ourselves to the terrible and beautiful upward reaching of the spirit, as we struggle to shape and to let be shaped our uniqueness of self, there are recurring places where the small lights of awareness are focused. These are Kierkegaard's "moments," when time and eternity intersect as two streams. We stand, as do the people here, at a White-Speck-of-Earth of emergence, bringing with us all the pain and suffering, the joy and love, which we have felt before. All their meanings flow around us and under us, and we are filled with the sound of them. And we are aware, even if through a mist, of where we have been and of something of what must be done now. (pp. 104–105)

"No one of you seems to be able to guess what these things are. I roam about and have little sense, but I have guessed all of them. You must all pay great attention to this ceremony since it concerns you all. This shall be Birth." Once more it is Coyote, the lowly, the despised, the restless wanderer, who is able to see what is at hand. Likewise in the myths of several California Indian groups, including Wishosk, Yurok, Karek, and Hupa, the culture-hero-trickster is responsible for the origin of birth. (Kroeber, 1905)

And the word must now be made flesh; the body must become the container for the spirit. Only individual carriers are able to realize the individuation process, or the centralization of the rhythmic inward life. To be an individual carrier involves a recognition of our own physical nature in all its superb design and its sorry limitations. Every child beginning to be aware of its differences, accumulating experience which leads to a sense of "I," is a process of becoming a conscious carrier of the unconscious mystery. Each of us as an adult, as we repeatedly renew acquaintance with a lost part, is a participant in the same process. The body and sex are basic and living factors in the architecture of the individual carrier, are as intrinsic to the fullness of self-recognition as the mind and the spirit. To forget this, to relegate the body and sex to inferior positions in the upward reach of emergence, is to walk certainly into the catastrophe of meaninglessness.

What of body and sex as psychological facts? According to Linda Fierz:

> The body is our first and last outward reality which defines and conditions our life experience and gives us personal identity and continuity. It is our roots, in the earth, the world, in outer life. It is our immediate reality and uniqueness, our first concrete mandala mirroring our peculiarities, and differences. It is the most expressive and faithful burden we have, and we must be kind to it, listen to it. We should be able to bear with our body, especially as we grow older, should deal with it with dignity. We must not project it into complexes and conflicts, but let it be a pure expression of ourselves. (Fierz, 1948)

Primitive man has a rich intuitive awareness of the inseparableness of mind and body—an awareness which modern civilized cultures have tragically lost. The bodily foundation of the personality, which functions irrationally and with a debonair disregard for the careful logic of the intellect, cannot be put into a category of nonessential fact, as contemporary man tries so earnestly to do. When the word is made flesh, both flesh and word must celebrate the individual nativity. Emotions and passions are birth pains, moving us forward to a new consciousness in the unconscious. They are not all of life; they are no *final* goal of satisfaction, to be sure. Yet they must be experienced and known. We must be conscious of them; only then can we decide whether to express them outwardly or inwardly, or both. (pp. 107–108)

Either repression or cheapening of instinctive drives, particularly of the sexual, can only lead to formation of various physical symptoms, to compulsions and addictions, to harmful judgments, and in general to a withering of the personality. These are some of the "dark games" played out when we do not "pay great attention" to this archetype of the Creation of Birth. On the other hand, when we do attend, great things shimmer in the air. (p. 109)

Only as we become conscious of the split within us, and conscious also of the desire to be one again, spirit and body, word and flesh, joining together in a single community, can we hear Coyote's words: "You must all pay great attention to this ceremony since it concerns you all. This shall be Birth." Then a fuller existence can begin, as it does in the Navaho myth. (p. 110)

Evil and good are thus contained in the same act. This is the burden of growing consciousness. When the word is thus made flesh, it is also confronted by mortality, upheaval, sin, and built. We face our limitedness and our loneliness. We sin against our limitation by trying to be whole; we sin against wholeness by forgetting to be conscious.

Growth and change seem always to breed upheaval. Most original ideas and revolutions have been condemned by guardians of the old as "sinful." (p. 111)

The body becomes an intense and awkward instrument in the life of the spirit, blundering its way outward into the world of irrational emotions. It is not yet supported by the collective consciousness and has no sense of direction or meaning, being impelled at first only by its own animal urges. As individuals held in the body substance, for good or for ill, we may not yet be cognizant of us. It reaches for us as the sea reaches for the shore. It surges against us with a powerful love in each rise and fall of our tides, in every error and risk we involve ourselves in. Once the creation of birth is undertaken by the gods, the suffering consciousness of every day is placed in our hands. (p. 113)

The sensitive poetry of the words of love is replaced time and again by the obscene joke. Sex is not to be discussed because it is "bad"—and so a perplexed promiscuity becomes the way people try to reach one another. Mother is glorified into "momism," and as a result men and women alike are caught in an infantile rebellion marked by whispers, giggles, sex play in backseats of autos, and growing cults of "sexual freedom." No one is being responsible for psyche and body as a total and rich unity. Our adolescent emergence is treated like a recalcitrant but unfortunately necessary ass, alternately beaten and doctored. (p. 113)

It is at first a puzzling fact that this myth, coming form a matriarchal people whose dominant orientation is feminine, places full blame for the separation between the sexes on the women. But it is precisely the deep feminine womb, the darkness of the fecund undifferentiated earth-water world, which was the source of what now has come to pass. Even as the first upward way had to be a separation from the primal vessel and a breaking up of this selfsame vessel into many pots, so now man must almost seem to disown the feminine if he is finally to relate to it. The Mother is elementary container without whom no life could be. The Mother is also, however, life-devouring. She is, so it seems, desirous of taking her children back into the darkness from whence she sent them forth. Day passes into night, summer into winter, life into death. If the human being is to proceed as a sentient part of eternal being, he must somehow succeed in getting a foothold in another dimension. Thus cyclic nature, the amoral substance is blamed for impeding the orderly march of events. Whereas in the beginning Mother Nature's vegetative prodigality was most evident, at this stage it is her inertia and indifference which loom large. (pp. 114–115)

Nonetheless to live out adolescence some way is always essential for any true wholeness and conscious unity of ourselves.

And it is always, as it is in the myth, a painful time of confusion and disorganization and rebellion. What forces the adolescent or the adolescent adult out of the unconscious world is the recognition that life does not mother eternally, but more and more frequently appears to be neglectful and indifferent, to care not at all about maintaining a comfortable orderliness of existence. This apparent difference is not true; but what is really lacking is the adolescent's own responsibility for life and for nurturance through his own efforts. The "other" can no longer be relied on to hold all the instruments of fulfillment. Seed and vessel, grinding and cooking, must be found as substances and processes belonging to oneself. Where this does not happen in adolescence, it happens later.

Every adult, whether man or woman, who is trying to achieve a more conscious balance between masculine and feminine can find in this episode of Wolf Chief and his wife clues for development. The man can learn that, while his rational ordering of his world seems to be proceeding satisfactorily, his feelings and emotions may be forgotten and so may begin to rebel. Perhaps he sleeps when he wants to be awake. Perhaps he gossips rather than works. Perhaps his only communication with wife or children is through irritability and impatience. The woman, too, needs to see what happens when masculine and feminine have no meeting. If, as in the myth, her unconscious and split-off masculine side commands her inner world, she is letting her real womanness be walked over. So she sinks into apathy, or makes chaos out of her relationships, or becomes compulsive about smoking, drinking, sex. For both sexes, therefore, a new discrimination between masculine and feminine is urgent if growth is to continue. Very often men and women are pushed, as are Wolf Chief and his wife, into unexpected ways because the heretofore repressed emotions erupt. The woman may find herself refusing all sexual advances, or being bored beyond endurance by household affairs, or expressing unbridled irritation toward husband and children. The man may wander away form home more frequently, or may spend hours talking of things that really hold no interest for him. In any case, if one or the other tips the carefully preserved balance, thus spilling emotions about in disorder, something must happen, as it does in the myth. (pp. 117–118)

Separation from the Mother is not to be undertaken in haste and without preparation. As with any mystery, there is need for contemplation, firm choice, and contact with the inward vision. (p.118)

This is the subjective confrontation of that destiny which is an inevitable consequence of discovering the polarized energy of male-female opposition in the psyche. In the process of becoming an individual, this separation from the mother attitude—which attitude can be both a desire to be "mothered" and an unthinking acceptance of things "just as they are"—needs much attention and careful preparing. All spiritual and psychological maturation must be concerned with this stage of shedding the "old man" and of orienting the "new man" to a genuine self-sufficiency. Outreaching consciousness needs to set itself over against seductive unconscious passivity, needs to pull away from the inertia and indifference which is so much a part of the negative feminine. Yet the masculine reach has its negative aspects, too, one of these being the impatient urge to get things done at once. So the urgency must be held back until it is somehow better related to its important task of crossing. (pp. 118–119)

The individual man, as long as the tension-opposition is inward, is torn between the downward pull of the Mother with her sedative and deceptively cradling effect and the growing urgency of his masculine need for discriminations and differences. The feminine side of him often tends to "dissolve the ego and consciousness in the unconscious," leaving the man in bondage to the mother. What the men of the myth, led by Wolf Chief, seem to be doing is trying to free themselves from dissolution in feminine negativity. They are propelled into the separation by the active hostility of the feminine. (pp. 122–123)

The masculine, as already indicated, has been reaching outward, thrusting forward since the first restless movements. But a principle of distinction, of differentiation, is necessary if the masculine outreach is not to become an overreach. In this sense, "domestication" of the hunting consciousness is imperative not only for primitive man but for modern man. This involves the interpenetration of outward action and inward feeling: in the myth the men learn the women's tasks, aided by Nadleh. The women, who are misusing their powers and becoming thereby impoverished, are then as an archetypal symbol the negative feminine cut off from creative purpose. Anyone, man or woman, who has had experience with this heavy purposelessness—autoerotic, self-pitying, and self-indulgent— know what the negative feminine principle can do.

Necessary as the separation into opposites is, however, there comes a time when the sundering reaches its limits and the alternatives are seen to be either complete dissolution or relationship on a new basis. Each movement of growth has its own particular ebb and flow, its shifting of the alignments of forces. These cannot be arrested. They can only be felt into, responded to, worked with. To forsake the comfortable mother-womb and walk into the exposed land of separateness, where reward and responsibility are inextricably linked, is one of the hardest tasks put upon man. It gives an exhilarating sense of accomplishment when the Glittering Shore is reached, and living is enriched and vitalized. Yet with it come added trials and frustrations, calling for still more comprehensive awareness. (pp. 126–127)

The masculine principle of growth, the urgent sense of purpose, for quite a time can thrust ahead and not suffer thereby; but when an extreme position of one-sidedness is reached, a new balance needs to be found.

This is as true for the woman as for the man, though the manifestations of each sort of one-sidedness will be different. The man may remain entirely unconscious of his feminine principle and only live it through projections on outer women, thus never really relating individually to any woman. The woman, likewise, unaware of her masculine principle, may seek its fulfillment in unconscious and un-individual projections. When the feminine is very little projected—that is to say, is allowed to dominate the interior world in larger or smaller degrees—the man is apt to become moody, sullen, childish, petulant, even lethargic. A woman ruled by an unconscious masculine may be dominating, judgmental, autocratic, hyperactive. Each sex needs eventually to be conscious of and to learn to use more creatively the contrasexual principle within; then real outer relationship can be achieved. But this can only happen first through projection, then through the withdrawal of projection (or "separation"), then through discouraging regressions which often follow, and finally through the reuniting. (p. 129)

Development does not proceed uniformly, but by climbs and falls, assemblings and disruptions, births, deaths, and rebirths. Whenever an extreme of fullness is reached, individuation pushes ahead by means of chaos and darkness. (p. 130)

Consciousness as a process of becoming more whole must involve the push upward and forward, the separation of one part from another, the resultant partialness that collapses under its own weight, guilt and sacrifice, then a fresh upward step. And the climb out of darkness is accomplished only if we stop to see what has happened, assume full responsibility for it, and willingly take whatever action is needed to correct it. (pp. 130–131)

The masculine principle must learn to "know" in the sense of the noncanonical statement, "Man, if thou knowest what thou doest, thou art blessed." A reversal of direction, a religious ritual descent, is the way to knowledge. (p. 131)

Each of us stands in the midst of a crumbling civilization and can salvage it only by finding in ourselves the missing man and performing over him the songs, prayers, and rituals of untying and renewing. (pp. 132–133)

In the elaborate and beautiful ceremonies following the finding of the lost, many offerings are made to the Holy Ones. Rigidity, arrogance, self-determination—all must be renounced. Rituals such as the untying of knots and the passing through hoops require a humble admission of tension and sterility and of the need for rebirth. (p. 133)

This is another portrayal of the distress of partialness which must be faced if relationship is to be achieved either within oneself or between oneself and the other. Every man and every woman can come to know where one-sidedness resides, can see where the deepest affections stir below the surface of life. Outer events or inner happenings push toward the separation, the parting of the road where the paths disappear into shadows and anxious obscurity. One can at that moment follow the way of healing, which is to stay with the aloneness and the hunger and the fear until excess forces change. Another way, tragically chosen too often by modern man, is to ignore the existence of incompleteness and to let the creative substance burn itself out in futile attempts of parts to fulfill the destiny of the whole. This is manifested in the increased straining after power, whether on highways or in places of learning, the increased use of alcohol and drugs, the emphasis on "success" as the criterion of a full life. The conflict is muted, forgotten; the potential growth inherent in conflict atrophies and dies. (pp. 133–134)

Such expressions of mystery, incorporated into ritual acts, seem to be essential for a final understanding of the nature of changelessness and change; because the need to unify and separate and unify again leads to the enunciation of rhythm itself as a meaningful mystery. (p. 136)

One way or another, man needs to celebrate his becoming. Not only birth, marriage, and death are peaks in a cycle, but so is each time of transition or confusion, of pain or progress, of desolation or fullness. These are all points of purpose. Each should be gathered into the circle of a life with songs and prayers, with sweat house and celebration, so that no possible meaning shall be left unhonored. The known reach of man's maturity is small enough at best and does not need the added constriction of disregard. On the other hand, the stretch of man's spirit is infinitely great, worthy of whatever beauty of symbol and ritual can be given to it. (p. 137)

The fecund feminine womb container, Mother-night-and-nature, benign and rich with unknown life in the beginning, repeatedly has exerted her deathly backward pull. Struggles for consciousness have been many, showing clearly how great must be the urge for spiritual progression if it is to overcome the enormous weight of primeval darkness.

This eternal battle in the psyche is there for modern man just as surely as for primitive man, because the law of psychological gravity is on the side of substance and nature. This is why we must be repeatedly reminded. Mothering darkness is, first of all, the shelter within which life is conceived, held, and nurtured, as it was evidenced n the early scenes of this myth. It is warm with possibility, seductive with dreams of what might be; but no responsibility attaches to this aspect of the mother principle. Only as the initial undirected desire for identity is felt and acted upon does the positive father thrust begin to emerge. And at this stage the mother shows her claws. The great She will not loose her children easily or willingly. (p. 139)

The unconscious individual sees his difficulties as arising from outside himself, and only as he becomes more conscious does he recognize the genesis as an inner one. The psyche of man is composed of manifold and varied parts, each having its own particular contribution to make to the prospective wholeness. That which we call "I" is generally, except in infants and psychotics, the most clearly defined and "known." As to other parts, they struggle along relatively "unhonored and unsung" until some constellation of outer or inner events forces recognition of them. It is very much as if that which was destined to become a democracy began and remained for a long time a dictatorship where all unorthodox and unfamiliar objects were at once clapped into prisons or concentration camps, or were otherwise outlawed. In a political system, this of course gives rise to innumerable "scapegoats" to be blamed for all sin and error and so to carry the burdens of the society's incompleteness.

The formation of personality, the journey to the self, is not far different. At first there is anarchy of a sort. Then, as the "I" or ego strengthens, a dictatorship emerges where all the negative, difficult, unorthodox, fallible elements are banished, one by one, into unconsciousness. And whatever evidence of these poor prisoners may be found by the "I," it is put into the "others" outside, who are made to carry the buried sense of incompleteness. So long as this condition lasts, there will be unhappiness in the ego-I and seething upheaval within. Constructive change is at hand when the ego-I begins to be able to see the "other" as inside and can at last work more creatively toward a psychological democracy. (pp. 141–142)

What he is required to do here is essentially what many such heroes have to do: to go to the place of the maternal water, to open the dark womb, and to call out the purposive male aspects which alone seem to have the power to exorcise those poisons springing form their own negative manifestations. (p. 144–145)

The magic egg, the virgin birth, the unknown foundling child, theft, flood—what an impressive array of cosmic archetypes is spread before us! The "child" at this point is not single but multiple, indicating that the individual "self"-consciousness has not yet been fulfilled. Jung has said that the plurality of the "child" image, if found in normal people, "is a case of the representation of an as yet incomplete synthesis of personality." (Jung and Kerenyi, 1949) The twins who burst forth, disappear, and reappear, the baby who is stolen and returned, are all harbingers of the final emergence after which a more complete synthesis and conscious unification will occur. (p. 147)

Man does so desire, in his better hours, to outwit the temporal and to transcend nature's rhythmic tides by illuminating both spirit and nature. (This comes later with the carrying of Sun and Moon by the "gourd twins.") But before man can be truly reborn in the fullness of his spirit, before he can emerge into the white world of a new day, he must deal again with his own incomplete and shadowed creatureliness, Coyote. (p. 148)

One of our omnipresent psychological dangers is that new values and resources, new indications of activity, as soon as they emerge from the unconscious levels of our personality, will be seized upon and either destroyed or misused. For example, when the awkward creaturely emotions too quickly try to force into action a new-found sense of meaning, the result is never happy. The waters begin to rise; the unconscious is enlivened, but it threatens to engulf the slowly emerging order in unconsciousness and confusion. This is always one of the critical times in the human growth process: when new values have been discovered, but a hasty seizing of them seems to be leading toward disaster. Is the only answer to flee the darkness and imminent inundation? This is never the way out.

  Part of the answer lies in the unappealing but healing recognition by each of us that our new psychological babies, have floated more or less helplessly within the reach of consciousness, are almost always stolen. That is to say, our very imperfection, so needful of new life, greedily takes over that life and tries to absorb it in the everlasting but futile struggle for perfection. (pp. 148–149)

This element of positive/negative—thus, polarized—humanness is omnipresent in the evolution of consciousness, whether at a personal or a cultural level. Coyote, with his virtuosity of manifestation, is the carrier of the temporal paradox of existence. He sins, he errs, he wanders, he scolds; yet withal he knows the mystery. So he can never quite be rendered univocal. (p. 149)

The animal energy alone, no matter how intense, is not adequate to break through to the place of transformation. It can only point the way and commence the task. Essentially we cannot use instincts to transcend instincts, but must turn toward those functions of the psyche which seem, in a manner of speaking, more unfamiliar and alien to our earth-boundness. (p. 151)

Each thing, each part system of the psyche, must eventually come full circle and fulfill its place in the emergence of individuation. (p. 151)

World 5: Individuation (pp. 155–183)

- Each individual must participate in creating his or her world wisely and compassionately

- Individuation as enlightened self-regulation and containment of rage and anger

- Emergent differentiation when encountering resistance

- Changeability, impermanence, and no-self as objects of higher consciousness

- The evolved feminine as the capacity to transform and release from the womb

- Mother of change presides over the making of man

Individually and personally this awareness of a time-space reality as well as of a spiritual unlimitedness is the mark of a mature and responsible human being. We must look "down" to the place of strange dreams to complement our upward desire. If we live solely n the realm of external facts and their clever manipulation, we are incomplete. (p. 157)

But through a recognition of his mortal domain man learns to discriminate more finely and to recognize the unconscious substratum of his existence as the very core of his divinity and immortality. To see the feminine principle as cave from which one emerges and to which one comes home, as pot which contains dreams and visions, as place of withdrawal and return, is also to see the feminine not as *all* but as *part* of becoming. This lets the masculine be released to function in its own right. (p. 157)

Conscious creation is here more imperatively present than ever before. In the dark beginning, the darkness itself seemed discontented and restless, the only creator being a dim sense of the need to move. No goal was known. It was as if an embryo, stirred by forces felt but not in any way comprehended, began the struggles leading to birth. And from that point on, the preforms of life have been working upward. The dim and errant vision of wholeness is, for man, the primal push. (pp. 157–158)

Above all, this White World marks the perception that consciousness is a necessary concomitant to life, that the masculine principle must become a creator planning for the future. (p. 158)

This is to say, unless man consciously chooses to be a part of creation, the divine foundations are held entirely within the nonhuman archetypal realm; and from the point of view of man's ultimate fulfillment, this is evil. When man says "Yes" to creation, however, the suprapersonal energies are made available to him. The tremendous Yeas and Nays of God are echoed in the Yeas and Nays of man. God and man work together as cooperators in creation if any real creation occurs. As archetype God seems to say both a Yea and a Nay to man's urgency toward creation and transformation. In this sense, God is good and evil. Man also speaks both a Yea and a Nay to his own urgency, thus bringing himself into the area of ambivalence and paradox, and also being both good and evil. He possesses the "good" of nature and the "evil" of unconsciousness if he does not choose to act toward a new creation. He possesses the "good" of goal direction and the "evil" of going against nature if he does choose. And God (or the gods), as man sees Him, is both for and against change, both wanting His creatures to stay as they are and wanting them to expand for His sake as well as their own. The transcendent aspects of God, the cosmic and ineffable divine ground within which man and the archetypes have their being, these are neither evil nor good, perhaps, but are. (p. 159)

The articulation and communication of the meanings of the universe belong to man; they are acts of his consciousness, imperfect though it be. How else can the knowledge of the sacred eternality be manifest except through the crying out of man who, like Coyote, carries within him the voices of all created things? The prodigal sweep of life remains forever unfathomed and thus useless unless the individual finds his unique speech to relate it to himself. When the scolding, goading, restless, and disturbing part of man's nature dares—and is permitted—to step forward and shout, all things move, and existence has meaning and worth. To dare this, to permit this, is always difficult because it is difficult to let the last be first, the lesser be greater. A kind of true innocence is required; and for all his brashness and slyness, Coyote preserves a forthright innocence enabling him to trust his immediate responses. And this is, despite man's frequent protests and strivings for perfection, a very basic part of Creation. (p. 163)

The relationship between human and archetypal meanings is double-edged. If we become enmeshed in the subjective and always immediately personal meanings of event, we never know the awesome and humbling mystery of the movements of the "eternal presences"; we never are filled with the life beyond our own, which carries the balm of sunlight and silent peaks and starlit sky.

On the other hand to be lost in contemplation of the heavens and so let the dinner burn is the second edge. Its cut is as sharp as the first edge, for it can sever us from the necessary tie to time and circumstance, can make us unrelated and intolerable. When the two youths assumed the weight of Sun and Moon, had the people and gods at that point been content with the beauty and wonder of the fixed creation, no word, no spirit, would have come to set things moving. In the famous Arthurian legends of the Holy Grail and of the various Knights of the Round Table, the fate of the Grail and its ineffable redemptive mystery lay in the hands of Parsifal, the "guileless fool." (Neumann, 1949) So with each individual life. Even though a great magnificence of substance is in place and recognized and discriminated, man's roguish human selfness must participate in setting *his* world moving through *his* space and time. This the gods cannot do. (p. 164)

But in the endings, the light has come into a focus, and the sound of accomplished creation rises in the silence. Endings, as completions of a cycle rather than as finality, are less shadowy, for consciousness has entered into their shaping. Endings are no more precise than beginnings, for each end has in it the germinating seeds of a new and unfamiliar beginning. (pp. 168–169)

Thus man's world must be upheld and structured by some purposive power beyond his own. He must live, psychologically speaking, eternally in time, always between the great Above and the great Below. Carl Jung (Jung, 1939), Erich Neumann (Neumann, 1955), and others (Baynes,

1949; Fromm, 1956; Northrop, 1946) have spoken at length of the bipolarities in man. These have been called the masculine and feminine principles, the great Mother and great Father, the Old Wise Man and Old Wise Woman, Eros and Logos, to name a few. These pairs are not equivalent, but are related psychologically. (p. 170)

Such is the repeated cycle, proceeding from unconscious unity to a new something reaching the threshold of consciousness, to a falling asunder or a "twinning" (psychological mitosis), and finally to an emergent differentiation. (p. 171)

It is as if man cannot really begin his own opus until he sees and experiences the creator-god in all greatness and littleness, until he lets himself be in the hands of the ambivalence of that which is not yet realized and yet is longing for realization. This ambivalence is the grandfather of all tangible things. (p. 172)

This can be realized only as the eternal presences are brought to earth, so to speak, are firmly rooted in the transitoriness of a single life span. To become is to become in time and space. Otherwise only the idea of wholeness exists, never the actuality. (p. 174)

It is of inestimable importance that the individual seeking self-fulfillment be deeply aware of this spiritual feminine principle and distinguish between it and the more archaic feminine. At the start of life the embryo rests in the womb of the mother. Likewise at the start of each psychic pregnancy, the unknown seeds of a later awareness rest in the containing darkness of Mother-night-and nature. This is as it should be and must be, for healthy growth depends on quiet and patient germination; the very young life needs to be protected and kept safe. This is the role of the archaic feminine, biologically and psychologically. But this aspect of the feminine principle must never become the ruler, else growth is arrested or even destroyed. Perhaps one possible distinction between the truly "primitive" and the truly "civilized"—whether culture or person—is the degree to which desire for containment in the archaic mother-vessel has been renounced.

To stay in the womb, or to want to return to and stay in the womb, is thus a stultifying action leading to ultimate death or disintegration. On the other hand, when issuance from the womb is followed by negation of all Eros and feminine elements, as is often the case psychologically, another sort of death threatens. The former death is from drowning, the latter from thirst. The first kind of disintegration can be seen either in cases of extremely dependent passive people who overtly demand the mother-womb from friends, psychotherapists, and material environment, or in cases where a seeming independence overlaps a desire for unconscious containment. Behavior patterns falling into the former class are infantilism, self-indulgence, conversion hysteria, indecision. In the covert "mother-seeking" groups are, among others, those whose independence is withdrawal-in-order-to-be sought, or those who retreat from reality into the undifferentiated world of unconscious fantasy. Those who are in danger of perishing from thirst are more likely to be cold, brittle, hostile, rationally refusing emotions, dominating, imaginatively impoverished. In both kinds of psychological death, the "mother-womb" is the clue; whether it be magnet or repellent, it is negative.

Changing Woman, however, is a personification of that benign and mediating feminine side of the godhead to which both men and women must relate if they are to find life. She is the mother in a transforming and releasing fashion. She is the divine and the eternal *within* the substance and the material. It is to her that one may turn for comfort and sustenance, but always to be thrust out again into the flux of things. One sees repeatedly how essential it is that the modern psyche find a living relationship to this aspect of the Great Mother. For contemporary man has been caught between a too rational masculine attitude toward the world and a compensatory and infantile search for "mother" in the small. He succeeds in splitting the atom, while the use of alcohol and drugs rises. His machine, his bridges, dams, cities, his space conquests, are evidences of a superb scientific mastery—at the same time he pollutes his environment, comforts himself with comic books, demands security, and is unable to tolerate any ambiguity or change. (pp. 178–180)

Thus the self is seen in full maturity. The ultimate task of each individual man is to realize vitally what it is to be created from everything, to become Man, to assume responsibility for a life lived. Each must move into the mystery. The mystery of Being—of being just what one truly is—cannot be experienced through theoretical knowledge and the verbal ability to describe processes and levels of behavior. Nor can it be known through the prevalent pattern of protective coloration labeled "adjustment." We can experience the mystery only by experiencing, to its resonant, painful depths, that which seems to be the not-mystery—our own frail, awkward, lonely, noble self in its joyous incompletion. In one variant of the Creation myth (Klah, 1942), when the people had come into their final world, with humble wisdom they asked, How can we learn to live here? They built the sweat house for purification, and there they sang the Song of the Holy Spirit of Darkness. They sang, "The world is beautiful and we will put the spirit into it." The vessel of each man's wholeness, the containment of the self—this is the sweat house. Man is *in* it; it is *his,* with God's help, through meditation, introversion, creation, and all the ways of inwardness.

This is not sung easily, this Song of the Holy Spirit of Darkness. This "requires us," as the poet Rilke said, requires us as intensely as we require the song. A call must go out, but man must answer in order to help the inner world of the forms and images of Man, the "eternal presences," become manifest. All may be there in us, everything may be ready for our healing, our redemption, our ability to move in our world. But if our initiative is lacking, nothing goes forward. We must take the way of the mystery. We must recognize that we have many aspects—the above, the below, the dark, the light, substance, spirit—which reflect the divine as well as the human. Unless we are connected with them, the cyclic rhythm of our full selfhood cannot be.

Each individual life is its own myth, filled with restlessness, struggle, emergence, danger, paradox, creation. Ancient myths, such as this Navaho Emergence myth, are valid to us insofar as they deal in symbolic language with our personal myth. For most of us, the individual life myth is not consciously serving us until we are willing to read it, until we are forced to embark on the hero journey of redeeming the lost. Whether or not we prefer it to be so, our life is a journey, and we must go forward or backward, up or down.

In this journey, inescapably, are incorporated all the levels and dimensions of the psychic structure: the instincts, basic drives, and urges; the ego level; social relationships; the differentiation of psychological maturity, the orientation toward both past and future, both oneself and others.

And what does this journey, this hero pilgrimage, require of us? The same thing the earth requires of each of her multitudinous forms of life: to fulfill our own destiny as creatures, to be as rich, as total in our unique humanness as a tree in its treeness. Yet one further step is needed from us which the tree does not have to take. For the tree has not lost itself, since form the beginning it has been humbly obedient to its particularity. Not so with us. We have become confused in the cerebral labyrinth of whence and whither. We have sought to be more than human—that is our greatness—but have insisted on our own definitions of how—and this is our littleness.

If we can but learn, as this myth shows, the simple and hard lesson of emergence, of going into the darker places to follow the restless longing upward, of letting no small thing stay forgotten and unhonored, then we shall be whole. Then we shall be related to the unconscious powers within us of life and God. This is redemption. (pp. 182–183)

CHAPTER 37

Stages of Shamanic Procedure

Besides that, the shamanistic techniques in themselves often cause the medicine-man a good deal of discomfort, if not actual pain. At all events, the "making of a medicine man" involves, in many parts of the world, so much agony of body and soul that permanent psychic injuries may result. His "approximation to the savior" is an obvious consequence of this, in confirmation of the mythological truth that the wounded is the agent of healing, and that the sufferer takes away suffering. (Jung, 1969)

Throughout this section of the book, I have attempted to define disease and illness, health, and healing in a spiritual context. This includes the way traditional cultures predate our Western cultural attempts at health and healing. This section of the book has merged findings in depth psychology, mythology, and cross-cultural healing into the new healing paradigm of biodynamic craniosacral therapy. Now, at the end of the book, I am proposing a sequence of events in the biodynamic therapeutic process to hold as a possibility for practitioners. Biodynamic practitioners may view the therapeutic process as shamanic because the practitioner places himself in a role that is by classical definition shamanic. The role is for the practitioner to remove himself from the immediate urban world and enter another domain of extrasensory perception. He travels to this dimension to invite the gods of healing into relationship with the client.

The domain of stillness and the void symbolically represent the archetypal realm of the gods or transpersonal energies. The biodynamic perceptual process frequently involves a dissociation from ordinary perception that is trans-sensory. There is a very strong somatic affect of awe and mystery that is larger than life's typical sensations outside the treatment room. The direct experience of the numinous is readily available in biodynamic sessions, by definition, since the biodynamic model is based on Dr. Sutherland's experience of the Breath of Life in a client's body. Along with trans-sensory experience comes potentially frightening imagery such as the body opening up and its contents being removed or animals appearing in and around the client's body during the session. Dream material is evoked that requires the practitioner to have the shamanic knowledge of another dimension beyond the worldly plane in order to hold the unconscious of the client as well as the client's soma. These aspects of the biodynamic process usually occur within the practitioner's perception and to a lesser extent within the client's perception. It occurs often enough that it must be taken seriously and included in the healing process.

> The shamans and mystics of primitive societies are considered—and rightly so—to be superior beings; their magicoreligious powers also find expression in an extension of their mental capacities. Hence the shaman becomes the exemplar and model for all those who seek to acquire power. The shaman is the man who *knows* and *remembers,* that is, who understands the mysteries of life and death; in short, who shares in the spirit condition. He is not solely an ecstatic but also a contemplative, a thinker. In later civilizations the philosopher will be recruited among these beings, to whom the mysteries of existence represent a passionate interest and who are drawn, by vocation, to know the inner life. (Eliade, 1958, p. 102)

Shamanism, as defined by Mircea Eliade (Eliade, 1964), is a "technique of ecstasy" (p. 4). Shamanism and its associated religious experience is the foundation for all Western religion. It employs ecstasy in that it is outside of the normal worldly states of sensation and feeling. Consequently, shamanism employs trans-sensory experiences that must necessarily include normal dissociation, trance states, and states similar to hypnotherapy. There is frequent misunderstanding about shamanism being related to magic, possession by evil spirits, and other phenomenal experiences. These distinctions are not relevant in this discussion of how a biodynamic craniosacral therapist fills the role of a shaman or a medicine man. Perhaps it is best to say that a shaman is more active in a session and a medicine man less active. These are labels given to the experience of the mystery of healing at a time during a session when the practitioner cannot possibly be cognitive.

> The shaman or the medicine man can be defined as a specialist in the sacred, that is, an individual who participates in the sacred more completely, or more truly, than other men. Whether he is chosen by Superhuman Beings or he seeks to draw their attention and obtain their favors,

the shaman is an individual who succeeds in having mystical experiences. In the sphere of shamanism in the strict sense, the mystical experience is expressed in the shaman's trance, real or feigned. The shaman is pre-eminently an ecstatic. Now on the plane of primitive religions ecstasy signifies the soul's flight to Heaven, or its wanderings about the earth or, finally, its descent to the subterranean world, among the dead. The shaman undertakes these ecstatic journeys for four reasons: *first,* to meet the God of Heaven face to face and bring him an offering from the community; *second,* to seek the soul of a sick man, which has supposedly wandered away from his body or been carried off by demons; *third,* to guide the soul of a dead man to its new abode; *fourth,* to add to his knowledge by frequenting higher beings. (Eliade, 1958, p. 95)

Typically, a traditional shaman is not recognized until she has received at least two types of teaching. The first teaching is specifically about the dissociative experience as it comes through different types of trances and dream states. As I mentioned in an earlier chapter, I discovered that as I started a craniosacral therapy session, I automatically put myself into a light trance by fixating my vision on an object inside or outside of the room for a brief time and simply spacing out. Even my grammar school teachers commented to me on the amount of time I spent staring out the window and not paying attention to the lesson on the blackboard. It is crucial for any practitioner to understand and become conscious of how he dissociates before, during, and after a session of biodynamic craniosacral therapy. Important information is coming through a different sensory channel. It is the direct experience of the deep mystery of life and what I call a midline experience. There is no interference or middle man interfering with this communion with the numinous. This requires a symbolic or, in ancient times, a literal stripping away of the body (ego) to get down to the skeleton or, in the case of a biodynamic therapy, to imaginally dissolve the contents of the soma so that all that remains is a three-dimensional, transparent living fluid body.

The second kind of teaching that a shaman receives relates to specific techniques, and in manual therapy, these techniques are limited to perceptual processes, visualizations, hand positions, and pressure gradients used with the hand positions. All sorts of symbols may be hanging from the walls of the practitioner's office, but in general, cross-cultural imagery is embodied by the practitioner in this day and age so as not to create fear in the client. It is just not acceptable to sacrifice a chicken in front of the client anymore. The media is already doing a splendid job of scaring the client by showing the killing fields in the Middle

East. The biodynamic shaman or medicine man needs to relate to a proper mythology which is that of the human embryo. The practitioner is attempting to harness the power of creation in every session. This is the key. He needs to have a coded language to talk to other shamans such as ignition, automatic shifting, the neutral, and so forth. He must know his spiritual lineage and which healing spirits and gods he calls upon for help. For example, there are many different names given to the cardinal directions, depending on which Native American group you study. The east can be represented by an eagle, a wolf, or other spirit figures, depending on the local culture. It is important that a shaman stick with one system of metaphors and mythology. Such healing processes are typically acquired in initiations, colored strongly by cultural complexes and traditions. The medicine woman does not choose her method of healing—it is revealed to her individually in her initiation.

The education of a shaman is complex and involves initiation rituals that are both ecstatic or outside the normal domains of human sensation and also didactic with the undertaking of a new language and system of thought related to how healing happens. This is how different societies prepare their healer-shamans to grow into their powers. The failure of some biodynamic foundation trainings is the lack of initiation for working with the power of creation. The great risk here is the practitioner getting overinflated or deflated when he leaves the training. The starting point for learning traditional healing ways is not as important as the technology itself and its underlying theory, transmitted through initiation. The first call to become a shaman may be through the family lineage or a previous illness. But the call can also be caused from a deep psychological disturbance and a predisposition to dissociation from the world, regardless of its origin.

The term *initiation* generally means a group of rituals and oral teachings whose purpose is to produce a decisive alteration in the religious and social status of the person to be initiated. Initiation creates a basic change in the life path and direction of the shaman. The shaman emerges from her ritual endowed with a totally different being from the one she possessed before her initiation; she has become *another* (Eliade, 1958). Initiation introduces the shaman into society and into the world of spiritual and cultural values. She learns the behavior patterns, the techniques, and the institutions of adults in her culture. More important, she learns the sacred myths and healing traditions of her tribe, the names of the gods, and the history of their creation; above all, she learns the mystical relations between the tribe and the gods of creation that were established at the beginning of time by experiencing them directly, not from a teacher didactically. This is the embryo. Primary Respiration introduces the initiate to the realm of the unseen power of creation in the universe. The visible embryo is the manifestation of the invisible act of incarnation. This education involves procedures and rituals that I have detailed throughout this book.

The shamanic initiation as applied to biodynamic craniosacral therapy sessions can be said to have seven phases, as outlined below.

Phase 1. Spiritual Disease

The shaman recognizes that all illness and disease is a spiritual problem first because of an alienation from the natural world. Contemporary Western culture leaves no choice for its population but to dissociate from the natural world. Yet the dissociation itself is a preexisting, inherent resistance to splitting away from the midline connection to the divine. It is healthy but unfocused. Dissociation in this light is a divine state of possession. I have detailed this in Chapter 34.

Alienation is a better description of the effects of speed and stress on the mind and soma of the client than is post-traumatic stress disorder. Alienation is a progressive withdrawal from the divine, nature, the body, and finally the mind. Alienation is the way the mind and body manages a fearful society. Healing must necessarily involve the technology that is capable of reconnecting those four worlds through and with a midline. The value of dissociation must be discovered and reframed as a movement toward the normalization of a reconnection to the natural world.

Phase 2. Sacred Space

> … how the boundaries that delimit the space are constituted and maintained or "stewarded." The issue should not be drawn as whether the practice is "society-wide" or not; it should be focused on the nature and permeability of the boundaries of the space involved and on the relative importance of the leadership of ritual elders or "technicians of the sacred" in making judgments as to the appropriate utilization of the space. (Schwartz-Salant and Stein (eds.), 1991, p. 23)

Healing must take place in a ritual container. Dissociative affect must be used and transformed into a more conscious distancing from contemporary society, rather than separation and alienation from the divine. It is the responsibility of the shaman to mark the space in which the session occurs and consecrate the container through whatever means she has learned. This ritual purification is a prayer first and foremost with the symbols of meditation, the lighting of a candle or the use of sage or cedar, to purify the room before the office opens and so forth. The intention of establishing sacred space is to clearly differentiate in the mind of the client that he is in a different world than the one he just came from.

It is, as Mircea Eliade calls it, the difference between the sacred and the profane (Eliade, 1959). Everyone who practices biodynamic craniosacral therapy would be well advised to read *The Sacred and the Profane* by Mircea Eliade.

Phase 3. Establishing a Midline

The shaman must establish a relationship first with her own midline, then the midline of stillness in the sacred space, and finally the client's midline. This is the actual work of biodynamic craniosacral therapy. I have written extensively about this process in Chapter 31 in Volume One. The central practice is establishing a relationship with dynamic stillness deep enough that one could experience a voidness or nondual state. I have suggested a meditation earlier in this book on going to the void in Chapter 13. The shaman must orient her attention completely to the stillness of the midline as a prerequisite for any healing effect from the session to occur. Again, this may require a dissociation from the mundane that, in this case, transports the perception of the shaman into the world of healing. The shaman has her feet in both worlds of the sacred and the mundane. There must, however, be a perceptual experience that grabs hold of the practitioner. Such perception is the doorway or threshold to a therapeutic process being governed by the forces of creation on the other side of the veil of ignorance worn by urban society. Often this can be simply boredom and irritation. It can also be anxiety or genuine feelings of compassion. The most important effect is heat and warmth. As the heat and feelings of the practitioner increase, another world is entered.

Phase 4. World Heart

Initiations by return to the womb have as their first aim the novice's recovery of the embryonic situation. From this primordial situation the various forms of initiations which we have reviewed develop in different directions, for they pursue different ends. That is, having symbolically returned to the state of "semen" or "embryo," the novice can do one of four things. He can resume existence, with all its possibilities intact. (This is the goal of the *hiranyagarbha* ceremonies and of "embryonic breathing," and the same motif is amply documented in archaic therapies.) Or he can reimmerse himself in the cosmic sacrality ruled by the Great Mother. … Or he can attain to a higher state of existence, that of the spirit …, or prepare himself for participation in the sacred. … Or, finally, he can begin an entirely different, a transcendent mode of existence, homologizable to that of the Gods (the goal of Buddhism). From all this, one common characteristic emerges—*access to the sacred*

and to the spirit is always figured as an embryonic gestation and a new birth.
(Eliade, 1958, p. 58)

The shaman gradually synchronizes her attention with the outside presence of Primary Respiration automatically shifting between the three embryonic fulcrums of the umbilicus, heart, and third ventricle to the horizon. It is the responsibility of the biodynamic craniosacral therapist at this point to generate a felt sense of heat, warmth, and compassion moving from her heart to the larger heart of nature and beyond. It is in this way that the two hearts of the client and practitioner are reunited to a larger spiritual principle contained in nature and possibly at or beyond the horizon. The shaman is always mediating information between the space of the session room and nature. It is in this process that different symbolic figures may appear in the consciousness of the practitioner or the client. These figures can span from being supernatural and mythic all the way to one's mother or father. The important job of the shaman is to discover the purpose and meaning for the appearance of such helpers through a nonverbal dialogue.

A visualization that sometimes occurs to me when I am in session is seeing the chest wall of the client open. I imagine a bloodless surgery as the skin subtly unzips from between the clavicles and the pubic bone. The skin, the muscles, and the bones are all pulled back, exposing the heart, the lungs, and all the organs. At this point, I imagine that all of these organs, one by one, are floating out of the body and slowly dispersing out into space on a wave of Primary Respiration toward the horizon. All that is left is a hollow, empty core of the client's body. I visualize the space being purified and cleansed with a bright light and then gradually the space being filled up with precious stones and precious metals, such as rubies, emeralds, diamonds, and gold. As these precious metals and stones fill the core of the client's body, they transmute into a rainbow of flowing, liquid forms permeating and surrounding every cell in the client's body. I then visualize the skin, the muscles, and the bones of the client in the front of the body closing. There is absolutely no scarring or marks left from this bloodless surgery. The movement and tempo of the removal of the organs and their being replaced with precious stones and metals takes place at the rate of Primary Respiration.

As an alternative, I might visualize the face of the client opening up all the way from the superior sagittal suture down through the hyoid bone to the sternoclavicular notch. In much the same way as above, all the nerves, the eyes, and finally the brain floats out of the cranial cavity. The same replacement process is used as a stream of liquid color, covering the full spectrum of the rainbow, is put back into the cranial cavity at the rate of Primary Respiration. Sometimes only one color will dominate the visualization. What's important is to allow the visualization to proceed with its own story line and process, rather than the practitioner dictating a memorized visualization. This is all under the guidance of Primary Respiration and stillness. It is extremely important to emphasize that practitioners do not know what is best for clients. The practitioner must be shown how and where to be in relationship with the client.

Phase 5. Client Focus

In order to facilitate a needed deconstruction of the old personality structure of the individual, the individual is offered an opportunity to surrender autonomy temporarily, to submit to a total process which has an autonomy of its own and which can enable the individual to maintain needed orientation and structure during this time of deconstruction. Built into the therapeutic process is the creation of a relatively safe psychosocial space in which this deconstruction and surrender of autonomy can occur. (Schwartz-Salant and Stein (eds.), 1991, p. 25)

Gradually through physical contact, the shaman pays attention to the movement of Primary Respiration in herself. Then the shaman allows her body to be moved by the Primary Respiration of the client. This is a whole-body response, as though the body was a single drop or sphere of living fluid breathing at the rate of Primary Respiration. The shaman may or may not be able to sense the unique movement of Primary Respiration inside the client's body. The focus is on the movement of the whole outside the body.

The typical sequence that I perceive is as follows: First, I orient my total and complete attention to a stillpoint. Sometimes I am able to do this by sensing the inside of my body, but more frequently, I must orient to a tree or a cloud outside of my body. I then wait to sense the movement of the outside presence of Primary Respiration moving back and forth from the horizon to my third ventricle. At this point, I may shift the fulcrum of perception of Primary Respiration down to my heart and/or umbilicus. I allow my attention to rest in the general space of my body on the surface of the skin between my clavicles and pubic bone. I wait to sense the Primary Respiration coming from the client and pushing my body away for fifty seconds and then drawing my body slightly back toward the client. I wait for this reciprocal relationship of Primary Respiration between me and the client to go through several cycles of 100 seconds each. Then I gradually bring my attention to my hands and wait for the movement of the client's whole fluid body and tidal body to move as one. Any other motion is disregarded. Only the motion of the whole gets my attention. I may visualize the client as being a sphere-shaped egg, such as prior to conception. This is the priority of treatment—to sense the movement of the whole in both self and other.

Phase 6. Regeneration

> The sun, plunging every evening into the darkness of death and into the primordial waters, symbol of the uncreated and the virtual, resembles both the embryo in the womb and the neophyte hidden in the initiatory hut. When the sun rises in the morning, the world is reborn, just as the initiate emerges from his hut. In all probability, burial in the embryonic position is explained by the mystical interconnection between death, initiation, and return to the womb. (Eliade, 1958, p. 59)

The presence of a benevolent spirit or being enters the room. This is the moment of conception or the starting place for renewal and restoration for the client. This benevolent "other pair of hands" is perceived to be assisting the biodynamic session (Jealous, 1998). Dr. Sutherland called it the presence of "Other." He also referred to the experience as the Breath of Life, which to him was like a flash of light in the night sky. This deeply shamanic figure, presence, image, or feeling either removes the illness from the soma of the client or has traveled in nature or beyond to retrieve that which was lost and replaces it into the soma of the client. Its intentions are frequently unknown to the practitioner. The practitioner has entered a deep stillpoint called a void state.

> And this will suffice to keep us from falling into the error of explaining all initiatory rites and symbols of return to the womb by the desire to prolong a merely biological existence. Such an existence is a quite recent discovery in the history of humanity—a discovery that was made possible precisely by a radical desacralization of nature. On the level on which our study is being conducted, life is still a sacred reality. (Eliade, 1958, p. 59)

Phase 7. Resolution

Healing and resolution occur through the felt sense of love in the client's mind and body. This may include a perception of connectedness to nature and spirit or may manifest through different dream material or perhaps initiating a divorce. As Carl Jung said, it is the affective experience of the archetypal world that is healing. The biodynamic practitioner waits to sense the heat and warmth of love as a felt sense around his heart breathing at the tempo of Primary Respiration between his heart and the heart of the client.

It is unlikely that all of this can occur in one session of biodynamic craniosacral therapy. The correct number of sessions for resolution is unknown. It may also involve help from other sources and, of course, time. I must again emphasize that the shamanic nature of the practitioner and of the biodynamic sessions comes about through an initiation from and by an "Other." Healing comes about through the felt sense of love and compassion as a permeating heat streaming through the body, not by what the practitioner needs and wants to have happen intuitively. Biodynamic practice is instinctual work. I believe that the statement below by Mircea Eliade is the essence of our embryonic nature, which is freedom from limitations.

> The desire for absolute freedom—that is the desire to break the bonds that keep him tied to earth and to free himself from his limitations—is one of man's essential nostalgias. And the break from plane to plane effected by flight or ascent similarly signifies an act of transcendence; flight proves that one has transcended the human condition, has risen above it, by transmuting it through an excess of spirituality. Indeed, all the myths, the rites, and the legends that we have just reviewed can be translated as the longing to see the human body act after the manner of a spirit, to transmute man's corporal modality into the spirit's modality. (Eliade, 1958, p. 101)

CHAPTER 38

I Hear You

By Sarajo Berman

Tell me the story of the Enoe
the tales you hold within your worn beauty
where supple newness meets substantial stalks blowing in the
    breezes,
wafted and graciously carried by the limbs of warrioresque
    trees in motion,
molded boulders and rocks.
A time when all that was heard were the sounds of animal
    feet lightly caressing your shaded shores,
your streaming waters
your covered trails leading to the sky.
And when the sound of fish flying out of the water toward
    dinner
splashing into their home again to feast was heard for miles,
when drops would splash on your surface and ripple out, and
    on for miles.
A time when only nature visited nature.
A story of your partnering with great storms,
fast rains, bulldozing winds, and days, months, years of
    drought,
always meeting the moment and going into the next
    unknowing with such grace.

I hear your sadness of lost waters, shrunken shores, and
    trampled trails
yet, what I feel most is your eagerness to remain in
    relationship.
Your trust of…

something will happen, will change, will move, will dance
will be with me...........always.

A soft breeze, liquid gold from the sky quenching my thirst.
those that swim with my currents and those that come to
    find power by ingesting my moving blood fulfills me as
    does,
the dying and birthing of years
to come.
And yes, moments of being seen and felt and heard
from an open
Heart.

August 11, 2007

Appendix A

CODE OF ETHICS

Shea Educational Group (SEG)

Preamble

The pursuit of wholeness and well-being requires dedication, discipline and vision. SEG believes in the dignity and worth of the individual human being. SEG is committed to increasing physical, spiritual and emotional well-being through the practice of compassion. While pursuing this endeavor, SEG is committed to having its students and staff protect the safety welfare of any person who may seek biodynamic craniosacral therapy. Students and staff do not use this professional relationship, nor knowingly permit their services to be used for purposes inconsistent with these values. As a school, SEG insists on freedom of inquiry and communication; accepts the responsibility this freedom confers, for competence where SEG claims it, for objectivity in the report of our findings, and for consideration of the best interest of our graduates and their clients, colleagues and of society. This Code of Ethics is a blueprint containing essential principles and an inherent code of conduct that may guide students, staff and graduates in the evolution of their personal and professional lives.

Principles

In the pursuit of these ideals the SEG subscribes to principles in the following areas: (1) responsibility; (2) competence; (3) moral and legal standards; (4) public statements; (5) confidentiality; (6) welfare of the consumer; (7) professional relationships; (8) practice management; and (9) sexual harassment policy.

481

Principle 1—Responsibility

In providing services whether they be teaching, research, administrative, or clinical, practitioners maintain the highest standards of this profession. They accept responsibility for the consequences for their acts and make every effort to ensure that their services are used appropriately. This responsibility extends to SEG approved teachers, their assistant instructors, co-instructors, administrative staff and any other person in a position of authority or power.

a. Teachers recognize their primary obligation to help others acquire knowledge and skill. They maintain high standards of scholarship and by presenting information objectively, fully and accurately. They continually study and evolve their teaching based on current information.

b. As clinicians, practitioners know that they have a social responsibility because their recommendations and professional actions may alter the lives of others. They are alert to personal, social, organizational, financial, or political situations and pressures that might lead to misuse of their influence. They excuse themselves from the possibility of a dual relationship especially in a decision making position.

c. As clinicians, practitioners show sensible regard for the social codes and moral expectations of the community in which they work, recognizing that violation of accepted moral and legal standards on their part may involve their clients and colleagues in damaging personal conflicts and injure their person reputation and the reputation of the profession and especially the client involved.

d. Practitioners accurately inform their clients, the client's primary care physician when appropriate, other health care practitioners, and the public of the scope and limitations of their knowledge and understanding of biodynamic practice as it relates to the individual client. They do not diagnose nor prescribe. They acknowledge limitations and contraindications for biodynamic craniosacral therapy and refer appropriately.

e. Practitioners who mix other modalities in their biodynamic practice such as massage therapy, provide draping and treatment that insures the safety, comfort and privacy of the client. Craniosacral therapists follow the rules for draping as provided under the regulation of their local and state licensure to professionally touch others. They inform the client of mixed modalities being used.

Principle 2—Competence

a. Practitioners accurately represent their competence, education, training, and experience. They claim as evidence for clinical and educational qualifications only those degrees and certifications obtained from institutions acceptable under the standards set forth by SEG and other professional associations of which the practitioner is a member.

b. Teachers perform their duties on the basis of careful preparation so that their instruction is accurate, current, and academically sound.

c. Practitioners recognize the need for continuing education and are open to new procedures and changes in biodynamic practice and theory over time. Practitioners consistently maintain and improve their professional knowledge and competence through regular assessment of personal and professional strengths and weaknesses by a qualified supervisor and by continuing education and training in approved programs of SEG or other SEG-approved programs.

d. Practitioners recognize differences among people, such as age, sex, socioeconomic, and ethnic backgrounds. When necessary, they obtain training, experience, research, or counsel to assure competent service to such persons or conditions that clients report.

e. Practitioners recognize that personal problems and conflicts may interfere with professional effectiveness. Accordingly, they refrain from undertaking any activity in which their personal problems are likely to lead to inadequate performance or harm to a client, colleague, student, or any other associate. If engaged in professional activity when they become aware of their personal problems, they seek competent professional assistance to determine whether they should suspend, terminate, or limit the scope of their professional activities. Biodynamic practitioners are committed to their own personal self-development.

f. Practitioners avoid deliberately provoking an emotional response in their clients with the use of release based cathartic techniques and/or other body centered psychotherapeutic techniques without an accredited academic degree or appropriate credentialed training, a supervised internship and ongoing supervision from an expert in the field of trauma resolution, a psychotherapist or a psychiatrist.

Principle 3—Moral and Legal Standards

a. Teachers are aware of the fact that their personal values may affect the selection and presentation of instructional materials. When dealing with topics that may give offense such as spirituality or sexuality, they recognize and respect the diverse attitudes that students may have toward such issues.

b. As employees or employers, teachers and practitioners do not engage in or condone practices that are exploitive or that result in illegal or unjustifiable actions. Such practices include but are not limited to those based on consideration of race, handicap, age, gender, sexual preference, religion, or national origin in hiring, promotion, or training. Dual relationships and conflict of interests are professionally acknowledged and recusal is used to withdraw from such conflict.

c. Practitioners are aware of their need for personal care and ongoing psychotherapy when working with psychological issues arising in their private practice between themselves and their clients. Practitioners strive to improve themselves not only through psychotherapy or other appropriate means but also psychological and or professional supervision from a qualified mental health counselor, receiving group support, body-centered therapy, and taking appropriate continuing education.

d. Practitioners follow all policies, guidelines, regulations, codes and requirements promulgated by local, state, and federal authorities governing their legal right to touch clients.

e. Practitioners receive informed consent for every specific technique or modality they intend to use with a client and the intended purpose of such. This includes the responsibility of informing the client during a session when the original contract has changed. Informed consent depends strongly on mutual trust, empathetic and compassionate attitudes, and behavior, as well as the capacity for clear communication.

f. Practitioners refuse any gifts or benefits in excess of acceptable gratuity which are intended to influence a referral, a decision, or a treatment.

Principle 4—Public Statements

a. When announcing or advertising professional services, practitioners may list the following information to describe their services: name, highest relevant academic degree earned from a regionally accredited institution, relevant certifications or diplomas from SEG-approved trainings, date, type, and level of certification, licensure or professional membership, address, telephone number, office hours, a brief listing of the type of modalities offered, and an accurate presentation of fee information, cancellation policy, foreign languages spoken, and policy with regard to third-party payments. Additional relevant or consumer information may be included if not prohibited by other rules and regulations in an individual's municipality, county, or state.

b. In announcing or advertising the availability of craniosacral therapy products, publications, or services, practitioners do not present their affiliation with any organization in a manner that falsely implies sponsorship or certification by that organization. Practitioners do not make public statements that are false, fraudulent, misleading, deceptive, or unfair. They do not misinterpret facts or make statements that are likely to mislead or deceive because in context it makes only a partial disclosure of relevant facts, especially comparing a style of craniosacral therapy to another with statements like "less invasive," "more forceful," or other statements that make another style of craniosacral therapy appear less than efficacious or the practitioner(s) in question as more than efficacious.

c. Practitioners do not use testimonials from clients regarding the quality of their clinical services nor do they use statements intended or likely to create false or unjustified expectations of favorable results such as suggesting their work is research-based (when it is not under the academic definition of accepted professional research), or can cure certain conditions when no such research exists; nor do they use statements implying unusual, unique, or one-of-a-kind abilities; nor do they use statements intended or likely to appeal to a client's fears, anxieties, or emotions concerning the possible results of failure to obtain their services such as, "Do you want your condition to drag on forever?" or "Without this kind of treatment you may experience more symptoms," etc.

d. Announcements or advertisements for classes, sessions, or clinics give a clear statement of purpose and a clear description of the service to be provided.

e. The education, training, and experience of the staff members are appropriately specified. Practitioners associated with the development or promotion of craniosacral therapy devices, books, or other products offered for commercial sale make reasonable efforts to ensure that announcements and advertisements are presented in a professional and factually informative manner.

f. Practitioners are guided by the primary obligation to aid the public in developing informed judgments, opinions, and choices.

g. Teachers ensure that statements in catalogs and course outlines are accurate and not misleading, particularly in terms of subject matter to be covered, basis for evaluating progress, the nature of course experiences, and who is actually teaching the course. Announcements, brochures, or advertisements describing workshops, seminars, or other educational programs accurately describe the eligibility requirements, educational objectives, and the nature of the materials to be covered. These announcements also accurately represent the education, training, and experience of the teacher(s) presenting the programs and any fees involved.

Principle 5—Confidentiality

a. Information obtained in the classroom, clinic, or consulting relationships or evaluative data concerning children, students, employees, and others is discussed only for professional purposes and only with those clearly concerned with such, and with the client's permission. Written and oral reports present only data germane to the purposes of the evaluation, and every effort is made to avoid undue invasion of privacy.

b. Practitioners who present information obtained during the course of professional work from other's writings, lectures, or other public forums either obtain adequate prior consent to do so or adequately disguise all identifying information when it concerns a case presentation of a client.

c. All classroom and clinical processes are considered confidential and all staff, instructors, and students are expected to honor and maintain the confidentiality of the classroom and the clinical setting.

d. Practitioners provide treatment only when there is reasonable expectation that it will be advantageous to the client.

e. Practitioners respect the client's right to refuse, modify, or terminate treatment regardless of prior consent given. Practitioners promote active verbal input by the client.

f. Practitioners respect the client's boundaries with regard to emotional expression, beliefs, and reasonable expectations of professional behavior. Practitioners respect the client's autonomy. The same is true for teachers of biodynamic craniosacral therapy and their student's autonomy.

Principle 6—Welfare of the Consumer

a. Practitioners are continually cognizant of their own needs and of their potentially influential position with clients, students, and subordinates. They avoid exploiting the trust and dependency of such persons. Practitioners make every effort to avoid dual relationships that could impair their professional judgment or increase the risk of exploitation. Examples of such dual relationships include, but are not limited to, socializing, doing research with, treating, or engaging in a fiduciary relationship with employees, students, supervisees, close friends, or relatives. Hiring a student, socializing with students, and hiring family members are some examples of dual relationships.

b. Sexual intimacies with clients and students are unethical and possibly immoral when predatory in nature.

c. Teachers and assistants must be cautious of dual relationships when doing private sessions with students during a training period, or between training modules. Unless a student is a client prior to the beginning of a training, private sessions between teaching team members and students during the three years of training are generally considered tutorial sessions rather than therapeutic sessions.

d. Practitioners have the right to refuse to accept prospective clients. However, once accepted, he or she owes the client complete loyalty, care, attention, and integrity. Practitioners strive to complete all necessary sessions with their clients. They will discontinue services only when self-respect, dignity, or other appropriate cause requires this action.

e. Practitioners terminate a clinical, teaching, or consulting relationship when it is reasonably clear that the consumer is not benefiting from it. He or she offers to help the consumer locate alternative sources of assistance.

Principle 7—Professional Relationships

a. Practitioners understand the areas of competence in related professions. They make full use of all the professional, technical, and administrative resources that serve the best interest of their clients. The absence of formal relationships with other professions and professional workers does not relieve the practitioner of the responsibility of securing for clients the best possible professional service, nor does it relieve the practitioner of the obligation to exercise foresight, diligence, and tact in obtaining the primary or complementary assistance needed by clients.

b. Practitioners know and take into account the traditions and practices of other professional groups, especially in the medical and osteopathic community and they work and cooperate fully with such groups. If a person is receiving similar services from another professional, practitioners do not offer their own services directly to such a person. If a practitioner is contacted by a person who is already receiving similar services from another professional, he or she carefully considers that professional relationship and proceeds with caution and sensitivity in regards to the therapeutic issues as well as the client's welfare. The practitioner is obligated to discuss these issues with the client so as to minimize the risk of confusion and conflict.

c. Practitioners do not exploit their professional relationships with clients, supervisees, students, employees, or others, sexually or otherwise.

d. When practitioners know of an ethical violation by another practitioner, and it seems appropriate, they initially attempt to resolve the issue by bringing the behavior to the attention of the practitioner. If the misconduct is of a minor nature and/or appears to be due to lack of sensitivity, knowledge, or experience, such an informal solution is usually appropriate. Such informal corrective efforts are made with sensitivity to any rights of confidentiality involved. If the violation does not seem amenable to an informal solution, or is of a more serious nature, practitioners bring it to the attention of the appropriate local, state, and/or the SEG management team.

e. As practitioners the client is considered the best and final authority about his or her own welfare. Practitioners seek at all times to further that understanding; at no time do they endeavor to assume that function for themselves. When a client is not competent to evaluate the situation (for example, in the case of a child), practitioners inform the person responsible for the client of the circumstances that may influence the relationship.

Principle 8—Sexual Harassment Policy

The SEG staff, students, and approved teachers reaffirm their commitment to the maintenance of study and work environments free of inappropriate and disrespectful conduct of a sexually harassing nature. This includes all practitioners and their relationships with their clients as well as assistants, co-instructors, administrative staff, or others in a position of authority and power. Sexual harassment—of any member of the SEG community by another or with any client or student of a practitioner—is damaging and furthermore may be interpreted to be in violation of the Title VII of the Civil Rights Act of 1964 and Title IX of the of the 1972 Education Amendments.

It is the policy of SEG that no member of SEG may sexually harass another person. Anyone who violates this policy will be subject to disciplinary action, which may include suspension or termination. Complaints of sexual harassment should promptly be reported to the office of the SEG. Every effort will be made to resolve the problem on an informal basis in such a way as to preserve the reputation, confidentiality, and integrity of every person involved. Disciplinary action will be taken toward the harasser if a complaint is determined to be valid. Complaints found to be motivated by the malicious intent of the person claiming to have been harassed rather than actual harassment will result in disciplinary action toward the accuser.

Sexual harassment refers to behavior that is not welcome, that is personally offensive, that debilitates morale, and that interferes with academic or work effectiveness of the receiver, and in the case of a student to the effectiveness of fellow students, staff, and instructors. It is usually imposed on a person in an unequal power relationship through abuse of authority but may also occur from friends and colleagues. Central to this concept is the use of implied reward or threat of deprivation in a coercive attempt to solicit sexual attention. Unwelcome sexual advances, requests for sexual favors, or other verbal or physical conduct of a sexual nature constitute harassment when:

a. Submission to such conduct is made, either explicitly or implicitly, a term or condition of an individual's employment or academic success;

b. Submission to, or rejection of such conduct by an individual, is used as the basis for employment or academic decisions affecting such individual; or

c. Such conduct has the purpose or effect of unreasonably interfering with an individual's (or group's) work or academic performance or creating an intimidating, hostile, or offensive working, clinical, or study environment. It is debilitating to the recipient's morale. Federal law states that "sexual harassment is clearly unwelcome by any reasonable person."

When there is a complaint against a member of the SEG with respect to ethics or any other matter, SEG pledges to respond to that complaint without delay and in a spirit of fairness and compassion for all parties. SEG does not consider that punitive action is the most just or efficacious form of discipline, seeking rather to heal the dispute and find ways of resolving the conflict between the two parties. SEG recognizes that competition, mistrust, or the spreading of rumors destroys the spirit of kindness and union, which is the heart of any human association. Whenever possible, students, staff, and approved SEG instructors will be given a single warning verbally or in writing prior to an official notice of dismissal.

Appendix B

RESOURCES

Michael J. Shea, PhD
13878 Oleander Ave.
Juno Beach, FL 33408-1626
Phone: 561-493-8080
Website: www.michaelsheateaching.com
Email: info@michaelsheateaching.com

Santa Barbara Graduate Institute
(MA and PhD programs in clinical, pre- and perinatal and somatic
psychology, and distance learning plus certificate programs)
Contact: Marti Glenn, PhD, martiglenn@sbgi.edu
Website: www.sbgi.edu
Phone: 805-963-6896

Castellino Prenatal and Birth Training
Contact: Sandra Castellino, MEd
1105 N. Ontare Rd.
Santa Barbara, CA 93105
Phone: 805-687-2897
Website: castellinotraining.com
Email: sandra@castellinotraining.com

Sarajo Berman, Body Therapist, MFA, CMT, LMT, RCST
2615 Cone Ave.
Durham, NC 27704
Phone: 919-688-6428
sjberman@mindspring.com

Wendy Anne McCarty, PhD, RN
Prenatal and perinatal psychology practice for all ages, supporting families and professionals, publications and information for individual support available at www.wondrousbeginnings.com
315 Meigs Road, A306
Santa Barbara, CA 93109
Email: wmcarty@wondrousbeginnings.com

Body Therapy Institute
Entry-level massage training, continuing education for massage, bodywork and somatic therapists, teacher training
Contact: Rick Rosen, MA, LMBT and Carey Smith, CSC
300 Southwind Road
Siler City, NC 27344
Phone: 919-663-3111
Website: www.massage.net
Email: info@massage.net

Carol A. Agneessens, MSc
Pacific School of Biodynamic Integration
Santa Cruz, CA
Phone: 831-662-3057
Website: http://www.biodynamicschool.com
Email: carolagneessens@mac.com

"What Babies Want"
Hana Peace Works
State of the art DVDs and books on birthing.
P.O. Box 681
Los Olivos, CA 93441
Website: www.whatbabieswant.com

International Affiliation of Biodynamic Trainings (IABT)
Offering two graduate designations: BCST (Biodynamic Craniosacral Therapist) with graduation from a recognized 700-hour biodynamic foundation training; Advanced Biodynamic Practitioner (ABP) with an additional 500 hours of postgraduate training and supervision.
Website: www.biodynamic-craniosacral.org

FROM BLUEPRINT TO STRUCTURE

I'm writing these books to change our sensibility and image of the human body and to effect a revision of the therapeutic relationship so that it is based in the metabolism of the human embryo and the physiology of the infant. The concept maps here summarize metaphors I've used for biodynamic practitioners to work with embryological growth and development. Perception of growth and development starts with the most fundamental movement processes of dynamic morphology, considered to be the most fundamental health in the soma. The ordering movements of the fluid body, especially the spiral that orients to points of stillness, are the characteristics of dynamic morphology as pointed out originally by Dr. Blechschmidt.

The next level of sensing and perception for the biodynamic practitioner involves the metabolic fields of the embryo—these interrelated areas of unique shape-changing in the early condensing of the fluid body. The differential rates of growth occurring around the cell clusters make up a single metabolic field. The eight fields arise almost sequentially in the developing embryo. Finally, as represented in the first concept map below, the ongoing process of molecular genetics contributes to what is called the "remodeling" of each of the systems of the body during growth and development. It is much like the insulation and dry wall installed in a new house over the electrical wiring and plumbing infrastructure.

In the later stages of embryonic development, metabolic fields contribute to the formation of the basic tissue, cartilage, and osseous structures of the body by the capacity to change shape under the guidance of a slow tempo and embodied stillness in the embryo. These fields are the scaffolding of the soma, or the "frame-out," continuing the metaphor of construction of a wood frame house. It must be remembered that the metabolic fields are a function of the fluid body and before genetic material is brought forward to fill in the gaps, the fluid body creates the perfect structure as a gelled shape in the fluid body called the extracellular matrix. Then the finished product can begin to be occupied by all the specialized genes necessary to support its molecular metabolism and proteins to "build out" the final structure. Molecular genetics generate operational physiological systems such as the cardiovascular system, where extensive remodeling is done throughout the embryonic, fetal, and perinatal cycles, and the entire lifespan.

Consequently, what we are shown by molecular genetics is that the final form of any structure or function of the body is very changeable and constantly undergoing a remodeling process that is rife with the possibility of defects. This is shown in the first chart, below.

DYNAMIC MORPHOLOGY	METABOLIC FIELDS	MOLECULAR GENETICS
1. Organizing	Differentiating	Remodeling
2. Growing	Structuring (developing)	Functioning
3. Tidal body—slow, still	Fluid body—medium slow	Soma—fast
4. Primary Respiration	Direct current and reciprocal tension potency	Cranial Rhythmic Impulses
5. Blueprint	Frame out, scaffolding	Finish-remodel
6. Radial-axial symmetry, spirals	Vectors and twisting	Looping, retraction, wedging
7. Choreographer	Repeatable pattern	Choreography
8. Wholeness, perfection	Perfection, normal	Imprinting, change orders
9. Nature, organism	Interpersonal kinetic metabolic relationship	Intrasystems physiology
10. Origin	Early	Middle-late
11. Fold-unfold	Congeal-shaping	Solidifying
12. Biodynamic	Biodynamic-biokinetic	Biokinetic-biomechanical
13. 4 stages	8 fields	23 Carnegie stages
14. Four-dimensional	Three-dimensional	Two-dimensional

Distinctions Between Dynamic Morphology and Metabolic Fields

The concept map here draws closer attention to the deeper and fundamental ordering and organizational forces in the fluid body of the embryo. It represents a three-dimensional pattern of growth and development that underlies or perhaps is more basic than the two-dimensional molecular genetics involved in the remodeling process.

DYNAMIC MORPHOLOGY	METABOLIC FIELDS
1. Four stages of growth	Eight phases of structuring the embryo
2. Growth is a process in the embryo of maintaining ordered wholeness through the phases of structuring.	Structuring of the embryo is a description of the initial phases of differentiation of tissues and organs.
3. Activity of the tidal body as it rhythmically expands and recedes in the different body planes	Catalytic activity of the tidal body condensing into a fluid body and the fluid body condensing into the frame-scaffolding of a soma
4. The tidal body is a relationship between Primary Respiration and Dynamic Stillness. The Dynamic Stillness is the fulcrum for Primary Respiration and automatically shifts between the horizon and the fulcrum or the midline of the fluid cavities.	The fluid body is a relationship between Primary Respiration, Dynamic Stillness, and tensegrity. Tensegrity is defined as the active compression-decompression breathing of the fluid body. This reciprocal tension fortifies the membrane boundaries of the embryonic cavities.
5. The Dynamic Stillness becomes the perception and/or image of stillness like a cloud or molecules of the soma shifting between the horizon of nature and the fulcrum or midline.	The Dynamic Stillness becomes an orienting stillpoint in each field as it is expanding and condensing. This is regional orientation for growth in and around the fluid body.
6. Principle of symmetry, both radial and axial (fulcrum and midline)	Principle of space, relationship, and shape-changing
7. Dynamic morphology also uses the principle of polarity, or ordered movement around a fulcrum or axis in the fluid body with respect to different gradients or densifications of fluid and temperature variations within those gradients.	Fields represent "a system with all its positional information specified with respect to the same fulcrum or midline(s)" (Haraway, 2004, p. 51). This means that fields change shape based on where they are located in the embryo and the nature of the neighboring field(s).
8. Autonomy of the embryo regarding its self-regulation	Interrelational dynamics of self-regulation
9. Dynamic morphology as a description of undifferentiated wholeness requires three-dimensional perception of both inside and outside the body all the way to the horizon of nature and back.	Metabolic fields as a description of differentiated wholeness requires three-dimensional perception of both inside and outside the body as far as the landscaping around your office and back.

It is my contention, along with others no doubt, that there is no such thing as a final form of a human being. We are perpetual embryos, so to speak. This is because human embryology demonstrates a constantly evolving change process carried forward or "conserved" through the lifespan. One reason is the ongoing complete remodeling at every level of existence, especially in the heart, as briefly described below. It can happen in a millisecond! Another reason is that the human embryo, more than in any other species, resists genetic specialization. Homo sapiens does not have a particular "breeding" characteristic in the way we gather food (without claws), eat food (without sharp teeth to eat raw flesh), walk with two legs, and so forth. In fact, we humans resist such specialization as much as possible for the sake of freedom, which is the defining characteristic of a late-stage human embryo. While other species "specialize" at the end of the embryonic period, human embryos resist specialization and maintain their embryonic characteristics throughout life. This resistance can be palpated as well.

In the embryonic heart and cardiovascular system we see all of these fundamental life processes and even deeper ones. This is especially true of the way cell death contributes to the remodeling process in the heart. Death is one way to get things to change, and the embryonic heart excels at it in the creation of itself. The heart is a spiritual master that "transdifferentiates" neighboring cells to fill the void left by the dead. Transdifferentiation is the immediate transmutation or transubstantiation (think of the Catholic mass and wine being converted into the blood of Christ) of a structure in the embryo being made into something else after it was already complete. A biodynamic practitioner holds the polarity of the necessity of death centrally in the heart and the womb imprint created by death, whether a lost twin, a previous miscarriage, or a part of the embryonic heart transforming itself.

Imagine the fluid body as a single spiral of transparent, living, viscous fluid occupying the entire space on the inside and outside of the soma, much like the soma being enclosed in a sphere or an egg. Primary Respiration is the biggest spiral radiating in and out in all directions from the central channel of stillness in and around the egg out to the horizon. Imagine the activity of the fluid body as a spiral emanating from the core of stillness that contains light, electrical activity, and the image of a flame. Finally, imagine the heart tube coming into existence as the *intention* of the spiral of the fluid body and the spiral of Primary Respiration.

The list below is my transition to Volume 3. I am drawn to invite the reader in my next volume on a journey of the heart from its remarkable beginnings in the embryo to the wide expanse of metaphors it represents. It is the most profound organ in the fluid body and soma.

The Heart—The Ninth Metabolic Field

- The heart field is the arising of three genetically marked areas. Two are in specific canalization zones of the fluid body and one is around the primitive node at the top of the primitive streak. The two fluid canals are laterally adjacent to the primitive streak between the roof of the ectoderm plate and the floor of the endoderm.

- Structuring of the heart begins with the center of the two tubes merging at the midline of the pharynx to form a singular tube. The two become one and the primitive node is the fulcrum at what is now C-3.

- The pharynx induces the heart tube to begin bending, looping, and rotating away from the pharynx. This gesture helps the tube form the letter "C." The letter "C" then inverts to a "U," and thus the tube turns itself downside up so the inflow and outflow tracks face each other.

- The sculpting of the "U" tube becomes the letter "S" so that the ends can connect to form an infinity symbol, which is the core myocardial template of the heart structure.

- The two primitive atria maintain their right-left symmetry from their original canals on either side of the primitive streak.

- Practically all remaining heart development is asymmetrical, originally relating to a shift in the cytoplasm of the newly fertilized egg.

- The embryonic heart constantly dies to itself as specific areas are developed only by cells dying and being replaced by cells from the outside of the heart or those immediately adjacent to the "dead zone" through the process of transdifferentiation.

- The embryonic heart is the most un-embryonic organ in the human body. The primordia of the heart chambers do not form its final anatomy. The final anatomy is a process of relationship and borrowing from all the surrounding structures of the heart mesoderm, ectoderm, and especially the endoderm tube.

Stay tuned for Volume 3!

BIBLIOGRAPHY

Achtenburg, J. 1985. *Imagery in Healing.* New York: Random House.

———. 1991. *Woman As Healer.* New York: Random House.

Adler, H. M. 2002. The Sociophysiology of Caring in the Doctor-Patient Relationship. *J Gen Intern Med* 17:883–890.

Amorok, T. 2007. The Eco-Trauma and Eco-Recovery of Being. *Shift: At the Frontiers of Consciousness* 15:28–31.

Arrien, A. 1993. *The Four-Fold Way: Walking the Paths of the Warrior, Teacher, Healer and Visionary.* San Francisco: Harper.

Barasch, M. 1994. *The Healing Path: A Soul Approach to Illness.* Los Angeles: Tarcher/ Putnam.

Basch, M. F. 1976. The Concept of Affect: A Re-Examination. *J of Amer Psychoanalytic Assoc* 24:759–777.

Bateman, W. L. 1990. *Open to Question—The Art of Teaching and Learning By Inquiry.* San Francisco: Jossey-Bass.

Bayley, H. 1952. *The Lost Language of Symbolism.* 4th ed. Vol. II. London: Williams and Norgate.

Baynes, H. 1949. *Mythology of the Soul.* London: Methuen.

Beck, C. J. 1993. *Nothing Special: Living Zen.* New York: HarperCollins.

Becker, R. 1963. Diagnostic Touch: Its Principles and Application. *Acad of Applied Osteopathy, 1963 Yearbook,* 32–40.

Becker, R. 1997. *Life in Motion.* Portland, Ore.: Rudra Press.

Begley, S. 2001. Religion and the Brain. *Newsweek,* May 7, 2001, 52–57.

Behnke, E. A. 1989. Edmund Husserl's Contribution to Phenomenology of the Body in Ideas, II. *SPPB Newsletter* Fall:5–17.

Benson, H. 1975. *The Relaxation Response.* New York: Random House.

Bergman, N., L. Linley, and S. Fawcus. 2004. Randomized Controlled Trial of Skin-to-Skin Contact from Birth Versus Conventional Incubator for Physiological Stabilization in 1200- to 2199-Gram Newborns. *Acta Paediatr* 93:779–785.

Bernstein, J. 2006. *Living in the Borderland: The Evolution of Consciousness and the Challenge of Healing Trauma.* New York: Routledge.

Biaggio, M. K. 1986. A Survey of Psychologists' Perspectives on Catharsis. *The Journal of Psychology* 121(3).

Black, I. 1993. *Rituals for Our Times.* San Francisco: Harper Collins.

Blatner, A. 1985. The Dynamics of Catharsis. *Journal of Group Psychotherapy, Psychodrama and Sociometry* 37(4):157–166.

Blechschmidt, E. 1961. *The Stages of Human Development Before Birth: An Introduction to Human Embryology.* Philadelphia: W. B. Saunders Company.

———. 1969. Die entstehung eines os frontale. *Image Roche* (Basel) 33:2–9.

———. 1973. *Die pränatalen organsysteme des menschen.* Stuttgart: Hippokrates Verlag.

———. 1974. *Humanembryologie, prinzipien and grundbegriffe.* Stuttgart: Hippokrates Verlag.

———. 1977. *The Beginnings of Human Life.* New York: Springer-Verlag.

———. 2004. *The Ontogenetic Basis of Human Anatomy: A Biodynamic Approach to Development from Conception to Birth.* Translated by B. Freeman. Berkeley: North Atlantic Books.

Blechschmidt, E., and R. Gasser. 1978. *Biokinetics and Biodynamics of Human Differentiation: Principles and Applications.* Springfield, Ill.: Charles C. Thomas.

Blonder, L. X., D. Bowers, and K. M. Heilman. 1991. The Role of the Right Hemisphere in Emotional Communication. *Brain* 114:1115–1127.

Bloom, S. 1997. *Creating Sanctuary: Toward an Evolution of Sane Societies.* New York: Routledge.

Booth, R. J., and K. R. Ashbridge. 1993. A Fresh Look at the Relationships Between the Psyche and Immune System: Teleological Coherence and Harmony of Purpose. *Advances* 9(2):4–23.

Born, G. 1883. Die plattenmodellirmethode. *Arch f Micr Anat* 22:584–589.

———. 1888. Noch einmal die plattenmodellirmethod. *Z Wis Mkr* 5:433–455.

Borod, J., B. A. Cicero, L. K. Obler, et al. 1998. Right Hemisphere Emotional Perception: Evidence Across Multiple Channels. *Neuropsychology* 12:446–458.

Bowlby, J. 1969. *Attachment.* Vol. 1: *Attachment and Loss.* New York: Basic Books.

Boyd, J. D. 1960. Development of Striated Muscle. In *Structure and Function of Muscle.* Vol. 1, Edited by G. H. Bourne. New York: Academic Press.

Brake, W. G., R. M. Sullivan, and A. Gratton. 2000. Perinatal Distress Leads to Lateralized Medial Prefrontal Cortical Dopamine Hypofunction in Adult Rats. *J Neurosci* 20:5538–5543.

Braun, B. G. 1988. The BASK Model of Dissociation. *Dissociation* 1:16–23.

Brent, L., and R. C. Resch. 1987. A Paradigm of Infant-Mother Reciprocity: A Reexamination of "Emotional Refueling." *Psychoanalytic Psychology* 4:15–31.

Broman, I. 1898. Ueber entwicklungsgeschichte der gehörknöchelchen beim menschen. *Anat Hefte* 11:509–661.

Broucek, F. J. 1982. Shame and Its Relationship to Early Narcissistic Developments. *Intl J of Psycho-Analysis* 63:369–378.

Bryce, T. H. 1923. Myology. In *Quain's Elements of Anatomy,* 11th ed., Vol. 4, Part 2, edited by E. S. Schafer, J. Symington, and T. H. Bryce. London: Longmans, Green Co.

Buber, M. 1971. *I and Thou.* New York: Charles Scribner's Sons.

Cahill, S., and J. Halpern. 1990. *The Ceremonial Circle.* San Francisco: Harper and Row.

Caldjii, C., B. Tannenbaum, S. Sharma, D. Francis, P. M. Plotsky, and M. J. Meaney. 1998. Maternal Care During Infancy Regulates the Development of Neural Systems Mediating the Expression of Fearfulness in the Rat. *Proc Natl Acad Sci USA* 95:5335–5340.

Campbell, J. 1949. *The Hero with a Thousand Faces.* Princeton, N.J.: Princeton University Press.

Carr, L., M. Iacoboni, M.-C. Dubeau, J. C. Mazziotta, and G. L. Lenzi. 2003. Neural Mechanisms of Empathy in Humans: A Relay from Neural Systems for Imitation to Limbic Areas. *www.pnas.org.*

Carter, C. S. 1998. Neuroendocrine Perspectives on Social Attachment and Love. *Psychoneurendocrinol* 23:779–818.

Cassidy, C. M. 1994. Unraveling the Ball of String: Reality, Paradigms and the Study of Alternative Medicine. *Advances* 10(1):5–31.

Chibon, P. 1964. Analyse par la méthode marquage nucléaire á la thymidine tritée des derivés de la crête neurale céphalique chez l'urodéle pleurodeles waltlii michah. *C R Adad Sc* (Paris) 259:3624–3627.

Chicchetti, D., and D. Tucker. 1994. Development and Self-Regulatory Structures of the Mind. *Develop Psychopathol* 6:533–549.

Chiron, C, I. Jambaque, R. Natbbout, R. Lounes, A. Syrota, and O. Dulac. 1997. The Right Brain Hemisphere Is Dominant in Human Infants. *Brain* 120:1057–1065.

Chown, M. 2007. Into the Void. *New Scientist* Nov. 24:34–37.

Cirulli, F., A. Berry, and E. Alleva. 2002. Early Disruption of the Mother-Infant Relationship: Effects on Brain Plasticity and Implications for Psychopathology. *Neurosci Biobehav Rev* 27:73–82.

Cofer, C. N., and M. H. Appley. 1964. *Motivation: Theory and Research.* New York: Wiley.

Contey, C., and D. Takikawa. 2007. *CALMS: A Guide to Soothing Your Baby.* Los Olivos, Calif.: Hana Peace Works.

Covey, S. R. 1989. *The Seven Habits of Highly Effective People.* New York: Simon & Schuster.

Crabbe, J. C., and T. J. Phillips. 2003. Mother Nature Meets Mother Nurture. *Nature Neuroscience* 6:440–442.

Cunningham, A. J. 1986. Information and Health in the Many Levels of Man: Towards a More Comprehensive Theory of Health and Disease. *Advances* 3(1):32–45.

———. 1991. Bringing the Mind into Medicine. *Today's Life Sciences* 11:8–13.

Dafter, R. E. 1996. Why *Negative* Emotions Can Sometimes Be Positive: The Spectrum Model of Emotions and Their Role in Mind-Body Healing. *Advances* 12(2):6–51.

Decety, J., and T. Chaminade. 2003. When the Self Represents the Other: A New Cognitive Neuroscience View on Psychological Identification. *Conscious Cognition* 12:577–596.

DeMause, L. 2002. *Emotional Life of Nations* New York: Other Press.

Demos, V., and S. Kaplan. 1986. Motivation and Affect Reconsidered: Affect Biographies of Two Infants. *Psychoanalysis and Contemporary Thought* 9:147–221.

Devinsky, O. 2000. Right Cerebral Hemisphere Dominance for a Sense of Corporeal and Emotional Self. *Epilep Behavior* 1:60–73.

Dillard, A. 1974. *Pilgrim At Tinker Creek.* New York: Harper Perennial.

Dimberg, U., and M. Petterson. 2000. Facial Reactions to Happy and Angry Facial Expressions: Evidence for Right Hemisphere Dominance. *Psychophysiology* 37:693–696.

Dixon, A. F. 1896. On the Developmnet of the Branches of the Fifth Cranial Nerve in Man. *Roy Dubline Soc, Sci Tr Ser 2,* 6:19–76.

Donaldson, R. 1971. Emotion As an Accessory Vital System. *Perspectives in Biology and Medicine* Autumn:46–71.

Edinger, E. F. 1972. *Ego and Archetype.* Boston: Shambhala Press.

Ekman, P., R. Levenson, and W. Friesen. 1983. Autonomic Nervous System Activity Distinguishes Emotions. *Science* 221:1208–1210.

Eliade, M. 1958. *Rites and Symbols of Initiation: The Mysteries of Birth and Rebirth.* New York: Harper and Row.

———. 1959. *The Sacred and the Profane: The Nature of Religion.* New York: Harcourt, Brace & World.

———. 1960. *Myths, Dreams and Mysteries.* London: Harvill Press.

———. 1963. *Myth and Reality.* New York: Harper and Row.

———. 1964. *Shamanism: Archaic Technique of Ecstasy.* Princeton, N.J.: Princeton University Press.

———. 1985. *Symbolism, the Sacred and the Arts.* New York: Crossroads.

Enlow, D. H., and J. A. McNamara. 1973. The Neurocranial Basis for Facial Form and Pattern. *Angle Orthod* 43:256–270.

Epstein, H. T. 2001. An Outline of the Role of Brain in Human Cognitive Development. *Brain Cognition* 45:44–51.

Feitis, R., and W. Schultz. 1997. *The Endless Web: Fascial Reality.* Berkeley: North Atlantic Books.

Feldenkrais, M. 1949. *Body and Mature Behavior.* Madison, Conn.: International Universities Press.

Fierz, L. 1948. Unpublished notes from a seminar given in 1948. Zurich: C. G. Jung Institute.

Fleming, A. S., D. H. O'Day, and G. W. Kraemer. 1999. Neurobiology of Mother-Infant Reactions: Experience and Central Nervous System Plasticity Across Development and Generations. *Neurosci Biobehav Rev* 23:673-685.

Fox, N. A., and R. J. Davidson. 1984. Hemispheric Substrates of Affect: A Developmental Model. In *The Psychobiology of Affective Development,* edited by N. A. Fox and R. J. Davidson. Hillsdale, N.J.: Erlbaum.

Freidman, N., and J. Lavender. 1997. On Receiving the Patient's Transference: The Symbolizing and Desymbolizing Countertransference. *J of Amer Psychoanalytic Assoc* 45:79–103.

Freud, S. 1910. *The Future Prospects of Psychoanalytic Therapy.* Standard ed., Vol. 11. London: Hogarth.

Fromm, E. 1956. *The Art of Loving.* 1st ed. New York: Harper.

Futamura, R. 1906. Über die entwicklung der facialismuskulatur des menschen. *Anat. Hefte* 30:433–516.

Gaensbauer, T. 1982. Regulation of Emotional Expression in Infants from Two Contrasting Caretaking Environments. *J of Amer Acady of Child Psychiatry* 21:163–171.

Gasser, R. F. 1967. The Development of the Facial Nerve in Man. *Annals of Otology, Rhinology, and Laryngology* 76(1):37–57.

———. 1967. The Development of the Facial Muscles in Man. *Amer J Anatomy* 120(2), March 1967.

———. 2006. Evidence that Some Events of Mammalian Embryogenesis Can Result from Differential Growth, Making Migration Unnecessary. *The Anatomical Record (Part B: New Anat)* 289B:53–63.

Gegenbaur, C. 1890. *Lehrbuch der anatomie des menschen.* Leipzig: Wilhelm Engelmann.

George, M. S., P. I. Parekh, N. Rosinsky, et al. 1996. Understanding Emotional Prosody Activates Right Hemispheric Regions. *Arch Neurol* 53:665–670.

Gershon, M. 1998. *The Second Brain: A Groundbreaking New Understanding of Nervous Disorders of the Stomach and Intestine* New York: HarperCollins.

Gluckman, P. D., and H. M. Adler. 2004. Living with the Past: Evolution, Development, and Patterns of Disease. *Science* 305:1733–1736.

Goleman, D. J. 1995. *Emotional Intelligence.* New York: Bantam.

Graham, Y. P., C. Heim, S. H. Goodman, A. H. Miller, and C. B. Nemeroff. 1999. The Effects of Neonatal Stress on Brain Development: Implications for Psychopathology. *Develop Psychopathol* 11:545–565.

Grossinger, R. 1998. Why Somatic Therapies Deserve As Much Attention As Psychoanalysis in The New York Review of Books, and Why Bodyworkers Treating Neurosis Should Study Psychoanalysis. In *The Body in Psychotherapy: Inquiries in Somatic Psychology,* edited by D. H. Johnson and I. J. Grand. Berkeley: North Atlantic Books.

Guggenguhl-Craig, A. 1971. *Power in the Helping Professions.* Dallas: Spring Publications.

Gunnar, M. R., and B. Donzella. 2002. Social Regulation of the Cortisol Levels in Early Human Development. *Psychoneuroendocrinol* 27:199–220.

Hagopian, S. 2001. On Becoming an Osteopath. *Alternative Therapies* 7(6):85–91.

Hanna, T. 1988. *Somatics.* New York: Addison-Wesley.

Haraway, D. J. 2004. *Crystals, Fabrics, and Fields: Metaphors that Shape Embryos.* Berkeley: North Atlantic Books.

Harman, W. 1995. Exploring the New Biology. *Noetic Sciences Review* Summer:29–33.

Heider, J. 1974. Catharsis in Human Potential Encounter. *J of Humanistic Psychology* 14(4):27–54.

Heller, W. 1990. The Neuropsychology of Emotion. In *Psychological and Biological Approaches to Emotion,* edited by N. Stein, B. Leventhal, and T. Trabasso. New York: Hillsdale.

Helmeke, C., W. Ovtscharoff, Jr., G. Poeggel, and K. Braun. 2001. Juvenile Emotional Experience Alters Synaptic Inputs on Pyramidal Neurons in the Anterior Cingulate Cortex. *Cerebral Cortex* 11:717–727.

Herman, J. L. 1992. *Trauma and Recovery: The Aftermath of Violence—From Domestic Abuse to Political Terror.* New York: Basic Books.

———. 1997. *Trauma and Recovery.* New York: HarperCollins.

Heuser, C. H. , and G. W. Corner. 1957. Developmental Horizons in Human Embryos: Description of Age Group X 4 to 12 Somites. *Contrib Embryol Carnegie Inst* 36:29–39.

Hillman, J. 1975. Abandoning the Child. In *Loose Ends: Primary Papers in Archetypal Psychology.* Dallas: Spring Publications.

———. 1997. *Emotion.* New York: Penguin.

His, W. 1889. Zur entwickelungsgeschichte des acustico-facialgebietes beim menschen u. *Entwickl: Arch. f Anat.*

Ho, M. W. 1998. *The Rainbow and the Worm: The Physics of Organisms.* 2nd ed. London: World Scientific.

———. 2004a. Is Water Special? *Science in Society* 23:47–48.

———. 2004b. The "Wholiness" of Water. *Science in Society* 23:48–49.

———. 2005. First Sighting of Structured Water. *Science in Society* 28:47–48.

Hoffman, Y. 1986. *Japanese Death Poems: Written by Zen Monks and Haiku Poets on the Verge of Death.* Rutland, Vt.: Charles E. Tuttle Company.

Hooker, D. 1952. The Prenatal Origin of Behavior. In *18th Porter Lecture.* Lawrence: University of Kansas Press.

———. 1958. Evidence of Prenatal Function of the Central Nervous System in Man. In *James Arthur Lecture on the Evolution of the Human Brain, 1957.* New York: The American Museum of Natural History.

Horowitz, S. L. 1970. Strategies within Hypnosis for Reducing Phobic Behavior. *Journal of Abnormal Psychology* 75(1):104–112.

Huber, E. 1931. *Evolution of Facial Musculature and Facial Expression.* Baltimore: The Johns Hopkins University Press.

Humphrey, T. 1964. Some Correlations Between the Appearance of Human Fetal Reflexes and the Development of the Nervous System. *Progr Brain Res* 4:93–135.

Iacoboni, M., I. Molnar-Szakacs, V. Gallese, G. Buccino, and J. C. Mazziotta. 2005. Grasping the Intentions of Others with One's Own Mirror Neuron System. *Public Library of Science Biology,* www.plosbiology.org.

Iffy, L., T. H. Shepard, A. Jakobovits, R. J. Lemire, and P. Kerner. 1967. The Rate of Growth in Young Human Embryos of Streeter's Horizons XIII to XXIII. *Acta Anat* 66:178–186.

Illich, I. 1976. *Medical Nemesis: The Expropriation of Health.* New York: Random House.

Immordino-Yang, M., and A. Damasio. 2007. We Feel, Therefore We Learn: The Relevance of Affective and Social Neuroscience to Education. *Mind, Brain and Education* (1).

Ingber, D. 2006. Mechanical Control of Tissue Morphogenesis During Embryological Development. *Intl J of Developmental Biol* 50:255–266.

Jackson, S. W. 1994. Catharsis and Abreaction in the History of Psychological Healing. *Psychiatric Clinics of North America* 17(3):471–491.

Jacob, J. 1977. The Linguistic Model in Biology. In *Roman Jakobson: Echoes of His Scholarship,* edited by D. Armstrong and C. H. Schoonefield. Lisse Peter de Ridder Press.

Jealous, J. 1993. Reciprocal Tensions. *The Cranial Letter* 46(1):7–9.

———. 1998. The Other Pair of Hands. *Alternative Therapies* 4(1):108.

———. 2002a. *The Embryonic Mind.* Compact disc recording, available from Long Tide Management Inc., 6501 Blackfin Way, Apollo Beach, FL 33572. www.biodo.com.

———. 2002b. *The Fluid Body:* Compact disc recording, available from Long Tide Management Inc., 6501 Blackfin Way, Apollo Beach, FL 33572. www.biodo.com.

Johnston, M. C. 1966. A Radiographic Study of the Migration and Fate of Cranial Neural Crest Cells in the Chick Embryo. *Anat Rec* 156:143–156.

Joseph, R. 1996. *Neuropsychiatry, Neuropsychology, and Clinical Neuroscience.* 2nd ed. Baltimore: Williams and Wilkins.

Jung, C. G. 1939. *Integration of the Personality.* New York: Farrar and Rinehart.

———. 1966. The Psychology of the Child Archetype. In *The Archetypes of the Collective Unconscious* (*Collected Works of C. G. Jung,* vol. 9), edited by M. Fordham and H. Read. Princeton, N.J.: Princeton University Press.

———. 1969. *Archetypes of the Collective Unconscious.* Edited by M. Fordham and H. Read, *Collected works of c.G. Jung, vol. 9.1.* Princeton, N.J.: Princeton University Press.

———. 1971. The Transcendent Function. In *The Portable Jung,* edited by J. Campbell. New York: Penguin.

———. 1976. Healing the Split. In *The Symbolic Life* (*Collected Works of C. G. Jung,* vol. 18), edited by W. McGuire. Princeton, N.J.: Princeton University Press.

Jung, C. G., and C. Kerenyi. 1949. *Essays on a Science of Mythology.* 1st ed., *Bollingen Series XXII.* New York: Pantheon.

Kabat-Zinn, J., L. Lipsworth, R. Burney, and W Sellers. 1987. Four-Year Follow-Up of a Meditation-Based Program for the Self-Regulation of Chronic Pain: Treatment Outcomes and Compliance. *The Clin J of Pain* 2:159–173.

Kalsched, D. 1996. *The Inner World of Trauma: Archetypal Defenses of the Personal Spirit.* New York: Routledge.

Keen, S. 1970. Sing the Body Electric. *Psychology Today* October:56–59.

———. 1992. *The Power of Stories Workshop.* Audiotapes, Sounds True Recordings, 735 Walnut Street, Boulder CO 80302.

Keenan, J. P., A. Nelson, M. O'Connor, and A. Pascual-Leone. 2001. A Self-Recognition and the Right Hemisphere. *Nature Neuroscience* 409:305.

Kerenyi, C. 1951. *The Gods of the Greeks.* 1st ed. London: Thames and Hudson, Ltd.

Kierkegaard, S. 1939. *Christian Discourses.* London: Oxford University Press.

Klah, H. 1942. *Navajo Creation Myth.* Santa Fe, N.M.: Museum of Navajo Ceremonial Art.

Kohut, H. 1971. *The Analysis of the Self.* New York: International Universities Press.

———. 1977. *The Restoration of the Self.* New York: International Universities Press.

Krampen, M. 1987. *Classics of Semiotics.* New York: Plenum Press.

Kroeber, A. 1905. Wishosk Myths. *J of American Folklore* 18:91.

Krystal, H. 1978. Trauma and Affects. *Psychoanalytic Study of the Child* 33:81–116.

Kurtz, R. 1990. *Body-Centered Psychotherapy.* Mendocino, Calif.: Life Rhythm.

Le Grand, R., C. Mondloch, D. Maurer, and H. P. Brent. 2003. Expert Face Processing Requires Visual Input to the Right Hemisphere During Infancy. *Nature Neuroscience* 6:1108–1112.

LeDoux, J. 1989. Cognitive-Emotional Interactions in the Brain. *Cognition and Emotion* 3:267–289.

Lemonick, D., and A. Park. 2007. The Science of Addiction. *Time Magazine,* July 16.

Lester, B. M., J. Hoffman, and T. B. Brazelton. 1985. The Rhythmic Structure of Mother-Infant Interaction in Term and Preterm Infants. *Child Develop* 56:15–27.

Levine, P. 1976. Accumulated Stress Reserve Capacity and Disease. PhD dissertation, University of California, Berkeley. Ann Arbor, MI: University Microfilms No. 77-15, 760.

———. 1990. The Body As Healer: A Revisioning of Trauma and Anxiety. *Somatics* 8(1, Autumn/Winter):13–21.

———. 1997. *Waking the Tiger: Healing Trauma.* Berkeley: North Atlantic Books.

Lewis, M., and J. Haviland, eds. 1993. *Handbook of Emotions.* New York: Guilford Press.

Long, S. Y., K. S. Larsson, and S. Lohmander. 1973. Cell Proliferation in the Cranial Base of A/J Mice with 6-AN-Induced Cleft Palate. *Teratology* 8:127–138.

Lorberbaum, J. P., J. D. Newman, A. R. Horwitz, et al. 2002. A Potential Role for Thalamocingualate Circuitry in Human Maternal Behavior. *Biol Psychiatr* 51:431–445.

Lowy, F. H. 1970. The Abuse of Abreaction: An Unhappy Legacy of Freud's Cathartic Method. *Canadian Psychiatric Assoc J* 15:557–565.

Luecken, I. J. 1998. Childhood Attachment and Loss Experiences Affect Adult Cardiovascular and Cortisol Function. *Psychosomat Med* 60:765–772.

Lyons, D. M., H. Afarian, A. F. Schatzberg, A. Sawyer-Glover, and M. E. Moseley. 2002. Experience-Dependent Asymmetric Maturation in Primate Prefrontal Morphology. *Exp Brain Res* 136:51–59.

MacLean, P. 1973. *A Triune Concept of the Brain and Behavior.* Toronto: University of Toronto Press.

Maitland, J. 1995. *Spacious Body: Explorations in Somatic Ontology.* Berkeley: North Atlantic Books.

Mall, F. P. 1918. On the Age of Human Embryos. *Amer J Anat* 23:397–422.

Manning, J. T., R. L. Trivers, R. Thornhill, et al. 1997. Ear Asymmetry and Left-Side Cradling. *Evol Human Behavior* 18:327–340.

Martin, J. E., and C. R. Carlson. 1988. Behavior Therapy and Religion: Integrating Spiritual and Behavioral Approaches to Change. In *Spiritual Dimensions of Health*

Psychology, edited by M. W. R. Miller and J. E. Martin. Newbury Park, Calif.: Sage Publications.

Matsuzawa, J., M. Matsui, T. Konishi, et al. 2001. Age-Related Changes of Brain Gray and White Matter in Healthy Infants and Children. *Cerebral Cortex* 11:335–342.

Matthews, S. G. 2002. Early Programming of the Hypothalamo-Pituitary-Adrenal Axis. *Trends Endocrinol Metab* 13:373–380.

Maunder, R. G., and J. J. Hunter. 2001. Attachment and Psychosomatic Medicine: Developmental Contributions to Stress and Disease. *Psychosomat Med* 63:556–567.

May, R. 1999. *Freedom and Destiny.* 2nd ed. New York: W. W. Norton.

McCraty, R. 2003. *Heart-Brain Neurodynamics: The Making of Emotions.* Boulder Creek, Calif.: HeartMath Research Center, Institute of HeartMath.

McPartland, J. M. 1996. Craniosacral Iatrogenesis. *J of Bodywork and Movement Therapies* 1(1):2–5.

———. 1997. Entrainment and the Cranial Rhythmic Impulse. *Alternative Therapies* 3(1):40–45.

Meadows, K. 1989. *Earth Medicine.* Rockport, Mass.: Element.

Meaney, M. J. 2001. Maternal Care, Gene Expression, and the Transmission of Individual Differences in Stress Reactivity Across Generations. *Annu Rev Neurosci* 24:1161–1192.

Meares, R. 1986. On the Ownership of Thought: An Approach to the Origins of Separation Anxiety. *Psychiatry* 49(1):80–91.

Menard, J. J., D. L. Champagne, and M. J. Meaney. 2004. Variations of Maternal Care Differentially Influence "Fear" Reactivity in Response to the Shock-Probe Burying Test. *Neuroscience* 129:297–308.

Moerman, D. 1983. Psychology and Symbols: The Anthropological Implications of the Placebo Effect. In *The Anthropology of Medicine, from Culture to Method,* edited by L. Romanucci-Ross, D. Moerman, and L. Tancredi. South Hadley, Mass.: Praeger Scientific.

Moore, T. 1993. *Care of the Soul.* San Francisco: HarperCollins.

Morrison, N. K. 1985. Shame in the Treatment of Schizophrenia: Theoretical Considerations with Clinical Illustrations. *Yale J of Biological Medicine* 58:289–297.

Neumann, E. 1949. *The Wagner Operas.* New York: Knopf.

———. 1955. *The Great Mother.* Princeton, N.J.: Princeton University Press.

NICHD Early Child Care Research Network. 2004. Affect Dysregulation in the Mother-Child Relationship in the Toddler Years: Antecedents and Consequences. *Develop Psychopathol* 16:43–68.

Nichols, M. P., and M. Zax. 1977. *Catharsis in Psychotherapy*. New York: Gardner Press.

Nitschke, J. B., E. E. Nelson, B. D. Rusch, A. S. Fox, T. R. Oakes, and R. J. Davidson. 2004. Orbitofrontal Cortex Tracks Positive Mood in Mothers Viewing Pictures of Their Newborn Infants. *Neuro Image* 21:583–592.

Northrop, F. 1946. *The Meeting of East and West*. 3rd ed. New York: Macmillan.

Nyima Rinpoche, C., and D. R. Shlim. 2004. *Medicine and Compassion: A Tibetan Lama's Guidance for Caregivers*. Boston: Wisdom Publications.

O'Rahilly, R. 1972. Guide to the Staging of Human Embryos. *Anat Anz* 130:556–559.

———. 1973. *Developmental Stages in Human Embryos, Part A: Embryos of the First Three Weeks (Stages 1 to 9)*. Washington, D.C.: Carnegie Institution of Washington.

O'Rahilly, R., and F. Muller. 2001. *Human Embryology and Teratology*. 3rd ed. New York: Wiley-Liss.

Odent, M. 1999. *The Scientification of Love*. New York: Free Association Books.

Ogden, P., K. Minton, and C. Pain. 2006. *Trauma and the Body: A Sensorimotor Approach to Psychotherapy*. New York: W. W. Norton.

Olausson, H., Y. Lamarre, H. Backlund, C. Morin, B. G. Wallin, G. Starck, S. Ekholm, I. Strigo, K. Worsley, A. B. Vallbo, and M. C. Bushnell. 2002. Unmyelinated Tactile Afferents Signal Touch and Project to Insular Cortex. *Nature Neuroscience* 5(9):900–904.

Overman, D. O., and D. R. Peterson. 1975. Brain-Palate Relationships in Induced Cleft Palate in Mice. *Anat Rec* 181:442.

Ovtscharoff, W., Jr., and K. Braun. 2001. Maternal Separation and Social Isolation Modulate the Postnatal Development of Synaptic Composition in the Infralimbic Cortex of *Octodon Degus*. *Neuroscience* 104:33–40.

Pauli, P., G. Wiedemann, and M. Nickola. 1999. Pain Sensitivity, Cerebral Laterality, and Negative Affect. *Pain* 80:359–364.

Paus, T., A. C. Collins, B. Leonard, and A. Zijdenbos. 2001. Maturation of White Matter in the Human Brain: A Review of Magnetic Resonance Studies. *Brain Res Bull* 54:255–266.

Payne, R., A. E. Bergin, and P. E. Loftus. 1992. A Review of Attempts to Integrate Spiritual and Standard Psychotherapy Techniques. *J of Psychotherapy Integration* 2(3):171–192.

Pearce, J. C. 2004. Nurturance: A Biological Imperative. *Shift: At the Frontiers of Science* (3):16–19.

Pearsall, P. 2007. In Awe of the Heart. *Alternative Therapies*. July-August:16–19.

Pearson, A. A. 1947. The Roots of the Facial Nerve in Human Embryos and Fetuses. *J Comp Neur* 87:139–159.

Perry, B. D., and R. Pollard. 1998. Homeostasis, Stress, Trauma and Adaptation: A Neuodevelopmetnal View of Childhood Trauma. *Child and Adolescent Psychiatric Clinics of North America* 7(1):33–51.

Perry, R. J., H. R. Rosen, J. H. Kramer, J. S. Beer, R. L. Levenson, and B. L. Miller. 2001. Hemispheric Dominance for Emotions, Empathy, and Social Behavior: Evidence from Right and Left Handers with Frontotemporal Dementia. *Neurocase* 7:145–160.

Pine, F. 1980. On the Expansion of the Affect Array: A Developmental Description. In *Rapprochement: The Critical Subphase of Separation-Individuation,* edited by S. B. R. Lax and J. A. Burland. New York: Jason Aronson.

Pink, D. H. 2005. *A Whole New Mind: Moving from the Information Age to the Conception Age.* New York: Riverhead Books.

Pipp, S., and R. J. Harmon. 1987. Attachment As Regulation: A Commentary. *Child Development* 58:648–652.

Plutchik, R. 1980. A General Psychoevolutionary Theory of Emotion. In *Emotion: Theory, Research and Experience,* edited by R. Plutchik and H. Kellerman. New York: Academic Press.

Popowsky, I. 1895. Zur entwicklungsgeschichte des n. Facialis beim menschen. *Morph Jahrb* 23:329–374.

Porges, S. W., J. A. Doussard-Roosevelt, and A. K. Maiti. 1994. Vagal Tone and the Physiological Regulation of Emotion. *Monographs of the Society for Research in Child Development* 59:167–186.

Rabl, K. 1887. Über das gebiet des nervus facialis. *Anat Anz* 2:219–227.

Reichard, G. 1944. Individualism and Mythological Style. *J of Amer Folklore* 57(223):20–22.

Remen, R. H. 1995. Health Reform in the Sacred: A Group Discussion. *Advances* 11(1):37–54.

Richie, D. 1996. *How to Be an Adult: Handbook on Psychological and Spiritual Integration.* New York: Paulist Press.

Ridley, C. 2006. *Stillness: Biodynamic Cranial Practice and the Evolution of Consciousness.* Berkeley: North Atlantic Books.

Rolf, I. P. 1978. *Ida Rolf Talks About Rolfing and Physical Reality.* Boulder: Rolf Institute.

Rosenzweig, M. R., and E. L. Bennett. 1996. Psychobiolby of Plasticity: Effects of Training and Experience on Brain and Behavior. *Behav Brain Res* 78:57–65.

Rubin, S. S., and D. L. Niemeier. 1992. Non-Verbal Affective Communication As a Factor in Psychotherapy. *Psychotherapy:*596–602.

Ruge, G. 1910. Verbindungen des platysma mit der tiefen musculature des halses beim menschen. *Morph Jahrb* 41:708–724.

Safran, J. D., and L. S. Greenberg. 1991. *Emotion, Psychotherapy and Change.* New York: Guilford Press.

Sandner, D. 1979. *Navaho Symbols of Healing.* New York: Harcourt Brace Jovanovich.

Sands, S. 1997. Self Psychology and Projective Identification—Whither Shall They Meet? A Reply to the Editors (1995). *Psychoanalytic Dialogue* 7:651–668.

Scaer, R. C. 2005. *The Trauma Spectrum: Hidden Wounds and Human Resiliency.* New York: W. W. Norton.

Schachter, S., and J. Singer. 1962. Cognitive, Social and Physiological Determinant of Emotional States. *Psychological Review* 69:379–399.

Schäfer, E. A., and J. Symington. 1909. Neurology. In *Quain's Elements of Anatomy,* edited by E. A. Schäfer, J. Symington, and T. H. Bryce. London: Longmans, Green.

Schafer, R. 1970. Requirements for a Critique of the Theory of Catharsis. *J of Consulting and Clinical Psychology* 35(1):13–17.

Scheff, T. J. 1979. *Catharsis in Healing, Ritual and Drama.* Berkeley: University of California Press.

Schimert, J. 1933. Zur entwicklungsgeschichte des musculus stapedius beim menschen. *Anat Anz* 76:317–332.

Schmidt, S., C. Nachtigall, O. Wuethrich-Martone, and G. Strauss. 2002. Attachment and Coping with Chronic Disease. *J Psychosomat Res* 53:763–773.

Schore, A. N. 1994. *Affect Regulation and the Origin of the Self: The Neurobiology of Emotional Development.* Mahwah, N.J.: Erlbaum.

———. 1996. The Experience-Dependent Maturation of a Regulatory System in the Orbital Prefrontal Cortex and the Origin of Developmental Psychopathology. *Develop Psychopathol* 8:59–87.

———. 2000. Plenary address: Parent-Infant Communications and the Neurobiology of Emotional Development. In *Proceedings of Head Start's Fifth National Research Conference, Developmental and Contextual Transitions of Children and Families. Implications for Research, Policy, and Practice.* Washington, D.C.: Department of Health and Human Services.

———. 2001a. The Effects of a Secure Attachment Relationship on Right Brain Development, Affect Regulation, and Infant Mental Health. *Infant Mental Health J* 22(1–2):7–66.

———. 2001b. The Effects of Early Relational Trauma on Right Brain Development, Affect Regulation, and Infant Mental Health. *Infant Mental Health J* 22(1–2):201–269.

———. 2002. Dysregulation of the Right Brain: A Fundamental Mechanism of Traumatic Attachment and the Psychopathogenesis of Post-Traumatic Stress Disorder. *Austral New Zeal J Psychiatr* 36:9–30.

———. 2003a. *Affect Regulation and the Repair of the Self.* New York: W. W. Norton.

———. 2003b. *Affect Dysregulation and Disorders of the Self.* New York: W. W. Norton.

Schulman, H. 1997. *Living At the Edge of Chaos: Complex Systems in Culture and Psyche.* Einsiedeln, Switzerland: Daimon.

Schwartz, G. E. 1986. Emotion and Psychophysiological Organization: A Systems Approach. In *Psychophysiology: Systems, Processes, and Applications,* edited by M. Coles, E. Dorchin, and S. W. Porges. New York: Guilford Press.

Schwartz, R. 1987. Our Multiple Selves. *Family Therapy Networker* (March-April).

Schwartz-Salant, N., and Stein, M. (eds.) 1991. *Liminality and Transitional Phenomena.* Wilmette, Ill.: Chiron Publications.

Sebeok, T. 1976. *Contribution to a Doctrine of Signs.* Bloomington: Indiana University Press.

Selye, H. 1976. *The Stress of Life.* New York: MaGraw-Hill.

Semrud-Clikeman, M., and G. W. Hynd. 1990. Right Hemisphere Dysfunction in Nonverbal Learning Disabilities: Social, Academic, and Adaptive Functioning in Adults and Children. *Psych Bull* 107:196–209.

Shamay-Tsoory, S. G., R. Tomer, B. D. Berger, and J. Aharon-Peretz. 2003. Characterization of Empathy Deficits Following Prefrontal Brain Damage: The Role of the Right Ventromedial Prefrontal Cortex. *J Cog Neurosci* 15:324–337.

Shea, M. 2007. *Biodynamic Craniosacral Therapy.* Vol. 1. Berkeley: North Atlantic Books.

Siegel, D. J. 1999. *The Developing Mind: Toward a Neurobiology of Interpersonal Experience.* New York: Guilford Press.

———. 2007. *The Mindful Brain: Reflection and Attunement in the Cultivation of Well-Being.* New York: W. W. Norton.

Sieratzki, J. S., and B. Woll. 1996. Why Do Mothers Cradle Babies on Their Left? *Lancet* 347:1746–1748.

Sills, F. 2001. *Craniosacral Biodynamics.* Rev. ed. Vol. 1. Berkeley: North Atlantic Books.

Slavson, S. R. 1951. Catharsis in Group Psychotherapy. *Psychoanalytic Review* 38:39–52.

Sontag, S. 1979. *Illness As Metaphor.* New York: Random House.

Spence, S., D. H. Shapiro, and E. Zaidel. 1996. The Role of the Right Hemisphere in the Physiological and Cognitive Components of Emotional Processing. *Psychophysiology* 33:112–122.

Spiegel, D., ed. 1994. *Dissociation: Culture, Mind and Body.* Washington, D.C.: American Psychiatric Press.

Spiegel, D., J. R. Bloom, and H. C. Kraemer. 1989. Effect of Psychosocial Treatment on Survival of Patients with Metastatic Breast Cancer. *Lancet* 2 (8668):888–891.

Sroufe, L. A. 1979. Socioemotional Development. In *Organization of Memory,* edited by E. T. W. Donaldson. New York: Academic Press.

Stevenson, M. C. 1901–1902. The Zuni Indians. In *23rd Annual Report of the Bureau of American Ethnology.* Washington, D.C.

Stone, L. J., and J. Church. 1968. *Childhood and Adolescence.* New York: Random House.

Streeter, G. L. 1907. On the Development of the Membranous Labyrinth and the Acoustic and Facial Nerves in the Human Embryo. *Am J Anat* 6:139–165.

———. 1945. Developmental Horizons in Human Embryos: Description of Age Groups XIII, Embryos 4 to 5 Millimeters Long, and Age Group XIV, Period of Indentation of the Lens Vesicle. *Contrib Embryol Carnegie Inst* 31:27–63.

———. 1948. Developmental Horizons in Human Embryos: Description of Age Groups XV, XVI, XVII, and XVIII. Being the Third Issue of a Survey of the Carnegie Collection. *Contrib Embryol Carnegie Inst* 32:133–203.

———. 1951. (Prepared for publication by C. H. Heuser and G. W. Corner.) Developmental Horizons in Human Embryos. Description of Age Groups XIX, XX, XXI, XXII, and XXIII. Being the Fifth Issue of a Survey of the Carnegie Collection. *Contrib Embryol Carnegie Inst* 34:165–196.

Stuss, D. T., and M. P. Alexander. 1999. Affectively Burnt In: One Role of the Right Frontal Lobe? In *Memory, Consciousness, and the Brain: The Talin Conference,* edited by E. Tulving. Philadelphia: Psychology Press.

Sullivan, R. M., and A. Gratton. 2002. Prefrontal Cortical Regulation of Hypothalamic-Pituitary-Adrenal Functions in the Rat and Implications for Psychopathology: Side Matters. *Psychoneuroendocrinol* 27:99–114.

Suomi, S. J. 2004. How Gene-Environment Interactions Can Influence Emotional Development in Rhesus Monkeys. In *Nature and Nurture: The Complex Interplay of Genetic and Environmental Influences on Human Behavior and Development,* edited by C. Bearer and R. Lerner. Mahwah, N.J.: Erlbaum.

Sutherland, W. G. 1998. *Contributions of Thought: The Collective Writings of William Garner Sutherland, DO.* 2nd ed. Portland, Ore.: Rudra Press.

———. 2002. Untitled talk. *AAO Journal* 12(4):10–17.

Tang, A. C., B. C. Reeb, R. E. Romeo, and B. S. McEwen. 2003. Modification of Social Memory, Hypothalamic-Pituitary-Adrenal Axis, and Brain Asymmetry By Neonatal Novelty Exposure. *J Neurosci* 23:8254–8260.

Teasdale, S. 1929. *Dark of the Moon.* 6th ed. New York: Macmillan.

Tembrock, G. 1975. *Biokommunkation.* Weisbaden: Vieweg Verlag.

Traer, C. 1992. Emotional Release During Treatment: How to Cope. *OMTA Newsletter* April/May:1–5.

Trevarthen, C. 1993. The Self Born in Intersubjectivity: The Psychology of an Infant Communicating. In *The Perceived Self: Ecological and Interpersonal Sources of Self-Knowledge,* edited by U. Neisser. New York: Cambridge University Press.

———. 1996. Lateral Asymmetries in Infancy: Implications for the Development of the Hemispheres. *Neurosci Biobehav Rev* 20:571–586.

Trevino, H. 1999. *The Tao of Healing: Meditations for Body and Spirit.* Revised ed. Novato, Calif.: New World Library.

Truex, R., and B. Carpenter. 1964. *Strong and Elwyn's Human Neuroanatomy* 5th ed. Baltimore: Williams and Wilkins.

Tulving, E. 1972. Episodic and Semantic Memory. In *Organization of Memory,* edited by E. T. W. Donaldson. New York: Academic Press.

Turner, J. A., R. A. Deyo, J. D. Loeser, M. von Korff, and W. E. Fordyce. 1994. The Importance of Placebo Effects in Pain Treatment and Research. *JAMA* 271(20):1609–1614.

Tzourio-Mazoyer, N., S. De Schonen, F. Crivello, B. Reutter, Y. Aujard, and B. Mazoyer. 2002. Neural Correlates of Woman Face Processing by 2-Month Old Infants. *NeuroImage* 15:454–461.

van der Kolk, B. A. 1996. The Body Keeps Score: Approaches to the Psychobiology of Post-Traumatic Stress Disorder. In *Traumatic Stress: The Effects of Overwhelming Experience on Mind, Body and Society,* edited by B. van der Kolk, A. C. McFarlane, and L. Weisaeth. New York: Guilford Press.

Van Toller, S., and M. A. Kendal-Reed. 1995. A Possible Protocognitive Role for Odor in Human Infant Development. *Brain Cognition* 29:275–293.

Vanaerschot, G. 1997. Empathetic Resonance As a Source of Experience-Enhancing Interventions. In *Empathy Reconsidered: New Directions in Psychotherapy,* edited by A. C. B. L. Greenberg. Washington, D.C.: American Psychological Association.

Varela, F. 1999. What a Relief! I Don't Exist: Buddhism and the Brain. *Enquiring Mind* 16(1):7–10.

Visscher, M. 2007. Signor Slow. *Ode* 5(7):57–59.

Vogler, H. 1987. *Human Blastogenesis: Formation of Extraembryonic Cavities.* New York: Karger.

von Franz, M. L. 1995. *Creation Myths.* Revised ed. Boston: Shambhala Press.

von Uexkull, T., W. Geigges, and J. M. Herrman. 1993. The Principle of Teleological Coherence and Harmony of Purpose Exists At Every Level of Integration in the Hierarchy of Living Systems. *Advances* 9(3):50–63.

Wade, J. 1998. Physically Transcendent Awareness: A Comparison of the Phenomenology of Consciouness Before Birth and After Death. *J of Near Death Studies* 16(4):249–275.

Warme, G. E. 1980. *Amer J of Psychiatry* 137:4.

Weaver, I. C. G., N. Cervoni, F. A. Champagne, et al. 2004. Epigenetic Programming By Maternal Behavior. *Nature Neuroscience* 7:847–854.

Weaver, I. C. G., A. D'Alessio, S. Brown, I. Hellstrom, S. Dymov, S. Sharma, M. Szyf, and M. J. Meaney. 2007. The Transcription Factor Nerve Growth Factor-Inducible Protein A Mediates Epigenetic Programming: Altering Epigenetic Marks By Immediate-Early Genes. *J of Neuroscience* 27(7):1756–1768.

Weller, A, and R. Feldman. 2003. Emotion Regulation and Touch in Infants: The Role of Cholecystokinin and Opiods. *Peptides* 24:779–788.

Wilber, K. 2000. *Integral Psychology: Consciousness, Spirit, Psychology, Therapy.* Boston: Shambhala Press.

Winnicott, D. W. 1960. The Theory of Parent-Infant Relationship. In *The Maturational Processes and the Facilitating Environment.* New York: International Universities Press.

Winston, J. S., B. A. Strange, J. O. O'Doherty, and R. J. Dolan. 2002. Automatic and Intentional Brain Responses During Evaluation of Trustworthiness of Faces. *Nature Neuroscience* 5:277–283.

Wittling, W. 1997. The Right Hemisphere and the Human Stress Response. *Acta Physiol Scand* 640 (suppl):55–59.

Wurmser, L. 1981. *The Mask of Shame.* Baltimore: Johns Hopkins University Press.

Yamada, H., N. Sadato, Y. Konishi, et al. 2000. A Milestone for Normal Development of the Infantile Brain Detected By Functional MRI. *Neurology* 55:218–223.

Zuckerman-Zicha, M. 1925. Sur le développement de la musculature des paupières chez l'homme. *Arch de Biol* 35:313–323.

A CLOSING THOUGHT

When it is said that beings are like the moon reflected in limpid water rippled by a gentle breeze, the reflection and its watery support are alike in being, at every moment, impermanent and empty in their nature. With this understanding, Bodhisattvas are overwhelmed by a compassion that sees beings immersed in the ocean of the view of the sense of "I," an ocean fed by the vast, dark rivers of ignorance. They perceive that in this ocean, agitated by the winds of discursive thought, the cause of so much harm, beings must confront the effects of their good and evil actions reflected in the ocean like the moon.

—Jamgon Mipham (1846–1912)

NOTES

1. This chapter was originally presented as a paper at the annual meeting of the Rolf Institute in 2006.

2. George Santayana, *The Life of Reason or The Phases of Human Progress: Reason in Common Sense* (2nd ed., New York: Charles Scribner's Sons, 1924, originally published in 1905 by Charles Scribner's Sons). The famous, often misquoted, sentence appears in Chapter 12, "Flux and Constancy in Human Nature," p. 284.

3. Bibliographical citations in this chapter are from Dr. Schore's original article, and have been modified only to be consistent with the style of this book. The sources cited are included here in the bibliography.

4. For a more extensive discussion of regulation theory and an index of the references of studies cited here, the reader is referred to two books by Schore: *Affect Regulation and the Repair of the Self* (Schore, 2003a) and *Affect Dysregulation and Disorders of the Self* (Schore, 2003b).

5. See Schore's *Affect Dysregulation and Disorders of the Self* (Schore, 2003b) for an extensive discussion of the neurobiology of psychopathogenesis.

6. This chapter originally appeared as an article in *Pediatrics in Review,* January 30, 2005. Editor's note from *Pediatrics in Review:* "This article is a departure from our usual review in that it discusses new frontiers in the correlation of brain, mind, and emotions in developing children as well as areas of collaboration between pediatrics and sister disciplines. Dr. Schore has adapted a substantial amount of technical information to the viewpoint of the pediatrician. At the same time, many readers will encounter perspectives and language that seem unfamiliar. We urge clinicians to invest the effort needed for a careful reading to appreciate exciting new ways to look at development and emotional coping mechanisms. Readers desiring an abbreviated version will find it in the print version.—LFN"

7. This chapter and the preceding one represent an attempt to bring forward the writing of Allan Schore to the community of biodynamic craniosacral therapists. The root texts I studied are from his *Affect Regulation and the Repair of the Self* (Schore, 2003a): Chapter 3, "Clinical Implications of a Psychoneurobiological Model of Projective Identification," and Chapter 5, "Early Superego Development: The Emergence of Shame and Narcissistic Affect Regulation in the Practicing Period." I am very grateful for his perseverance in spreading this vital knowledge of relationship building.

8. The original micrographs from Dr. Gasser's article were not able to be reproduced for this chapter. Only the line drawings are shown.

9. This chapter originally appeared as Chapter 2 in *Symposium on Development of the Basicranium,* edited by James F. Bosma (U.S. Dept. of Health, Education, and Welfare, National Institutes of Health, DHEW Publication no. NIH 76-989, 1976).

10. This article originally appeared in *The American Journal of Anatomy,* Volume 120, No. 2, March 1967. Permission to reprint from Dr. Gasser. Published in the original article: "Submitted in partial fulfillment of the requirements of the degree of Doctor of Philosophy in the Department of Anatomy in the Graduate School of the University of Alabama, University, Alabama, 1965. Aided in part by grant HD-00230, National Institutes of Child Health and Human Development, National Institutes of Health to Dr. Tryphena Humphrey. Appreciation is expressed to Dr. Tryphena Humphrey, Dr. E. C. Sensenig, and to the late Dr. Davenport Hooker for making their collections of human embryonic material available during this investigation."

11. This article originally appeared in *Annals of Otology, Rhinology and Laryngology,* March 1967, Vol. 76, No. 1, pp. 37ff. Copyright 1967, Annals Publishing Company. Reprinted with permission from Dr. Gasser. Published in the original article: "This work was submitted in partial fulfillment of the requirements for the degree of Doctor of Philosophy in the Department of Anatomy in the Graduate School of the University of Alabama, University, Alabama, 1965. Aided in part by grant HD-00230, National Institutes of Child Health and Human Development, National Institutes of Health to Dr. Tryphena Humphrey. Appreciation is expressed to Dr. Tryphena Humphrey, Dr. E. C. Sensenig, and the late Dr. Davenport Hooker for making their collections of human embryonic material available. The author is especially indebted to Dr. Sensenig and Dr. Humphrey who graciously gave their time, encouragement, and valuable suggestions throughout this investigation."

12. This chapter is based on original text from *The Tao of Healing: Meditations for Body and Spirit* by Haven Trevino (Trevino, 1999).

13. Kathleen Martin, LMT, BCST, is a practicing biodynamic craniosacral therapist in Santa Barbara, California, and a graduate of the Shea Educational Group Foundation Training.

14. From *Japanese Death Poems* (Hoffman, 1986, p. 105).

15. From *A Magic Dwells* by Dr. Sheila Moon.

16. From *A Magic Dwells* by Dr. Sheila Moon.

COPYRIGHT ACKNOWLEDGMENTS

INDEX